HEALTH CARE ISSUES, COSTS AND ACCESS

HANDBOOK OF FATIGUE IN HEALTH AND DISEASE

HEALTH CARE ISSUES, COSTS AND ACCESS

Additional books in this series can be found on Nova's website under the Series tab.

Additional E-books in this series can be found on Nova's website under the E-books tab.

HEALTH CARE ISSUES, COSTS AND ACCESS

HANDBOOK OF FATIGUE IN HEALTH AND DISEASE

HOWARD S. SMITH
EDITOR

Nova Science Publishers, Inc.
New York

For permission to use material from this book please contact us:
Telephone 631-231-7269; Fax 631-231-8175
Web Site: http://www.novapublishers.com

Additional color graphics may be available in the e-book version of this book.

LIBRARY OF CONGRESS CATALOGING-IN-PUBLICATION DATA

Handbook of fatigue in health and disease / editor, Howard S. Smith.
p. ; cm.
Includes bibliographical references and index.
ISBN 978-1-61761-920-5 (hardcover)
1. Fatigue--Handbooks, manuals, etc. I. Smith, Howard S., 1956-
[DNLM: 1. Fatigue. WB 146]
RB150.F37H365 2010
613--dc22
2010043904

Published by Nova Science Publishers, Inc. † New York

Contents

PREFACE

Fatigue is the most common and frequent symptom that people experience, yet the field of medicine has not paid all that much attention to it until the past decade or so. One can appreciate the relative lack of "coverage" for fatigue if one contrasts the number of texts on pain to the number of texts on fatigue. Isolating a patient's specific etiology of fatigue may be exceptionally difficult because of a multitude of contributing factors which may be involved. In fact, I personally experienced significant fatigue multiple times in putting together this text. This text intended to familiarize the reader with the physiologic/pathophysiologic mechanisms, assessment and treatments of fatigue.

Unfortunately, the pathophysiology of fatigue still remains uncertain. Factors which may contribute to fatigue likely include both central and peripheral mechanisms. Mediators such as cytokines, neurotransmitters, and/or neurohormones may promote or contribute to fatigue. Mediators of stress may lead to decreased brain derived neurotrophic factor (BDNF). The treatment of fatigue is still in its infancy. Therapeutic approaches which enhance the binding of serotonin to 5-HT_{2A} receptors in the brain may ameliorate fatigue. Exercise conceivably may help fatigue via dual mechanisms. Firstly, exercise may lead to adrenergic induced lipolysis of free fatty acids resulting in increased free tryptophan in blood due to liberation from albumin with consequent higher free tryptophan uptake into the brain [1] and enhanced serotonin biosynthesis. Secondly, voluntary exercise may increase mRNA levels of brain derived neurotrophic factor (BDNF) as it has in rats [2]. The increase in BDNF may regulate 5-HT_{2A} receptors, leading to an increase in 5-HT_{2A} receptor levels. The combination of increased serotonin and increased 5-HT_{2A} receptors should promote enhanced binding, which may ameliorate fatigue. Several antidepressant treatments may also increase the mRNA levels of BDNF [3].

Recently, Tanaka and colleagues established an animal model of fatigue. The fatigued animals showed reduced 2-[(18)F] fluoro-2-deoxy-D-glucose uptake in their brain, although their blood glucose level did not differ from that of the control animals. The study also measured regional cerebral blood flow, ATP level, and the ability of mitochondria to produce ATP in the brain of the fatigued and control rats. The fatigued animals showed almost equal regional cerebral blood flow, a significantly higher ATP level, and almost equal mitochondrial ability to produce ATP. These data suggest that decreased energy utilization in the brain may be a feature of fatigue [4].

Novel assessment tools may be utilized in the future to evaluate mental fatigue. The work of Shen et al. demonstrates the feasibility of an automatic EEG method for assessing and monitoring of mental fatigue [5]. Furthermore, it appears that muscle pain is perceived by acid-sensing ion channel #3 (ASIC3). Moreover, lactic acid and extracellular ATP (acting via binding to the P2X7 purinergic receptor) increases the sensitivity of ASIC3 to protons. Thus, ASIC3 essentially functions as a "coincidence detector" of three molecules (lactic acid, ATP, and protons) to "sense" to muscle discomfort/pain. Similarly, ASIC3 may function as a fatigue "sensor/receptor" for peripheral muscle; warning the body that pain may be next if the subject doesn't rest. Novel treatments of fatigue are increasingly becoming appreciated, get matching treatment to the specific etiologies/mechanisms primarily contributing to fatigue in an individual patient remains vitally important. It appears that agents with antioxidant effects such as (-)-epigallocatechin gallate (EGCg) (the major catechinconstituent of green tea) [6] or Applephenon® (an apple polyphenol extract produced commercially from unripe apples, and used as a food additive to prevent oxidation of food and beverage components) may be beneficial in the treatment of fatigue [7].

The text has eleven chapters. Chapter one serves as an introduction chapter and as a broad background for "Fatigue 101". The second chapter covers evaluation tools in the assessment of fatigue. Subsequent chapters deal with barriers to the communication of fatigue, and then the clinical significance of fatigue. The next six chapters cover fatigue and various pathophysiologic mediators/states/conditions/diseases related to fatigue. Finally, chapter eleven presents strategies of the management of fatigue.

References

[1] Kalman, D., & Villani, L.J. (1997). Nutritional aspects of cancer-related fatigue. J Am Diet Assoc, 97,650-654.

[2] Adlard, P.A., & Cotman, C.W. (2004). Voluntary exercise protects against stress-induced decreases in brain-derived neurotrophic factor protein expression. Neuroscience, 124,985-992.

[3] Rosel, P., Arranz, B., San, L., Vallejo, J., Crespo, J.M., Urretavizcaya, M., & Navarro, M.A. (2000). Altered 5-HT(2A) binding sites and second messenger inositol trisphosphate (IP(3)) levels in hippocampus but not in frontal cortex from depressed suicide victims. Psychiatry Res, 30;99,173-181.

[4] Tanaka, M., & Wantanabe, Y. (2008). Reduced Energy Utilization in the Brain is a Feature of an Animal Model of Fatigue. Int J Neurosci, 188,683-692.

[5] Shen KQ, Li XP, Ong CJ, Shen KQ, Li XP, Ong CJ, Shao SY, Wilder-Smith EP. EEG-based mental fatigue measurement using multi-class support vector machines with confidence estimate. Clin Neurophysiol. 2008 Jul;119(7):1524-33.

[6] Tanaka, M., Baba, Y., Kataoka, Y., Kinbara, N., Sagesaka, Y.M., Kakuda, T., & Watanabe, Y. (2008). Effects of (-)-epigallocatechin gallate in liver of an animal model of combined (physical and mental) fatigue. Nutrition, 24,599-603.

[7] Ataka, S., Tanaka, M., Nozaki, S., Mizuma, H., Mizuno, K., Tahara, T., Sugino, T., Shirai, T., Kajimoto, Y., Kuratsune, H., Kajimoto, O., & Watanabe, Y. (2007). Effects of Applephenon® and ascorbic acid on physical fatigue. Nutrition, 23,419-423.

In: Handbook of Fatigue in Health and Disease
Editor: Howard S. Smith
ISBN 978-1-61761-920-5

Chapter 1

FATIGUE IN HEALTH AND DISEASE

Howard S. Smith*

Associate Professor of Anesthesiology, Internal Medicine, and Physical Medicine and Rehabilitation
Academic Director of Pain Management
Albany Medical College
Department of Anesthesiology
47 New Scotland Avenue; MC-131
Albany, New York 12208, USA

ABSTRACT

Fatigue is the most common symptom experienced by humans. It is likely that every human at some point in time has experienced some form of fatigue. Clinicians need to listen to their patients' complaints and avoid minimizing complaints about fatigue. Health care providers should accurately assess fatigue the distress it leads to, and its impact on quality of life. The use of interdisciplinary "fatigue clinics" may minimize barriers to effective communication regarding the fatigue. Although the precise mechanisms that contribute to fatigue remain uncertain, general treatment strategies may be beneficial. Pharmacologic and non-pharmacologic treatment strategies should both be employed. Future therapeutic efforts may be able to target multifactorial mechanisms that may be involved in contributing to pain in a particular patient.

* Phone: 518-262-4461
Fax: 518-262-2671
smithh@mail.amc.edu

Introduction

Fatigue is a universal and daily phenomenon and is ranked third on the list of most reported problems in the general practitioner's surgery [1]. Fatigue is without question--- the most frequent symptom experienced by humans. It is essentially omni-prevalent--- in the sense that essentially every human at some point in time can state that they experienced some type of "fatigue" (and typically more than once). Yet, although it is exceedingly common--- the definition, assessment, and treatment approaches to fatigue have not received anywhere near as much attention as other symptoms.

Fatigue remains an ill-defined mysterious symptom and/or disease which is an unique personal experience, --- perceived and experienced differently by different people. It often tends to be ignored, (especially relative to other symptoms) --- by patients, family, colleagues, and health care providers. Fatigue may vary dramatically in its scope, severity, duration, course, and effects on life/performance. Busy clinicians all too often reflexly ignore the complaint of fatigue which may be associated with virtually every known diagnostic condition, although some condition tend to be closely linked with significant fatigue. Currently, there exists little basic science research purely focused on fatigue predominantly due to the lack of any useful animal models.

Fatigue (especially cancer-related fatigue) may exhibit temporal variation. Richardson et al. found that fatigue in patients receiving chemotherapy varied throughout the day, more frequently occurring in the afternoon and early evening [2]. Cancer-related fatigue can be pervasive, and may begin with treatment, continuing throughout therapy, and improving somewhat after the completion of treatment. However, frequently even after treatment is over, fatigue may persist at a higher-than-baseline level--- possibly even for several years, in a patient with no apparent disease [3].

Often there exists poor correlation between the subjective fatigue and physiologic (e.g. performance-based or objective fatigue-ability) fatigue. A patient who describes severe subjective physical fatigue may exhibit essential normal performance decrement on muscular and/or cardiovascular physiologic testing, whereas, another patient who describes mild subjective physical fatigue may exhibit significant performance decrement on muscular and/or cardiovascular physiologic testing.

Furthermore, although often subjective fatigue and/or physiologic fatigue translates directly into expected low-level, depressed behavioral manifestations, there may also be poor correlation with behavior (i.e. a patient who describes severe subjective fatigue may carry on relatively routine life activities [e.g. holding down a job, doing recreational activities with friends]), while another patient who describes mild subjective fatigue may be a "couch potato".

Fatigue Taxonomy

Since widely accepted fatigue taxonomy does not exist, the following discussion has not stood the test of time or been "ratified" by consensus. **Fatigue** can be defined as a sensory and emotional experience associated with actual or potential sensations within physical (e.g. "tired", "weak"), mental "exhaustion" (e.g. "feeling wiped out") and/or emotional (e.g.

"drained") domains; --- with the perception that a state or potential state exists of impaired performance/efficiency, diminished capacity/energy, decreased endurance, and/or less motivation/inertia with respect to usual activities/states in one or more of these domains [4].

In 1921, Muscio [5] advised that the term fatigue was vague and should be banished from scientific discussion and therefore "attempts to obtain a fatigue test should be abandoned" [5]. Various authors have employed the broader term asthenia which includes fatigue but is less commonly used. It appears that the term fatigue has stood the test of time in the medical literature as well as in clinical and common jargon.

Fatigue has been difficult to define in a clinically useful manner which is universally accepted--- partly perhaps because different disciplines may look at and/or assess fatigue differently, and partly perhaps because of lay terminology used to describe fatigue. Fatigue has been described in terms such as decreased motivation, a sense of lassitude, a sense of exhaustion, tiredness, weariness, or a decreased physical or mental endurance. Lezak stated that fatigue required no definition [6]; --- however, in order to make progress in the basic and clinical sciences of fatigue there should be an accepted definition and taxonomy.

In a healthy person, fatigue occurs as a sensation which accompanies and perhaps signals and/or protects against "over exertion", --- and prompts the desire to rest. The Multiple Sclerosis (MS) Council for Clinical Practice Guidelines (1998) published the following definition of fatigue: "A subjective lack of physical and/or mental energy that is perceived by the individual or caregiver to interfere with usual and desired activities" [7]. The Oxford American Dictionary defines fatigue as "extreme tiredness after exertion" or "a reduction in the efficiency of a muscle, organ, etc. after prolong activity." Although, this clearly pertains to "physical" fatigue (or "physiologic" fatigue), it appears that repetitive cognitive tasks/activities requiring a "high level of intellectual functioning" may lead to cognitive or mental fatigue or repetitive "emotionally draining" experiences may lead to "affective fatigue" or "psychologic fatigue". "Seasonal Fatigue" should prompt a careful evaluation for underlying or unrecognized "seasonal depression".

Fatigue can be considered as a multidimensional perceived lack of "energy" to initiate or complete necessary or desired tasks/activities (e.g. a sensation that one cannot muster enough effort to attempt a necessary/desired activity). Fatigue may be perceived as a physical tiredness or exhaustion, a need for reduced activity, reduced motivation, and/or mental fatigue [8]. Patients may report "everything is an effort". Physiologically, fatigue can be considered as the inability to maintain power output, and is perceived as a sensation of weakness (even when the muscle is not active) and/or a sense of greater effort required to complete an activity/task (e.g. effort tolerance). Mental fatigue can be considered as a reduced capacity for attention, concentration, and learning, as well as disturbance in short-term memory [9]. Mental fatigue, with decreased concentration capacity, is common in neuroinflammatory and neurodegenerative diseases, often appearing prior to other major mental or physical neurological symptoms [9]. Rönnbäck and Hansson have presented the hypothesis that the proinflammatory cytokines tumor necrosis factor-alpha, IL-1beta and IL-6 could be involved in the pathophysiology of mental fatigue through their ability to attenuate the astroglial clearance of extracellular glutamate, their disintegration of the blood brain barrier, and effects on astroglial metabolism and metabolic supply for the neurons, thereby disturbing glutamate regulation (potentially leading to reduced filtration of information) [9]. Magnusson et al. suggested that negative aspects of perfectionism may cause maladaptive coping strategies which predispose individuals to fatigue [10].

Fatigue Classifications

There are ten major ways fatigue subtypes can be categorized:

1. Fatigue Subtypes based on Fatigue Duration

Acute fatigue generally refers to fatigue lasting three months or less. Subacute fatigue refers to fatigue which has lasted between three and six months. Chronic fatigue refers to persistent fatigue lasting more than 6 months or significant long-term transient episodes of fatigue which abate spontaneously and recur over 15 days a month.

2. Fatigue Subtypes based on Associated Diagnosis/Etiologies

Example: Cancer-related fatigue. Note: two or more classifications may be combined (e.g. chronic cancer-related fatigue.

3. Fatigue Subtypes based on Body System Involved

Example: cardiac-related fatigue, renal-related fatigue.

4. Fatigue Subtypes based on Severity

i.e. mild, moderate, severe.

5. Fatigue Subtypes based on Predominate Domain Affected

Example: physical or mental [(cognitive) vs. emotional (affective).

Fatigue may be tied to inefficient information processing perhaps secondary to neuronal hypoactivity in several brain and spinal cord regions. Mental fatigue may be related to suboptimal noradrenergic or impaired dopaminergic functioning in the prefrontal cortex. Physical fatigue may be related to deficient noradrenergic functioning or deficient dopaminergic functioning in the striatum nucleus a hypothalamus, and descending spinal cord projections.

Physical fatigue may be further subdivided into muscular physical fatigue and non-muscular physical fatigue. Cognitive fatigue may correlate with scores on the Attentional Function Index (AFI). Examination of validity indicated that the scores on the AFI showed expected correlations with established measures of ability to concentrate, cognitive failures, states of confusion, and mental fatigue [11].

6. Fatigue Subtypes based on Characteristics

Example : reactive fatigue, "Major" fatigue.

"Major fatigue" or "Endogenous fatigue"can be considered to be "pathologic" fatigue which is abnormal and not solely due to the surrounding circumstances or environmental conditions, functional state, or activities preceding the fatigue state (HIV-related fatigue).

"Reactive fatigue" can be considered to be "physiologic" and not necessarily pathologic fatigue which may be essentially normal and expected in view of various circumstances (e.g. the mental fatigue experienced after taking a school exam or the physical fatigue experienced after running a marathon--- are expected--- and therefore although the intensity may be severe and the duration may last days or weeks--- these would be examples of reactive fatigue.

Currently the use of fatigue subtype categories based on mechanisms involved (e.g. cytokine-related fatigue) or based on treatment responsiveness (e.g. exercise-responsive fatigue) are not well developed or utilized.

7. Fatigue Subtypes based on Normal vs. Abnormal Physiologic Mechanisms

Physiologic Fatigue vs. Pathologic Fatigue

8. Fatigue Subtypes based on Fatigue

Being the sole diagnosis ("Primary Fatigue") vs. fatigue being secondary to/associated with other diagnoses ("Secondary Fatigue").

Primary fatigue by medical convention may be considered a condition where the "diagnosis" of fatigue embodies the condition (e.g. chronic fatigue syndrome) whereas secondary fatigue might then be considered conditions where significant fatigue is often associated with the primary diagnosis (e.g. rheumatoid arthritis).

The criteria for the diagnosis of "primary fatigue" [chronic fatigue syndrome] includes: long-standing (six months or longer) fatigue that is not explained by an existing medical or psychiatric diagnosis, is not substantially alleviated by rest, and causes considerable disabilities in professional, social, and for personal functioning (at least 50 percent reduction in baseline level) [12]. Clearly "secondary" fatigue syndromes (i.e. those that are explained by an existing medical or psychiatric diagnosis [e.g. cancer-related fatigue]) may equally affect quality of life and thereby satisfy the duration, severity characteristics that are used for chronic fatigue syndrome.

9. Subtypes based on Pathophysiologic Mechanisms

Neuropathic Fatigue vs. Non-Neuropathic Fatigue

Neuropathic fatigue has been considered fatigue which is caused by primary neural mechanisms initiated by specific biological mechanisms (e.g. disease activity of a condition such as multiple sclerosis). Non-neuropathic ("visceral" or "somatic") fatigue can then be considered to be fatigue which is perpetuated or exacerbated by general mechanisms such as deconditioning, sleep, disturbances, stress/anxiety/depression, and pain.

10. Fatigue Subtypes based on Fatigue-associated Sources

Peripheral vs. Central Fatigue

Fatigue has been divided into "peripheral" and "central" components. Clearly there exist multiple classification of fatigue [4] (See Figure 1).

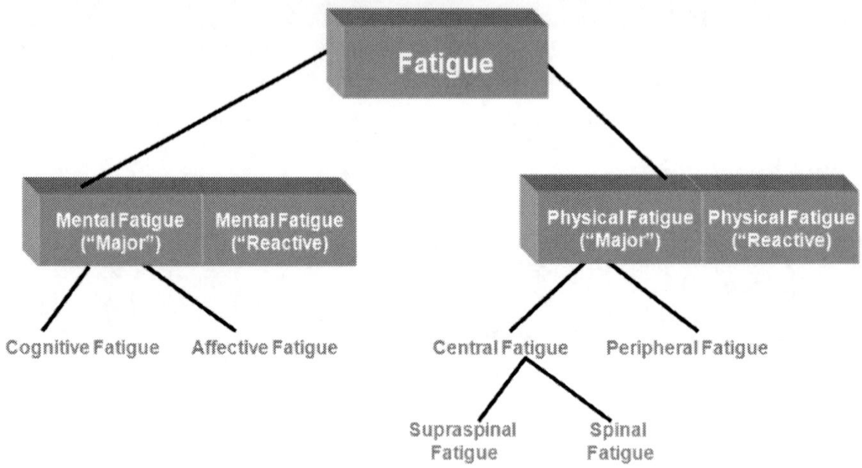

Figure 1. Fatigue Classifications.

Peripheral Fatigue

Peripheral fatigue has been defined as the inability to sustain a specified force or level of activity because of physical limitations of the muscles, nerves (e.g. peripheral nervous system), or cardiovascular system [13]. Peripheral fatigue, which largely originates in the neuromuscular junctions, muscle, and soft tissues and related structures (e.g. tendons, joints), results in the inability of the peripheral neuromuscular apparatus to perform a task in response to central stimulation. Reduced adenosine triphosphate concentration and/or efficiency of adenosine triphosphate generation, may contribute to peripheral fatigue. (ATP and the accumulation of metabolic by-products have been implicated in peripheral fatigue as well as any condition/insult which perturbs optimal functioning of the neuromuscular apparatus). However, there are at least 5 metabolic causes of fatigue, a decrease in the phosphocreatine level in muscle, proton accumulation in muscle, depletion of the glycogen store in muscle, hypogylcemia and an increase in the plasma concentration ratio of free trytophan/branched-chain amino acids [14].

CENTRAL FATIGUE

Central fatigue, largely originates in the central nervous system (CNS), from the progressive inability to optimally transmit motor neuron impulses [15]. Chaudhuri and Behan consider central fatigue as difficulty in the initiation or maintenance of voluntary activities and define central fatigue as the failure to initiate and/or sustain attentional tasks (mental fatigue) and/or physical activities (physical fatigue) requiring self-motivation and/or internal cues (as opposed to external stimulation) [in the absence of demonstrable cognitive dysfunction or motor dysfunction [13]]. The term "supraspinal fatigue" has been defined [15-17] as opposed to "spinal fatigue". It refers to that component of central fatigue that is due to failure to utilize available output from the motor cortex, and it can be demonstrated with transcranial motor cortical stimulation (TMS) [18].

As supraspinal fatigue develops with exercise, there are dramatic changes within the motor cortex [17, 19] and also in corticospinal "connectivity" with motoneurons [20]. The electromyogram (EMG) silent period after corical stimulation lengthens (a reflection of intracortical inhibition) and the initial excitatory EMG response [motor evoked potential (MEP)] increases during fatiguing contractions, and there are depressions in MEPs and cervicomedullary evoked potentials (a test of corticomotoneuronal function) after exercise [15, 20, 21].

Magnetic and electrical stimulation at different levels of the neuraxis show that supraspinal and spinal factors limit force production in maximal contractions, motoneurons become less responsive to synaptic input in put and descending drive becomes supoptimal [22]. Exercise-induced activity in group III and IV muscle afferents acts supraspinally to limit motor cortical output does not alter motor cortical responses to transcranial magnetic stimulation [22].

Less is known about precise mechanisms in the central nervous system which lead to fatigue. It is generally recognized that the feeling of fatigue may be significantly affected by psychological factors (e.g. mood, personality, motivation) [23]. "Seasonal Fatigue" should prompt a careful evaluation for underlying or unrecognized "seasonal depression".

Posttraumatic fatigue (PTF) may result from a myriad of causes. One subtype of PTF which may differ from many other causes of PTF, is traumatic brain injury (TBI)-induced fatigue. TBI begins with a disruption, typically via shearing forces, of the central nervous system (CNS) structures maintaining arousal. TBI-related central fatigue can be conceptualized as a higher-order deficit resulting from altered levels of neurotransmitters release by more caudal structures [24]. The interaction of the ARAS and basal ganglia is well-know and may play a significant role in PF. This conceptual framework dovetails with the concept of the ARAS as mediating not only arousal but also the ability to "phasically" turn on cortical tissue efficiently [24]. This, the increases "fatigue-ability" after brain injury may be conceptualized as a decreased ability not only to activate specific brain region which may be relatively "silent at baseline", but also to efficiently sustain cortical tissue [24].

Subtle problems of perplexity, distractibility, and fatigue accompany all kinds of brain injury for they appear to result from disruption of accustomed neural pathways and loss or change of mental function. Emotional disturbances may mask these subtle problems, but they can also result from them [25]. Some of the emotional distress after brain insult may result from less obvious problems than those impairing mobility, strength, or competency and Counseling may reduce the patient's vulnerability to the psychologically crippling effects of perplexity, distractibility, and fatigue [25].

The epidemiology incidence and prevalence of fatigue is not especially well documented. However, there is general consensus that the prevalence of fatigue symptoms in the general population is high. Efforts to determine the prevalence of fatigue in specific populations (i.e. among cancer patients) is complicated by this high prevalence of fatigue symptoms in the general population [26].

The impact or extent of how drastically fatigue affects or interferes with an individual's quality of life may vary dramatically--- even with the same severity of fatigue. The degree to how highly motivated an individual is to engage in various activities may factor in significantly. Additionally, although it has only been studied with chronic pain (and not with fatigue), --- the concept of three distinct subgroups of chronic fatigue patients based on cluster analyses of patient responses to the Multidimensional Pain Inventory [27] [e.g. dysfunctional, interpersonally distressed, adaptive copers] may have utility in fatigue as well as pain.

Although the epidemiology of fatigue is not known among the healthy--- it is conceivable that essentially every human has experienced some form of the spectrum of fatigue at some point in time. There are numerous conditions/etiologies associated with fatigue including: psychiatric (e.g. depression); medical--- endocrine disturbances (e.g. thyroid), immunologic (e.g. rheumatoid arthritis), infectious (e.g. HIV-related conditions), cardiovascular disease (e.g. congestive heart failure), pulmonary disease (e.g. emphysema), renal dysfunction (e.g. chronic kidney/disease/end-stage renal disease), hematologic/oncologic (e.g. anemia/breast cancer), gastrointestinal (e.g. hepatic dysfunction); neurologic (e.g. multiple sclerosis, parkinsonism, dementia, cerebral vascular accidents); other conditions (e.g. hemochromatosis, gaucher's disease) and trauma (e.g. traumatic brain injury). Treatments which lead to better sleep quality and/or duration with increased "restful" restorative sleep and improved sleep architecture also appear to improve symptoms of fatigue in patients with suboptimal sleep.

Aside from numerous pathologic states/conditions which may contribute to fatigue (e.g. chronic inflammation), many treatment approaches may contribute to fatigue as well pharmacologic (e.g. Beta Blockers, "statins"), chemotherapy, immunotherapy, physical therapy, radiotherapy, and surgery).

Magnusson and colleagues in 1995 mailed questionnaires to 442 Swedish registered nurses and reported (with a 49% response rate) that nurses regarded fatigue as the most common symptom in cancer patients, however, few established nursing interventions existed and overall nurses wanted further education and tools for evaluation of fatigue, it's causes and treatment [28].

Cancer-related fatigue can be defined as a complex syndrome, with physical mental, and emotional component and diverse causes, characterized by a chronic and abnormal/unusual whole-body experience of tiredness, decreased capacity for physical and mental work, or persistent exhaustion that is disproportionate or unrelated to exertion and not relieved by rest

[12, 29]. Even in patients with cancer who may have many significant symptoms, fatigue remains a debilitating symptom [30]. The National comprehensive cancer network (NCCN) has addressed the evaluation and management of cancer-related fatigue in 2000 [31, 32] and 2007 [33]. Cancer-related fatigue is the most prevalent symptom of cancer, occurring in 60-90% of patients [34]. The University of Texas M.D. Anderson Cancer Center developed a fatigue specialty clinic in efforts to improve our patients' quality of life by decreasing fatigue; educate health care providers, patients, and patients' families about cancer-related fatigue; develop an appropriate clinical and diagnostic evaluation for this symptom; correlate objective measures of fatigue with its clinical evaluation; and develop innovative treatment plans for cancer-related fatigue [34]. The nurse practitioner in the Fatigue Clinic has a special role in the management of these patients [30].

The European Association of Palliative Care has developed a working definition [35] of Cancer-Related Fatigue (CRF) on the basis of the European Organization for Research and Treatment of Cancer Quality of Life Questionnaire (EORTC QLQ C30). This defines fatigue as a subjective feeling of tiredness, weakness or lack of energy. The Fatigue Symptom Inventory (FSI) [36] is a 13-item scale that was originally validated in a breast cancer population. A subsequent validation study involved 342 mixed cancer patients [37]. It has reasonable psychometric properties but there is a question over its test–retest reliability [38].

Some cancer states are associated with significant increases in a variety of cytokines (e.g. tumor necrosis factor – related weak inducer of apoptosis). Li and colleagues demonstrated that tumor necrosis factor-related weak inducer of apoptosis (TWEAK) augments matrix metalloproteinase 9 (MMP-9) production in skeletal muscle through the activation of nuclear factor-kappaB-inducing kinase and p38 mitogen-activated protein kinase [39]. Li et al thus proposed TWEAK-induced expression of MMP-9 in cancer related cachexia fatigue.

Mittal and colleagues found that in denervation-induced skeletal muscle atrophy in mice expression of the TWEAK receptor Fn14 (fibroblast growth factor-inducible receptor 14) and not the cytokine itself is significantly increased in muscle upon denervation, demonstrating an unexpected inside-out signaling pathway; the receptor up-regulation allows for TWEAK activation of nuclear factor kappaB, causing an increase in the expression of the E3 ubiquitin ligase MuRF1 [40]. This study reveals a novel mediator of skeletal muscle atrophy and indicates that the TWEAK-Fn14 system may be an important target for preventing skeletal muscle wasting [40].

The Anatomy of Fatigue

Three predominant areas in the brain which are thought to play a major role in fatigue and its associated behavior include: a.) the motor coordination centers (basal ganglia and mesencephalofrontal activating system [MFAS]) (The MFAS is a separate dopaminergic system projectin from the ventral tegmental area (VTA) of the midbrain to the frontal lobe (especially including the cingulated gyrus), which drives internal states toward motivated behaviors, b.) the executive and motor planning areas (frontal circuits), and c.) the internal motivational neuronal network (hypothalamus and limbic structures) [13].

Associated brain circuitry/projections/pathways which may be important in maintaining attention) [41]; striatocortical fibers that channel motivational influences into the motor system; fibers that "transfer" thalamic activity to suppress frontal activation striato-corticofrontal [13]; and the hypothalamic-pituitary-adrenal (HPA) axis [42].

The ascending reticular activating system (ARAS) is the fundamental structure responsible for maintaining arousal--- and is also part of a larger and more complex system that integrates sensory attention and tonic arousal. The ARAS may also have a key role in "phasically" and effectively activating cortical tissue.

The ARAS may interact with the basal ganglia and dysfunction of these systems may contribute to fatigue in certain circumstances. Chaudhuri and Behan postulated that basal ganglia dysfunction--- especially disruption of function in the striatothalamocortical fibers is responsible for central fatigue following neurologic injury [13].

Import projections and pathways exist which tightly connect the basal ganglia with limbic signaling in the amygdala. The limbic system provides a route for channeling spontaneous, unconscious, emotionally driven motivational forces into the motor system, influencing the likelihood of initiating and sustaining goal-directed action [43].

Although fatigue and apathy may exhibit a clinical overlap of behavioral similarities, apathy and fatigue are distinct entities. Apathy may be defined as a quantified and observable behavioral syndrome consisting of a quantitative reduction of voluntary (or goal-directed) behaviors, and occurs when the systems that generate and control voluntary actions are altered [44]. These systems are mostly represented by the different subregions embedded in the prefrontal cortex (PFC) and in the basal ganglia regions that are closely connected with the PFC [44].

It appears that brain regions may be essentially silent until they are activated and persist activated by the appropriate neurotransmitter(s) [45]. Elovic and colleagues proposed that the increased "fatigue-ability" after brain injury may be conceptualized a decreased ability not only to activate but also to efficiently sustain recruited cortical tissue [24].

Roelcke et al. utilized positron emission tomography (PET) scanning to compare multiple sclerosis (MS) patients with subjective fatigue versus MS patients without subjective fatigue [46]. They found that MS patients with subjective fatigue had diminished glucose metabolism especially in the frontal lobes and basal ganglia [46].

Electrophysiologic and other data also revealed frontal lobe dysfunction in fatigued versus nonfatigued MS patients using transcranial magnetic stimulation [47] and electroencephalography (EEG) [48]. The more pronounced the EEG abnormalities--- the more intense was the subjective feeling of fatigue [48].

Filippi and colleagues utilized functional magnetic resonance imaging (fMRI) to compare 15 MS patients with subjective fatigue to 14 MS patients with no fatigue performing a simple motor task [49]. MS patients with fatigue demonstrated significantly lower activation in cortical and subcortical regions involved in motor planning execution than MS patients without fatigue [49].

Brain cytokines (e.g. interferon–alpha) appear to contribute to fatigue, perhaps via effects at the 5-HT (1A) receptor [50]. The basal gangli nuclei may be a primary site of action for interferon-alpha-induced fatigue [51]. The nucleus accumbens and its communications seem to be important in the regulation of effort-based processes [52]. Many cortical structures are activated during tasks of voluntary muscular force perception [53]. A voluntary force perception appears to be primarily related to a sense of effort (and not through a sense of intramuscular tension), however, sensory input contributes significantly to effort awareness [53].

The basal ganglia may support the coherence of cortical activity during voluntary muscular tasks [53]. Niepel et al. demonstrated significantly longer T1 relaxation times of two deep gray matter structures (thalamus and the putamen), in relapsing-remitting multiple sclerosis patients with fatigue when compared to healthy volunteers [54]. The median T1 in the thalamus and the putamen were significantly higher in the patients with relapsing-remitting multiple sclerosis than in healthy controls [54]. There was a significant correlation between fatigue severity scale and the T1 of the thalamus (rho=0.418; p-0.014) [54]. Also, the median T1 in the thalamus was significantly higher in patients with fatigue compared with those without fatigue (0=0,018) supporting a role for subcortical gray matter structures in the pathogenesis of multiple sclerosis-related fatigue [54].

The basal ganglia and its multiple projections are involved in a number of functions (e.g. cognition, emotional, motor tasks). Any insult or pathology which perturbs certain pallido-thalamo-cortical pathways may result in reduced motivation, and the subsequent perception of "central-type" fatigue [55]. Fatigue is extremely common in conditions predominantly involving the basal ganglia (e.g. Parkinson's disease) and may be the initial and/or most severe symptoms [56]. Patients with bilateral lesions of the basal ganglia especially the globus pallidus, appear apathetic and demotivated without any motor symptoms [57]. The globus pallidus magnetization transfer ratio (MTR), a quantifiable tissue characteristic that may be abnormal in the presense of normal magnetic resonance imaging, was significant reduced in precirrhotic primary bilary cirrhosis patients compared with healthy controls [58].

These measurements correlated with blood manganese levels and were more abnormal in the more fatigues patients [58]. Magnetic resonance experiments with manganese chloride phantoms have demonstrated a strong inverse linear relationship between mangese concentration in various brain regions and MTR [55]. Manganese deposition in brain structures may result in loss of neuronal and/or glial function leading to alterations in neurotransmission and intracerebral cytokine release [59]. Forton and colleagues hypothesized that the fatigue experienced by patients with primary biliary cirrhosis could be partially explained by impaired biliary excretion of manganese leading to significantly increased managanese levels in the globus pallidus with subsequent globus pallidus dysfunction and resultant fatigue perception [58]. Thus, basal ganglia appear to be one of the key brain regions which may contribute to the perception of fatigue. Furthermore, it appears that dopaminergic agonists may improve fatigue and contrariwise; that many D_1 and/or D_2 dopamine receptor antagonists, may lea to fatigue (as an adverse effect) after long-term administration. These, multiple studies point to the frontal lobes and basal ganglia (as well as the links between these two areas) as key areas of the brain involved in fatigue. Chaudhuri and Behan have proposed that central fatigue may be the result of "failure in the integration of limbic input and motor functions within the basal ganglia affecting the striatal-thalamic-frontal cortical system" [13].

In a study by Tedeschi et al. [60] a multivariate analysis showed that white matter (WM) and grey matter (GM) volume losses were the "final" factors related to fatigue, which confirms the association found between fatigue and progression of brain atrophy in an eight-year follow up study of patients with RRMS with mild clinical disability [61]. The association between GM loss and fatigue fits with previous data showing a relationship between damage of deep GM nuclei and this symptom [54, 62-64], and further supports the theory of a central origin of MS-related fatigue [65]. Tedeschi and colleagues did not explore the relation between T2- and T1-lesion loads and atrophy of the different brain compartments or the regional distribution of macroscopic visible lesions, with particular focus on the involvement of GM structures [60], thus leaving unanswered the question as whether MS-related fatigue is largely due to a damage of GM or to a disconnection of specific WM pathways secondary to the presence of T2-visible lesions or to a combination of the two [65].

Although the biochemistry of fatigue cannot be simplified into raising or lowering levels of one or two neurotransmitters, --- there are some neurotransmitter concentrations which seem to influence fatigue status. For instance, it appears that acetylcholine and catecholamine agents act as stimulants--- (e.g. donepezil and methylphenidate may increase these neurotransmitter levels respectively) and thereby may improve symptoms of fatigue. Additionally, dopaminergic agonists may improve symptoms of fatigue and dopaminergic antagonists may promote fatigue after long-term administration.

Alternatively, higher levels of serotonin (5-HT) may lead to increased fatigue. Blomstrand published that human performance was diminished when 5-HT was elevated and that rats ran more efficiently when 5-HT levels were lowered [66]. Furthermore, Blomstrand et al. revealed that sustained exercise to the point of fatigue resulted in an increase in typtophan levels (a precursor to serotonin) by 36% across various brain regions [67].

Administration of branched-chain amino acids (BCAA) reduced perceived exertion and mental fatigue during exercise and improved cognitive performance after exercise thought to be a secondary to diminishing typtophan levels [and therefore 5HT levels] via competitive binding for tryptophan transport proteins [66]. When BCAAs were supplied to human subjects during a standardized cycle ergometer exercise their ratings of perceived exertion and mental fatigue were reduced, and, during a competitive 30-km cross-country race, their performance on different cognitive tests was improved after the race [68].

Malaguarnera et al. suggested that the administration of acetyl-L-carnitine (ALC) may reduce both physical and mental fatigue in older persons improving cognitive status and physical functions [69]. Maes et al. has advocated for the use of antioxidants in the treatment of fatigue based on some preliminary evidence that chronic fatigue syndrome is accompanied by an activation of the inflammatory response system and by increased oxidative and nitrosative stress [70]. Nuclear factor kappa beta (NF-kB) is the major upstream, intracellular mechanism which regulates inflammatory and oxidative stress neduatirs [70]. Maes and colleagues examined the production of NFkappabeta p50 in unstimulated, 10 ng/mL TNF-alpha (tumor necrosis factor alpha) and 50 ng/mL PMA (phorbolmyristate acetate) stimulated peripheral blood lymphocytes of 18 unmedicated patients with CFS and 18 age-sex matched controls. The unstimulated ($F=19.4$, $df=1/34p=0.0002$), TNF-alpha-($F=14.0$, $df=1/34$, $p=0.0009$) and PMA-($F=7.9$, $df=1/34$, $p=0.008$) stimulated production of NFkappabeta were significantly higher in CFS patients than in controls [70]. There were significant an positive correlations between the production of Nuclear Factor-kappa beta (NF-kB) and the severity of illness as measured with the FibroFatigue scale and with symptoms, such as aches and pain, muscular tension, fatigue, irritability, sadness, and the subjective feeling of infection [70].

Sleep and Fatigue

The association between sleep and fatigue is intuitively obvious. However, they remain separate but intimately related entities. Fatigue may be present without sleepiness and sleepiness may be present without fatigue. The presences if sleepiness depends on the balance of activity between ascending wakefulness-promoting and sleep-promoting and sleep-promoting pathways. Disorders with problems related to attention, concentration, focus, or vigilance may be more in the realm of sleep medicine than fatigue. It appears that fatigue is related to dysfunction of circuitry linking the cortex to the basal ganglia.

The prominence of hyperarousal in the genesis of sleep disorders resulting in fatigue suggests that cortical hyperarousal of specific circuits involving the basal ganglia may generate fatigue with marked dysfunction of subcortical circuits [71].

Ancoli-Israel et al. have proposed that some degree of cancer-related fatigue experienced during the day may relate to sleep/wake cycles or to the quality and quantity if sleep obtained at night. Different components or dimensions of fatigue (physical, attentional/cognitive, emotional/affective, etc.) are probably associated in some way with disrupted sleep and desynchronized sleep/wake rhythms [72].

Fatigue Assessment

Assessment tools for fatigue remain suboptimal. The Piper Fatigue Scale (Piper) was an early multidimensional tool attempting to subdivide the experience of pain into several distinct domains, but it seems to be too cumbersome to be used in clinical practice. The Schwartz Cancer Fatigue Scale which has four subscales (physical, emotional, cognitive, and temporal) was developed specifically for the cancer patient [73]. Routine clinical assessment of fatigue can be performed utilizing a numerical rating scale (NRS-11), --- with zero being no fatigue and ten being the worst fatigue imaginable. Fatigue assessment tools should allow for detection of temporal changes in the level of distress caused by fatigue. Agasi-Idenberg et al. evaluated thirty-five articles with cancer-related fatigue self-report questionnaires that described 18 questionnaires. The mean item count was 20.8 (range: 3-83). They argued in favor of repeatedly reassessing psychometric properties of even established questionnaires to ensure they comply with evermore increasing stringent quality criteria [74].

It is crucial to appreciate that fatigue has a significant impact on the quality of life and functionality not only of patients, but also of their caregivers, family, and partners/significant others/friends. Therefore, assessment and treatment of fatigue in the caregivers/family is vitally important [24, 75]. When the role demands of the caregiver exceed caregiver resources, fatigue may ensue and may compromise care giving. Teel and Press contrasted perceptions of fatigue among 92 older adults caring for spouses with Alzheimer's disease, Parkinson's disease, or cancer with a control group of 33 older adults whose spouses did not require extra care [76]. Care giving elders reported more fatigue, less energy, and more sleep difficulty than did controls [69]. Teel and Press suggested that health care providers can support older caregivers in monitoring their own health and recognizing the need for services that support the caregiving role [76].

Clinical Fatigue

Fatigue in health is generally transient (i.e. acute fatigue) and be termed "reactive fatigue" as it is usually the "executed" result of work, exertion, activities/stressors, or expending energy in physical, mental, or emotional domains [4]. "Reactive fatigue" tends to improve with rest or sleep and it may be perceived as a pleasant experience by some as it may be intimately associated with a "feeling of fulfillment, satisfaction or accomplishment." Examples may include finishing a marathon or finishing final exams after staying up all night studying.

"Major or endogenous fatigue" refers to fatigue that is generally chronic in nature and disproportionate or unrelated to work, exertion, activities or expending energy in physical, mental and emotional domains [4]. "Major fatigue" is not typically relieved with rest or sleep and is usually perceived as an unpleasant experience. Examples may include cancer-related fatigue or the fatigue associated with renal disease.

There are so many contributing etiologies to fatigue that it is beyond the scope of this book to cover all causes. Most chronic diseases especially in their advanced stages can contribute to fatigue. Pain and fatigue appear to be somewhat related--- co-existing in many advanced chronic illnesses [77]. Although other symptoms (e.g. nausea, sigultus, pruritis, dyspnea) have not been implicated as contributing to fatigue--- it is likely that they can in certain circumstances.

However, interest in fatigue appears to be growing. The second edition of the Oxford Text book of Palliative Medicine devotes a chapter to asthenia, although the 1st edition did not dedicate a specific chapter to any fatigue-related topic [78]. Simon and Zittoun [79] found that a Medline search of the National Library of Medicine combining the key words "fatigue" and "cancer" produced 72 entries in 1989 as opposed to the same search in 1999 producing 248 entries [79].

In 1999, cancer-related fatigue was accepted as a diagnosis in the International Classification of Diseases; Tenth Revision, Clinical Modification (ICM-10-CM) [80]. Exhaustion and tiredness are subsumed under the diagnosis of cancer-related fatigue in this revision [81].

Physical exercise which generates mechanical energy affects the equilibrium of the internal environment. Depending on the form of exercise, sooner or later sensations of fatigue and exhaustion will occur. Because of these sensations the subject will adapt their exercise strategy and at some point reduce or stop exercising. The relationship between physical exercise and fatigue has been the scope of interest of many researchers for more than a century and is very complex [82]. Physical exercise affects the biochemical equilibrium within the exercising muscle cells [82]. Furthermore, the contracting muscle fibers release cytokines, which in their turn create many effects in other organs, including the brain [82]. Voluntary muscle fatigue is a progressive process. A recent study demonstrated the energy of both EEG and EMG signals decreased significantly with muscle fatigue [83].

Energy is largely supplied bu mitochondia and mitochondrial dysfunction may contribute to or affect fatigue sensations. Mitochondria may adapt to a well designed exercise program with improved efficiency. The specificity of an endurance-exercise stimulus is reflected by the signature of the transcriptome response after muscle work [84]. A quantitative match in mitochondrial transcript adjustments and mitochondrial volume density after endurance training suggests that the gradual accumulation of expressional microadaptations underlies the promotion of fatigue resistance with training [84]. Contrariwise, mitochondrial function may be adversely affected by multiple factors included perhaps some involved with physiologic aging.

Skeletal muscle accounts for approximately 30% of resting energy expenditure, and physical activity can increase energy utilization by 10% to 60%. The systemic delivery of myostatin results in extreme muscle wasting in mice [85]. Myostatin, a member of the transforming growth factor- b (TGF b) superfamily, is a well-conserved and powerful negative regulator of muscle mass, which has emerged as a potential therapeutic target for improving muscle health [86]. Myostatin is highly expressed in skeletal muscle and undergoes a complex and regulated process of posttranslational modification to generate a bioactive dimer [87]. Le Brasseur et al. examined the effects of physical exercise and a neutralizing antibody to myostatin, PF-354, on clinically relevant performance and metabolic outcomes in aged mice. LeBrasseur and colleagues suggest that even in advanced age, myostatin significantly affects muscle health and its short-term (4 weeks) blockade significantly increases muscle mass [88]. This is especially significant given the diminished responsiveness of aged skeletal muscle to a host of other progrowth interventions, for example, contractile activity [89], essential amino acids [90], and insulin-like growth factor-1 [91]. These improvements were associated with increased PGC-1 a , a powerful regulator of oxidative phosphorylation and mitochondrial biogenesis in skeletal muscle [92] that is repressed in states of inactivity [93] and type 2 diabetes mellitus (T2DM) [94]. A short-term intervention comprised of physical exercise and myostatin inhibition mediated significant improvement in clinically relevant measures of physical function and all treatment groups demonstrated more than 30% reductions in muscle fatigue [88].

Somewhat of a paradox for therapy is that one of the treatments for fatigue and most conditions where fatigue plays a major role (e.g. fibromyalgia) is to initiate a slow gradual aerobic exercise program. In addition to traditional physical therapy and exercise programs, other aerobic physical activities may be beneficial as well. Yoga and sports climbing (SC) might improve some of the MS symptoms and should be studied in the future as possible complementary treatments [95].

Muscle Fatigue

Essentially, all people who have undergone prolonged exercise have experienced muscle fatigue. The complex nature of voluntary muscle contraction involves the central nervous system (CNS), the peripheral nerve, the neuromuscular junction, and the skeletal muscles. For contraction force levels less than 15% of maximum voluntary contraction (MVC) level, people could maintain the target level indefinitely (>45 minutes) [96]. However, as the force increases ---- the endurance time (which some regard as the opposite of a muscle fatigue measure) rapidly decreases [e.g. at 25% MVC→endurance time (ET) is roughly 3.75 minutes, 50% MVC→ET roughly 20-30 seconds] [96].

Bigland-Ritchie and colleagues compared the average firing rate of fast muscles (e.g. biceps brachii) to slow muscles (e.g. soleus) and found that firing rates varied in proportion to the relative speeds of the two muscles [97, 98]. This, it appeared that firing rates are tailored to muscle contractile properties. They also measured single muscle fiber action potentials in human adductor pollicis longus muscles during MVCs and found that as fatigue ensues and muscle force declined during the MVC; the average motor firing rate decreased from approximately 30 Hz to about 15 Hz [97, 98].

Following the time course of the muscle twitch during fatigue, they found that the muscle contracted and relaxed more slowly, with the time-to-peak tension (TPT) and half-relaxation time (HRT) significantly increasing [97, 98]. Slower muscles generate higher forces at lower frequencies because the muscle is not able to keep up with incoming impulses, much as a slow-contracting muscle shows titanic fusion at lower frequencies than a fast muscle. If firing rate decreased and TPT and HRT increased, then the muscle contraction force and same degree of fusion would be maintained.

As muscle contraction proceeds, adenosine triphosphate (ATP) levels begin to drop (but are initially replenished as creatine phosphate levels drop) and cellular glycogen and fat stores become mobilized to replenish energy stores.

Creatine Phosphate + ADP $\rightarrow$ Creatine + ATP

Hultman studied glycogen content in muscle biopsies obtained from the vastus lateralis muscles of cross-country skiers and found that muscle glycogen dropped dramatically with increasing exercise [99]. Furthermore, the amount of time the skiers could pedal a bicycle ergometer at an intense level was directly related to the amount of glycogen in their muscles [99].

Muscle differs with respect to endurance. One method to ascertain various endurance differences in muscle fibers is the motor unit fatigue index [100]. The original fatigue index test involved stimulation of the motor unit at roughly 40 Hz (generating about half-maximum tension) for one-third of a second and then allowing muscles to relax for two-thirds of a second, allowing the muscle to relax for two-thirds of a second, and repeating the sequence so that every second the motor unit receives a burst of 40 Hz pulses [100]. After two minutes of this protocol, the muscle tension was measured [100]. If the tension dropped significantly (compared to the initial tension) the motor unit was regarded as highly fatigable and if the tension was unchanged or dropped (compared to the initial tension) slightly; the motor unit was regarded as poorly fatigable [100]. Motor units then were classified as:

- Highly fatigable (defined as units that generated less than 25% of the initial tension after two minutes); fatigue resistant (units that generated over 75% of the initial tension after two minutes); and fatigue intermediate (units that generated between 25% and 75% of the initial tension after two minutes) [100].
- Highly fatigable or fast fatigable motor units have predominantly fast glycolytic muscle fibers.
- Fast fatigue-resistant motor units have predominantly fast oxidative glycolytic muscle fibers.
- Slow motor units have predominantly slow oxidative muscle fibers.

Warmolts et al. suggested that Type-II muscle fiber (e.g. FG) atrophy may be a systematic effect of cancer even in the early and non-metastatic stages [101]. Additionally, Bruera and colleagues demonstrated impaired maximal strength, decreased relaxation velocity, and increased fatigue after electrical ulnar nerve stimulation of the abductor pollicis muscle in patients with breast cancer versus healthy controls [102].

Intracellular acidification of skeletal muscles has been commonly thought to contribute to muscle fatigue. However, intracellular acidosis may act to preserve muscle excitability when muscles become depolarized, which occurs with working muscles. This process may be mediated by decreased chloride permeability, which enables action potentials to still be propagated along the internal network of tubules in a muscle fiber (the T system) despite muscle depolarization; and thus, intracellular acidosis of muscle may have protective effects during muscle fatigue [103].

During intense exercise, potassium flows out of the cells and accumulates, which reduces muscle contractions. Lowering pH to a level typical of a hard-working muscle counteracts potassium's reduction of muscle contractions. The acidity does this by reducing the dampening effect of chloride ions, probably by stemming their flow in and out of the muscle cell, which would normally inhibit spontaneous muscle contractions [104]. This phenomenon may also explain why warming up helps an athlete's performance, if this boosts acid levels in the muscles.

It is conceivable that a mitochondrial factor that is released when ATP production is incapacitated and that reduces t-tubular membrane excitability [105]. The concept that fatigue is related at least in part to a failure of membrane excitability has important implications not only for understanding factors limiting muscle force/power but also for cellular Ca^{2+} homeostasis and energy metabolism [106]. Muscle fatigue acts to preserve cellular integrity via regulation of $[Ca^{2+}]i$ and ATP levels, and thus survival. At least three membrane components are sensitive to either ATP or Ca^{2+}: *1)* the ATP-sensitive K^+ channel, *2)* the CLC-1 Cl^- channel [107], and *3)* the Ca^{2+}-sensitive K^+ channel [106, 108].

Marked perturbations in each of $[Na^+]_i$, $[K^+]_i$, and $[K^+]_{int}$ occur during fatiguing exercise in humans and during electrical stimulation in in-vitro preparations, with less well established changes in $[Na^+]_{int}$, $[Cl^-]_i$, and $[Cl^-]_{int}$ [106]. In unfatigued muscle, these ionic changes depress force, but under some conditions they can also enhance force or alleviate the fatigue effect; i.e., the effects of these ions are more complex than originally thought [106]. It is proposed that these enhancing or alleviating effects are important early in exercise, whereas their depressing effects are dominant later and directly contribute to development of muscle fatigue [106]. Similarly, exercise results in an early and sustained increase in NKA activity, which potentiates contractility, whereas later in exercise or after intense contractions a decline in maximal NKA activity occurs and contributes to fatigue [106].

The causes of muscle fatigue after extreme activity (e.g. marathon runners) are elusive. For more than 80 years, physiologists blamed lactic acid, which is produced during exercise and which they believed interfered with muscles' contractile proteins. But in the early 2000s, researchers found that at realistic body temperatures, very little acid accumulates inside muscle cells--and the bit that does may even improve endurance. Instead, suspicions have turned to the way muscle cells control the movement of calcium.

During normal muscle function, a nerve cell triggers the release of calcium within a muscle cell; the calcium, in turn, prompts the muscle cell to contract. A protein called calstabin is a subunit of the ryanodine receptor which binds to calcium channels and stabilizes the closed state of the ryanodine receptor/calcium-release channel. Lehnart et al. [109] and Huang et al. [110] reported that, in mice with heart failure and some forms of exercise-induced cardiac death, calstabin exhibits diminished binding affinity to the ryanodine receptor. This causes the channels to leak and depletes the supply of calcium needed to trigger contraction, resulting in heart exhaustion. The same mechanism was theorized to also be behind muscle fatigue.

Bellinger et al. put a group of mice on an intense marathon-scale training regimen, swimming for two 90-minute sessions every day for 2 weeks. Control mice went for only two 15-minute swims per day. Several muscle samples were obtained from the mice and it was found that, just as in failing heart muscle, the calcium channels of the more athletic mice had undergone changes that made them chronically leaky and required days of rest to recover [111].

Bellinger and colleagues analyzed the calcium-channel structure in human muscle samples from 12 elite athletes before and after a series of intense cycling sessions, their calcium channels had begun to undergo changes that were similar to what had happened in the mice [111]. During exercise in mice and humans, the major Ca^{2+} release channel required for excitation–contraction coupling (ECC) in skeletal muscle, the ryanodine receptor (RyR1), is progressively PKA-hyperphosphorylated, *S*-nitrosylated, and depleted of the phosphodiesterase PDE4D3 and the RyR1 stabilizing subunit calstabin1 (FKBP12), resulting in "leaky" channels that cause decreased exercise tolerance in mice [111]. Mice with skeletal muscle-specific calstabin1 deletion or PDE4D deficiency exhibited significantly impaired exercise capacity [111]. A small molecule (S107) which serves as a calcium channel stabilizer that prevents depletion of calstabin1 from the RyR1 complex improved force generation and exercise capacity, reduced Ca^{2+}-dependent neutral protease calpain activity and plasma creatine kinase levels [111]. Taken together, these data suggest a possible mechanism by which Ca^{2+} leak via calstabin1-depleted RyR1 channels leads to defective Ca^{2+} signaling, muscle damage (largely via calpain activation), and impaired exercise capacity [111]. S107 is thought to work by making calstabin bind more tightly to calcium channels. Rodents administered S107, the high-exercise mice could run 10% to 20% longer on a treadmill than controls could, the researchers report, even after 3 weeks of extreme exercise [111].

Work led by geneticist Kathryn North has shown highly significant associations between ACTN3 genotype and athletic performance [112]. The gene ACTN3 codes for the protein alpha-actinin-3, which is made mostly by fast fibers, and has been implicated in their capacity for rapid force generation. It appears that if ACTN3 is absent or mutated, alpha-actinin-3 is not produced, and as a result, fast muscle fibers turn into slow fibers.

Macarthur et al. found that mice lacking a functional ACTN3 gene had fast fibers containing much higher levels of aerobic metabolism, suggesting that the absence of alpha-actinin-3 caused the fast fibers to work more like slow fibers with a shift in muscle metabolism toward the more efficient aerobic pathway and an increase in intrinsic endurance performance [113].

These mice without alpha-actinin-3 could run about 33% farther than control mice suggesting an association of the ACTN3 mutation and endurance [113]. Macarthur and co-workers found that the region surrounding the mutant version of the genes showed less variability than did other parts of the genome, a sign of positive natural selection (i.e. the mutation might have had an evolutionary advantage) [113]. Macarthur et al. proposed that the 577X allele has been positively selected in some human populations owing to its effect on skeletal muscle metabolism [113]. It is unknown if humans with different ACTN3 genotypes performing various activities/tasks will also differ in the severity, duration and occurrence of fatigue.

More women than men suffer with significant fatigue and chronic widespread musculoskeletal pain, suggesting potential gender differences in the development of fatigue. Testosterone increases intracellular calcium in myocytes producing increases in phosphorylation and transcription factors through a G protein-linked receptor [114], and when administered to myocytes; it decreases the action potential threshold and increases synaptic facilitation resulting in an enhancement of synaptic efficiency in the flexor carpi radialis muscle of the frog [115]. Burnes and colleagues hypothesized that testosterone, through intracellular signaling pathways, increases efficacy of ASIC3 and/or increases production of ASIC3 to reduce fatigue, allowing myocytes to contract with a lower motor neuron output [116].

Burnes et al. suggested that H^+ ions play a critical role in fatigue and recovery from fatigue through activation of ASIC3 on muscle fibers. Excitability of muscle fibers is modified by the Na^+-K^+ cotransporter and depends on extracellular K^+ concentration [117], however the Na^+-H^+ contransporter may play a role as well. The Na^+/K^+ gradient across the membrane is critical for generation of action potential amplitude [117]. By mimicking extracellular sodium decreases and potassium increases seen in exercising muscle, thus reducing the gradients for Na^+ and K^+, there is a reduction in the M-wave similar to that observed with fatiguing contractions [118]. Restoring the sodium gradient through activation of ASICs could potentially improve the Na^+/K^+ gradient to reduce fatigue [116].

Muscle fatigue is common in multiple chronic pain conditions, including fibromyalgia, osteoarthritis, and rheumatoid arthritis [119-128]. As many as 76% of people with chronic widespread musculoskeletal pain report fatigue and as many as 94% of people with chronic fatigue syndromes report muscle pain [109, 116, 123, 128]. In an animal model of pain, induced by intramuscular injections of acidic saline, exercise increases nociceptive responses in mice during a long-duration fatigue task [129]. These data suggest an overlap between fatigue and pain such that fatigue plays a significant role in the development of pain, and that pain is enhanced in response to fatigue [116]. Since both fatigue and muscle pain appear ro involve ASIC3, Burnes and colleagues have theorized that a common pathway may occur in the periphery to generate the pain and fatigue associated with chronic muscle pain conditions [116].

The Impact of Fatigue

Fatigue affects more cancer patients and more persistently than any other symptoms and it is regarded by many patients as being more distressing than pain, nausea, vomiting or depression [130, 131]. Vogelzang et al in a tri-part assessment survey of cancer patients found that--- 78% of patients experienced significant fatigue (defined as a general feeling of debilitating tiredness or loss of energy) during the course of their disease and treatment, care givers reported observing fatigue in 86% of patients, and oncologists perceived that 76% of their patients experienced fatigue [132].

Oncologists believed that pain adversely affected their patients to a greater degree than fatigue 61% versus 37%), however, patients felt that fatigue adversely affected their daily lives more than pain (61% versus 19%) [132]. Eighty percent of oncologists believed that fatigue is overlooked or under treated, and the majority of patients (74%) felt that fatigue was a symptom to be endured [132]. Fifty percent of patients did not discuss treatment options with their oncologists, and only 27% answered that their oncologists recommended any treatment for fatigue [132]. It appears that fatigue is appreciated as a commonly experience symptom--- however, it seems that the level of "symptom distress" caused by fatigue and the effectiveness of treatments may be underappreciated.

Fatigue may be a predominant determinant of quality of life in patients without cancer, in patients with cancer, and among cancer survivors. Cancer-related fatigue has detrimental effects on a cancer patient's quality of life and ability to sustain their usual personal, professional, and social relationships. In a study of sixty-one women with breast cancer, Broeckel et al. reported that former adjuvant chemotherapy patients reported more severe fatigue and worse quality of life because of fatigue as compared to women without cancer [133]. Servaes et al. found that 19% of 85 adult disease-free (off treatment for at least six months) cancer patients in their study were severely fatigued [134]. Their fatigue experience was comparable to that of patients with chronic fatigue syndrome [134]. Severe fatigue was associated with problems of concentration and motivation, reduced physical activity, and emotional health problems [134]. Additionally, fatigue has been shown to be an independent predictor of impaired quality of life in multiple sclerosis (MS) [135]. The 22-item Unidimensional Fatigue Impact Scale (U-FIS) provides an index of the impact of fatigue on patients with multiple sclerosis (MS) [136].

The National Institute of Health Consensus Development Panel concluded that quality of life needs to be evaluated in selected randomized clinical trials to examine the impact of the major acute and long-term side effects of adjuvant treatments, particularly fatigue, premature menopause, weight gain, and mild memory loss [137].

A Glimpse at Approaches to Improving Fatigue

Aside from general therapeutic measures for fatigue (e.g. aerobic exercise), specific conditions with associated fatigue may respond to specific treatment strategies. Frailty is a geriatric syndrome characterized by muscle weakness, sarcopenia, and fatigue, and is associated with several adverse health outcomes, including disability [138]. Carnitine is vital to fatty acid metabolism due to its crucial role in the translocation of long chain acylCoA across the inner mitochondrial membrane. Thus, carnitine is important for optimal mitochondrial functioning and energy production in skeletal muscles. There seems to be a negative correlation between advancing age and muscle carnitine levels [138]. Carnitine deficiency may therefore contribute to geriatric frailty and fatigue. Age-associated carnitine deficiency from a variety of etiologies, including organic cation transporter (OCTN2) mutation [OCTN2 mediates the cellular uptake of carnitine] and carnitine palmitoyltransferase II (CPT) deficiency [CPT II mediates the transport of carnitine esters across the inner mitochondrial membrane and their reconversion to CoA esters], may potentially explain the relationship between carnitine-associated mitochondrial dysfunction and geriatric frailty [138]. Serum free carnitine levels were lower after physical fatigue inducing sessions than those after the relaxing sessions [139].

Although some evidence exists that treatment with carnitine "replacement"/ administration may be beneficial with respect to fatigue [140-142], Tejani and colleagues demonstrated that there is insufficient evidence that carnitine for the treatment of MS-related fatigue offers a therapeutic advantages over placebo or active comparators [143].

In multiple sclerosis, axonal demyelination with subsequent activity-dependent conduction block (ADCB) of nerve function may contribute to fatigue. Na^+/K^+ pump dysfunction may induce a depolarizing conduction block associated with inactivation of Na^+ channels. Resultant normal Na^+ concentrations may, via reverse operation of the $Na^+ - Ca^{++}$ exchanges, lead to increase intracellular Ca^{++}. Investigators have postulated that strategies aimed at restoring normal conduction in demyelinated axons (e.g. selective channel blockers) [144]may improve fatigue [144] Two randomized trials have shown that body cooling significantly reduces fatigue [145, 146] .Cooling may impact on fatigue by reducing the activity of Na^+/K^+ ATPase so limiting the extent of hyperpolarizing ADCB, and by slowing Na+ channel kinetics, thereby improving the safety factor of transmission in critically impaired axons [147, 148]. In addition, cooling has been reported to be associated with a 41% reduction in mean leukocyte nitric oxide [NO] production [145]. Given that NO can induce conduction failure in myelinated axons [149], it was suggested that cooling may impact on fatigue by reversing conduction block. The hypothesis that ADCB contributes to symptoms of fatigue in MS provides therapeutic options such as 4-diaminopyridine [3,4-DAP], which block (juxta-)paranodal F and I K+ currents in the peripheral nerve [see above], improve conduction in demyelinated axons by prolonging the duration of the action potential and thereby improving the safety factor of impulse transmission [150]. Trials of both 4-aminopyridine [151-155] and 3,4-diaminopyridine [152, 153, 156, 157] have demonstrated benefit for both fatigue and other neurological symptoms, such as weakness.

Conclusion

In summary, fatigue assessment, evaluation, and management remain suboptimal and as a result may lead to significant impairment of patient quality of life. It is becoming clearer that fatigue is not "just a mildly annoying symptom" that patients "need to live with." In efforts to optimize the existing state of the art fatigue knowledge/practices--- the use of interdisciplinary "fatigue clinics" may be a useful option (at least in terms of minimizing barriers to effective communication regarding fatigue). Future research designed to develop new tools for the assessment, evaluation of fatigue allowing mechanism-based treatment approaches is needed in efforts to improve patient care.

References

[1] Lamberts, H. (1991). In het huis van de huisarts. Verslag van het Transitieproject. Meditekst,.

[2] Richardson. A., Ream, E., & Wilson-Barnett, J. (1998). Fatigue in patients receiving chemotherapy: patterns of change. *Cancer Nurs*, 21,17-20.

[3] Morrow, G.R., Andrews, P.L., Hickok, J.T., Roscoe, J.A., & Matteson, S. (2002). Fatigue associated with cancer and its treatment. *Support Care Cancer*, 10,389-398.

[4] Smith, H.S. (2007). Fatigue Revisited. Presented at the Capital District New York Pain Research Meeting. Albany, NY.

[5] Muscio, B. (1921). Is a fatigue test possible? *British Journal of Psychology*, 12,31-46.

[6] Lezak, M.D. (1995). Neuropsychological assessment. 3rd Edition. New York: Oxford University Press.

[7] Multiple Sclerosis Council for Clinical Practice Guidelines. (1998). Fatigue and multiple sclerosis: Evidence-based management strategies for fatigue in multiple sclerosis. Washington DC: Paralyzed Veterans of America.

[8] Ahsberg, E., & Furst, C.J. (2001). Dimensions of fatigue during radiotherapy---An Application of the Swedish Occupational Fatigue Inventory (SOFI) on cancer patients. *Acta Onocologica*, 40,37-43.

[9] Rönnbäck, L., & Hansson, E. (2004). On the potential role of glutamate transport in mental fatigue. *J Neuroinflammation*, 1,22.

[10] Magnusson, A.E., Nias, D.K. & White P.D. (1996). Is Perfectionism associated with fatigue? *J Psychosom Res*, 41,377-383.

[11] Cimprich. B., Visovatti, M., & Ronis DL. (2010). The Attentional Function Index-a self-report cognitive measure. Psychoncology, In press.

[12] Patarca-Montero, T. (2004). Handbook of Cancer-related Fatigue, The Haworth Medical Press. Binghamton, NY

[13] Chaudhuri A., & Behan, P.O. (2000). Fatigue and basal ganglia. *J Neurol Sci*, 179,34-42.

[14] Newsholme, E.A., Blomstrand, E., & Ekblom, B. (1992). Physical and mental fatigue: metabolic mechanisms and importance of plasma amino acids. *Br Med Bull*, 48,477-495.

[15] Gandevia, S.C. (2001). Spinal and supraspinal factors in human muscle fatigue. Physiol Rev, 81,1725–1789.

[16] Gandevia, S.C., Allen, G.M., Butler, J.E., & Taylor, J.L. (1996). Supraspinal factors in human muscle fatigue: evidence for suboptimal output from the motor cortex. *J Physiol*, 490,529–536.

[17] Taylor, J.L., Allen, G.M., Butler, J.E., & Gandevia, S.C. (2000). Supraspinal fatigue during intermittent maximal voluntary contractions of the human elbow flexors. *J Appl Physiol*, 89,305–313.

[18] Gandevia, S.C., & Taylor. J.L. (2006). Spuraspinal fatigue: the effects of caffeine on human muscle performance. *J Appl Physiol*, 100,1749-1750.

[19] Taylor, J.L., Butler, J.E., Allen, G.M., & Gandevia, S.C. (1996). Changes in motor cortical excitability during human muscle fatigue. *J Physiol*, 490,519–528.

[20] Petersen, N.T., Taylor, J.L., Butler, J.E., & Gandevia, S.C. (2003). Depression of activity in the corticospinal pathway during human motor behavior after strong voluntary contractions. *J Neurosci*, 23,7974–7980.

[21] Butler, J.E., Taylor, J.L., & Gandevia, S.C. (2003). Responses of human motoneurons to corticospinal stimulation during maximal voluntary contractions and ischemia. *J Neurosci*, 23,10224–10230.

[22] Taylor, J.L., & Gandevia, S.C. (2008). A comparison of central aspects of fatigue in submaximal and maximal voluntary contractions. J Appl Physiol, 104,542-550.

[23] Wessely, S. (2001). Chronic fatigue: symptom and syndrome. Ann Intern Med., 134,838-843.

[24] Elovic, E.P., Dobrovic, N.M., & Fellus, J.L. Fatigue after traumatic brain injury. In: Deluca, J., editor. Fatigue as a window to the brain: Cambridge, Massachusetts: MIT Press; 2005.

[25] Lezak, M,D. (1978). Subtle sequelae of brain damage. Perplexity, distractibility, and fatigue. *Am J Phys Med*, 57,9-15.

[26] Cella, D., Lai, J.S., Chang, C.H., Peterman, A., & Slavin, M. (2002). Fatigue in cancer patients compared with fatigue in the general United States population. *Cancer*, 94,528-538.

[27] Kerns, R.D., Turk, D.C., & Rudy, T.E. (1985). The West Haven-Yale Multidimensional Pain Inventory (WHYMPI). Pain, 23,345-356.

[28] Magnusson, K., Karlsson, E., Palmblad, C., Leitner, C., & Paulson, A. (1997). Swedish nurses' estimation of fatigue as a symptom in cancer patients--- Report of a questionnaire. *European Journal of Cancer Care*, 6,186-191.

[29] Tavio, M., Milan, I., & Tirelli, U. (2002). Cancer-related fatigue (review). *International Journal of Oncology*, 21,1093-1099.

[30] Valdres, R.U., Escalante, C., & Manzullo, E. (2001). Fatigue: a debilitating symptom. *Nurs Clin North Am*, 36,685-694.

[31] Mock, V., Atkinson, A., Barsevick, A., Cella, D., Cimprich, B., Cleeland, C., Donnelly, J., Eisenberger, M.A., Escalante, C., Hinds, P., Jacobsen, P.B., Kaldor, P., Knight, S.J., Peterman, A., Piper, B.F., Rugo, H., Sabbatini, P., Stahl, C., & National Comprehensive Cancer Network. (2000). NCCN Practice Guidelines for Cancer-Related Fatigue. *Oncology*, 14,151-161.

[32] Mock, V. (2001). Fatigue management: Evidence and guidelines for practice. *Cancer*, 92, 1699-1707.

[33] Mock, V., Atkinson, A., Barsevick, A.M., Berger, A.M., Cimprich, B., Eisenberger, M.A., Hinds, P., Kaldor, P., Otis-Green, S.A., & Piper, B.F. (2007). Cancer-related fatigue. *J Natl Compr Canc Netw*, 5,1054-1078.

[34] Escalante, C.P., Grover, T., Johnston, B.A., Harle, M., Gui, H., Mendoza, T.R., Rivera. E., Ho, V., Lee, E.L., & Cleeland, C.S. (2001). A fatigue clinic in a comprehensive cancer center: Design and experiences. Cancer, 92, 1708-1713.

[35] Radbruch, L., Strasser, F., Elsner, F., Gonçalves, J.F., Løge, J., Kaasa, S., Nauck, F., Stone, P.; & Research Steering Committee of the European Association for Palliative Care (EAPC). (2008). Fatigue in palliative care patients—an EAPC approach. *Palliat Med*, 22,13–32.

[36] Hann, D.M., Jacobsen, P.B., Azzarello, L.M., Martin, S.C., Curran, S.L., Fields, K.K., Greenberg, H., & Lyman, G. (1998). Measurement of fatigue in cancer patients: development and validation of the Fatigue Symptom Inventory. *Qual Life Res*, 7,301–310.

[37] Hann, D.M., Denniston, M.M., & Baker, F. (2000). Measurement of fatigue in cancer patients: further validation of the Fatigue Symptom Inventory. *Qual Life Res*, 9,847–854.

[38] Minton, O., & Stone, P. (2009). A systematic review of the scales used for the measurement of cancer-related fatigue (CRF). *Ann Oncol*, 20,17-25.

[39] Li, H., Mittal, A., Paul, P.K., Kumar, M., Srivastava, D.S., Tyagi, S.C., & Kumar, A. (2009). Tumor necrosis factor-related weak inducer of apoptosis augments matrix metalloproteinase 9 (MMP-9) production in skeletal muscle through the activation of nuclear factor-kappaB-inducing kinase and p38 mitogen-activated protein kinase: a potential role of MMP-9 in myopathy. *J Biol Chem*, 284,4439-4450.

[40] Mittal, A., Bhatnagar, S., Kumar, A., Lach-Trifilieff, E., Wauters, S., Li, H., Makonchuk, D.Y., Glass, D.J., & Kumar, A. (2010). The TWEAK-Fn14 system is a critical regulator of denervation-induced skeletal muscle atrophy in mice. *J Cell Biol*, 188,833-849.

[41] Bruno, R.L., Creange, S.J., & Frick, N.M. (1998). Parallels between post-polio fatigue and chronic fatigue syndrome: a common pathophysiology? *The Amer J Med*, 105,66S-73S.

[42] Franceschini R., Tenconi G.L., Zoppoli F., & Barreca, T. (2001). Endocrine abnormalities and outcome of ischaemic stroke. *Biomedicine and Pharmacotherapy*, 55,456-465.

[43] Coutureau, E., & Killcross, S. (2003). Inactivation of the infralimbic prefrontal cortex reinstates goal-directed responding in overtrained rats. *Behav Brain Res*, 146,167-174.

[44] Levy, R., & Czernecki, V. (2006). Apathy and the basal ganglia. *J Neurol*, 253,VII54-61.

[45] Heilman, K.M., & Valenstein, E. Clinical Neurophyscology, 4th ed. Oxford, UK: Oxford University Press; 2003.

[46] Roelcke, U., Kappos, L., Lechner-Scott, J. Brunnschweiler, H., Huber, S., Ammann, W., Plohmann, A., Dellas, S., Maguire, R.P., Missimer, J., Radü, E.W., Steck, A., & Leenders K.L. (1997). Reduced glucose metabolism in the frontal cortex and basal ganglia of multiple sclerosis patients with fatigue: a 18F fluorodeoxyglucoise positron emission tomography study. *Neurology*, 48,1566-1571.

[47] Sheean G.L.; Murrary N.M.; Rothwell J.C.; Miller DH, Thompson AJ. An electrophysiological study of the mechanism of fatigue in multiple sclerosis. *Brain*. 1997, 120(Pt 2), 299-315.

[48] Leocani, L., Colombo, B., Magnani, G., Martinelli-Boneschi, F., Cursi, M., Rossi, P., Martinelli, V., & Comi, G. (2001). Fatigue in multiple sclerosis is associated with abnormal cortical activation to voluntary movement-EEG evidence. *Neuroimage*, 13,1186-1192.

[49] Filippi, M., Rocca, M.A., Colombo, B., Falini, A., Codella, M., Scotti, G., & Comi, G. (2002). Functional magnetic resonance imaging correlates of fatigue in multiple sclerosis. *Neuroimage*, 15,559-567.

[50] Katafuchi, T., Kondo, T, Take, S., & Yoshimura, M. (2006). Brain cytokines and the 5-HT system during poly 1:C-induced fatigue. *Ann NY Acad Sci*, 1088,230-237.

[51] Capuron, L., Pagnoni, G., Demetrashvili, M.F., Lawson, D.H., Fornwalt, F.B., Woolwine, B., Berns, G.S., Nemeroff, C.B., & Miller, A.H. (2007). Basal Ganglia Hypermetabolism and Symptoms of Fatigue during Interfron-alpha Therapy. *Neuropsychopharmacology*, 32,2384-2392.

[52] Salamone, J.D., Correa, M., Farrar, A., & Mingote, S.M. (2007). Effort-related functions of nucleus accumbens dopamine and associated forebrain circuits. *Psychopharmacology* (Berl), 191,461-482.

[53] Larfargue, G., & Sirigu, A. (2006). The nature of the sense of effort and its neural substrate, *Rev Neurol* (Paris), 162,703-712.
[54] Niepel, G., Tench, C.R., Morgan, P.S., Evangelou, N., Auer, D.P., & Constantinescu, C.S. (2006). Deep gray matter and fatigue in MS. A T1 relaxation time study. *J Neurol*, 253,896-902.
[55] Iwasa, M., Kinosada, Y., Nakatsuka, A., Watanabe, S., & Adachi, Y. (1999). Magnetization transfer contrast of various regions of the brain in liver cirrhosis. *AJNR Am J Neuroradical*, 20,652-654
[56] Córdoba, J., Alonso, J., Rovira, A., Jacas, C., Sanpedro, F., Castells, L., Vargas, V., Margarit, C., Kulisewsky, J., Esteban, R., & Guardia, J. (2001). The development of low-grade cerebral edema in cirrhosis is supported by the evolution of (1)H-magnetic resonance abnormalities after liver transplantation. *J Hepatol*, 35,598-604.
[57] Laplan, D., Baulac, M., Widlovher, D. & Dubois, B. (1984). Pure psychic akinesia with bilatral lesions of basal ganglia. J Nerurol Neurosurg Psychiatry, 47,377-385.
[58] Forton, D.M., Patel, N., Prince, M., Oatridge, A., Hamilton, G., Goldblatt, J., Allsop, J.M., Hajnal, J.V., Thomas, H.C., Bassendine, M., Jones, D.E., & Taylor-Robinson, S.D. (2004). Fatigue and primary biliary cirrhosis: association of globus pallidus magnetisation transfer ratio measurements with fatigue severity and blood manganese levels. *Gut*, 53,587-592.
[59] Chen, C.J., & Liao, S.L. (2002). Oxidative stress involves in astrocytic alterations induced by manganese. *Exp Neurol*, 175,216-225.
[60] Tedeschi, G., Dinacci, D., Lavorgna, L., Prinster, A., Savettieri, G., Quattrone, A., Livrea, P., Messina, C., Reggio, A., Servillo, G., Bresciamorra, V., Orefice, G., Paciello, M., Brunetti, A., Paolillo, A., Coniglio, G., Bonavita, S., Di Costanzo, A., Bellacosa, A., Valentino, P., Quarantelli, M., Patti, F., Salemi, G., Cammarata, E., Simone, I., Salvatore, M., Bonavita, V., & Alfano, B. (2007). Correlation between fatigue and brain atrophy and lesion load in multiple sclerosis patients independently of disability. *J Neurol Sci*, 263, 5–19.
[61] Marrie, R.A., Fisher, E., Miller, D.M., Lee, J.C., & Rudick, R.A.(2005). Association of fatigue and brain atrophy in multiple sclerosis. *J Neurol Sci*, 228,161–166.
[62] Tartaglia, M.C., Narayanan, S., Francis, S.J., Santos, A.C., De Stefano, N., Lapierre, Y., & Arnold, D.L. (2004). The relationship between diffuse axonal damage and fatigue in multiple sclerosis. *Arch Neurol*, 61, 201–207.
[63] Colombo, B., Martinelli Boneschi, F., Rossi, P., Rovaris, M., Maderna, L., Fillippi, M., & Comi, G. (2000). MRI and motor evoked potential findings in nondisabled multiple sclerosis patients with and without symptoms of fatigue. *J Neurol*, 247,506–509.
[64] Inglese, M., Park, S.J., Johnson, G., Babb, J.S., Miles, L., Jaggi, H., Herbert, J., & Grossman, R.I. (2007). Deep gray matter perfusion in multiple sclerosis: dynamic susceptibility contrast perfusion magnetic resonance imaging at 3 T. *Arch Neurol,* 64,196–202.
[65] Filippi, M., & Rocca, M.A. (2007). Toward a definition of structural and functional MRI substrates of fatigue in multiple sclerosis. *J Neurological Sci*, 263,1-2.
[66] Blomstrand, E. (2001). Amino acids and central fatigue. Amino Acids, 20,25-34.
[67] Blomstrand,E., Perrett, D., Parry-Billings, M., & Newsholme, E.A. (1989). Effect of sustained exercise on plasma amino acid concentrations and on 5-hydroxytryptamine metabolism in six different brain regions in the rat. Acta Physiol Scand, 136,473-481.

[68] Blomstrand, E.(2006). A role for branced-chain amino acids in reducing central fatigue. *J Nutr*, 136,544S-547S.

[69] Malaguarnera, M., Gargante, M.P., Cristaldi, E., Colonna, V., Messano, M., Koverech, A., Neri, S., Vacante, M., Cammalleri, L., & Motta, M. (2008). Acetyl l-carnitine (ALC) treatment in elderly patients with fatigue. *Arch Gerontol Geriatr*, 46,181-190.

[70] Maes, M., Mihaylova, I., & Bosmans, E. (2007). Not in the mind of neurasthenic lazybones but in the cell nucleus: patients with chronic fatigue syndrome have increased production of nuclear factor kappa beta. *Neuro Endocrinol Lett*, 28,456-462.

[71] Duntley, S.P. Fatigue and Sleep. In*:* Fatigue as a Window to the Brain. DeLuca, J., Editor. Cambridge, Massachusetts: MIT Press; 2005.

[72] Ancoli-Israel, S., Moore, P.J., & Jones, Y. (2001). The relationship between fatigue and sleep in cancer patients: A review. *European Journal of Cancer Care*, 10 245-255.

[73] Schwartz, J.E., Jandorf, L., & Krupp, L.B. (1993). The measurement of fatigue: A new instrument. *Journal of Psychosomatic Research*, 37,753-762.

[74] Agasi-Idenberg, C. Velthuis, M., & Wittink, H. (2010). Quality criteria and user-friendliness in self-reported questionnaires on cancer-related fatigue: a review. *J Clin Epidemiol*, In Press.

[75] Winningham, M.L. (2001). Strategies for managing cancer-related fatigue syndrome: A rehabilitation approach. *Cancer*, 92,988-997.

[76] Teel, C.S., & Press, A.N. (1999). Fatigue among elders in caregiving and noncaregiving roles. *Western Journal of Nursing Research*, 21,498-514.

[77] Kaasa, S., Loge, J.H., Knobel, H., Jordhøy, M.S., & Brenne, E.(1999). Fatigue: Measures and relation to pain. *Acta Anaesthesiologica Scandinavica*, 43, 939-947.

[78] Oxford Textbook of Palliative Medicine. Doyle, D., Hanks, G.W.C., & Macdonald, N., Editors. Third Edition. . Oxford, UK: Oxford University Press; 2003.

[79] Simon, A.M., & Zittoun, R. (1999). Fatigue in cancer patients. *Current Opinions in Oncology*, 11,224-249.

[80] Portenoy, R.K., & Itri, L.M. (1999). Cancer-related fatigue: Guidelines for evaluation and management. *Oncologist*, 4,1-10.

[81] Zahner, J., Meran, J., & Karthaus, N. (2001). [Exhaustion and fatigue--- A neglected problem in hematologic oncology]. Wien Medizinische Wochenschrift, 151,89-93.

[82] Ament, W., & Verkerke, G.J. (2009). Exercise and fatigue. *Sports Med*, 39,389-422,

[83] Yang, Q, Siemionow, V., Yao, W. Sahgal, V., & Yue, G.H. (2010). Single-Trial EEG-EMG Coherence Analysis Reveals Muscle Fatigue-Rellated Progressive Alterations in Corticomuscular Coupling. IEEE Trans Neural Syst Rehabil Eng, In Press.

[84] Flueck, M. (2009). Tuning of mitochondrial pathways by muscle work: from triggers to sensors and expression signatures. Appl Physiol Nutr Metab, 34,447-453.

[85] Zimmers, T.A. , Davies, M.V. , Koniaris, L.G. , Haynes, P., Esquela, A.F., Tomkinskon, K.N., McPherron, A.C., Wolfman, N.M. & Lee, S.J. (2002). Induction of cachexia in mice by systemically administered myostatin . *Science*, 296,1486 – 1488.

[86] McPherron, A.C. , Lawler, A.M., & Lee, S.J . (1997). Regulation of skeletal muscle mass in mice by a new TGF-beta superfamily member. Nature, 387,83 – 90 .

[87] Lee, S.J. (2004). Regulation of muscle mass by myostatin . *Annu Rev Cell Dev Biol*, 20,61 – 86 .

[88] LeBrasseur, N.K., Schelhorn, T.M., Bernardo, B.L., Cosgrove, P.G., Loria, P.M., & Brown, T.A. (2009). Myostatin inhibition enhances the effects of exercise on

performance and metabolic outcomes in aged mice. *J Gerontol A Biol Sci Med Sci*, 64,940-948.

[89] Parkington, J.D., LeBrasseur, N.K., Siebert, A.P., & Fielding, RA . (2004). Contractionmediated mTOR, p70S6k, and ERK1/2 phosphorylation in aged skeletal muscle . *J Appl Physiol*, 97,243–248 .

[90] Cuthbertson, D., Smith, K., Babraj, J., Leese, G., Waddell, T., Atherton, P., Wackerhage, H., Taylor, P.M., & Rennie, M.J. (2005). Anabolic signaling defi cits underlie amino acid resistance of wasting, aging muscle . *FASEB J*, 19,422–424.

[91] Dardevet, D. , Sornet, C. , Attaix, D. , Baracos, V.E. , & Grizard, J . (1994). Insulin-like growth factor-1 and insulin resistance in skeletal muscles of adult and old rats. *Endocrinology*, 134,1475–1484.

[92] Wu, Z., Puigserver, P., Andersson, U., Zhang, C., Adelmant, G., Mootha, V., Troy, A., Cinti, S., Lowell, B., Scarpulla, R.C., & Spiegelman, B.M. (1999). Mechanisms controlling mitochondrial biogenesis and respiration through the thermogenic coactivator PGC-1. *Cell*, 98,115–124.

[93] Timmons, J.A., Norrbom, J., Scheele, C., Thonberg, H, Wahlestedt, C., & Tesch P. (2006). Expression profiling following local muscle inactivity in humans provides new perspective on diabetes-related genes. *Genomics*, 87,165–172.

[94] Mootha, V.K., Lindgren, C.M., Eriksson, K.F., Subramanian, A., Sihaq, S., Lehar, J., Puigserver, P., Carlsson, E., Ridderstråle, M., Laurila, E., Houstis, N., Daly, M.J., Patterson, N., Mesiroy, J.P., Golub, T.R., Tamavo, P., Spiegelman, B., Lander, E.S., Hirschorn, J.N., Altshuler, D., & Groop, L.C.. (2003). PGC-1alpha-responsive genes involved in oxidative phosphorylation are coordinately downregulated in human diabetes. *Nat Genet*, 34,267–273.

[95] Velikonja, O., Curić, K., Ožura A., & Jazbec, S.S. (2010). Influence of psorts climbing and yoga on spasticity, cognitive function, mood and fatigue in patients with multiple sclerosis. *Clin Neurol Neurosurg*, In Press.

[96] Rohmert, W. (1960). Ermittung von Erholungspausen für statische Arbet des Menschen. *Phsyciologust*, 18,123-130.

[97] Bigland-Ritchie, B., Johansson, R, Lippold, O., & Woods, J.J. (1983). Contractile speed and EMG changes during fatigue of sustained maximal voluntary contractions. *Journal of Neurophysiology*, 50,313-324.

[98] Bigland-Ritchie, B., Johansson, R., Lippold, O., Smith, S., & Woods, J.J. (1983). Changes in motoneurone firing rates during sustained maximal voluntary contractions. *Journal of Neurophysiology* (London), 340,335-346.

[99] Hultman, E. (1967). Physiological role of muscle glycogen in man, with special reference to exercise. *Circulation Research*, 21,I99-I112.

[100] Lieber, R.L. Skeletal Muscle Physiology. In: Lieber, R.L editor. Skeletal Muscle Structure, Function, & Plasticity. The physiologiocal basis of rehabilitation. Second Edition. Philadelphia, Pennsylvania: Lippincott Williams & Wilkins; 2002.

[101] Warmolts, J.R., Re, P.K., Lewis, R.J., & Engel, W.K. (1975). Type II Muscle Fiber Atrophy (II – Atrophy): An Early Systemic Effect of Cancer. Neurology, 2,374.

[102] Bruera, E., Jackson, F., Michaud, M., Jackson, P.I., & MacDonald, R.N. (1988). Muscle Electrophysiology in Patients with Advanced Breast Cancer. *Journal of the National Cancer Institute*, 80,282-285.

[103] Pedersen, T.H., Nielsen, O.B., Lamb, G.D., & Stephenson, D.G. (2004). Intracellular Acidosis Enhances the Excitability of Working Muscle. *Science*, 205,1144-1147.

[104] Nielsen, O.B., & de Paoli, F.V. (2007). Regulation of Na+-K+ homeostasis and excitability in contracting muscles: implications for fatigue. *Appl Physiol Nutr Metab*, 32,974-984.

[105] Ørtenblad N., & Stephenson, D.G. (2003). A novel signaling pathway originating in mitochondria modulates rat skeletal muscle membrane excitability. *J Physiol*, 548,139–145.

[106] McKenna, M.J., Bangsbo, J., & Renaud, J.M. (2008). Muscle K+, Na+, and Cl disturbances Na+-K+ pump inactivation: implications for fatigue. *J Appl Physiol*, 104,288-295.

[107] Bennetts, B., Rychkov, G.Y., Ng, H.L., Morton, C.J., Stapleton, D., Parker, M.W., & Cromer, B.A. (2005). Cytoplasmic ATP-sensing domains regulate gating of skeletal muscle ClC-1 chloride channels. *J Biol Chem*, 280,32452–32458.

[108] Kristensen, M., Hansen, T., & Juel, C. (2006). Membrane proteins involved in potassium shifts during muscle activity and fatigue. *Am J Physiol Regul Integr Comp Physiol*, 290,R766–R772.

[109] Lehnart, S.E., Terrenoire, C., Reiken, S., Wehrens, X.H., Song, L.S., Tillman, E.J., Mancarella, S., Coromilas, L., Lederer, W.J., Kass, R.S., Marks, A.R. (2006). Stabilization of cardiac ryanodine receptor prevents intracellular calcium leak and arrhythmias. *Proc Natl Acad Sci USA*, 103, 7906-7910.

[110] Huang, F., Shan, J., Reiken, S., Wehrens, X.H., & Marks, A.R. (2006). Analysis of calstabin2 (FKBP12.6)-ryanodine receptor interactions: rescue of heart failure by calstabin2 in mice. *Proc Natl Acad Sci USA*, 103,3456-3461.

[111] Bellinger, A.M., Reiken, S., Dura, M., Murphy, P.W., Deng, S.X., Landry, D.W., Nieman, D., Lehnart, S.E., Samaru, M., LaCampagne, A., & Marks, A.R. (2008). Remodeling of ryanodine receptor complex causes "leaky" channels: a molecular mechanism for decreased exercise capacity. *Proc Natl Acad Sci USA*, 105,2198-2202.

[112] Yang, N., MacArthur, D.G., Gulbin, J.P., Hahn, A.G., Beggs, A.H., Easteal, S., & North, K. (2003). ACTN3 genotype is associated with human elite athletic performance. *Am J Hum Genet*, 73,627-631.

[113] Macarthur, D.G., Seto, J.T., Raftery, J.M., Quinlan, K.G., Huttle, G.A., Hook, J.W., Lemckert, F.A., Kee, A.J., Edwards, M.R., Berman, Y., Hardeman, E.C., Gunning, P.W., Easteal, S., Yang, N., & North, K.N. (2007). Loss of ACTN3 gene function alters mouse muscle metabolism and shows evidence of positive selection in humans. *Nat Genet*, 39,1261-1265.

[114] Estrada, M., Espinosa, A., Müller, M., & Jaimovich, E. (2003). Testosterone stimulates intracellular calcium release and mitogen-activated protein kinases via a G protein-coupled receptor in skeletal muscle cells. *Endocrinology*, 144,3586–3597.

[115] Nagaya, N., & Herrera, A.A. (1995). Effects of testosterone on synaptic efficacy at neuromuscular junctions in a sexually dimorphic muscle of male frogs. *J Physiol*, 483,141–153.

[116] Burnes, L.A., Kolker, S. J., Danielson, J.F., Walder, R.Y.,& Sluka, K.A. (2008). Enhanced muscle fatigue occurs in male but not female in ASIC3-/-mice. *Am J Physiol Regul Integr Comp Physiol*, 294,R1347-R1355.

[117] Nielsen, O.B. & Overgaard, K. (1996). Ion gradients and contractility in skeletal muscle: the role of active Na^+, K^+ transport. Acta Physiol Scand, 156,247–256.

[118] Overgaard, K., Nielsen, O.B, Flatman, J.A., & Clausen, T. (1999). Relations between excitability and contractility in rat soleus muscle: role of the Na^+-K^+ pump and Na^+/K^+ gradients. *J Physiol*, 518,215–225.

[119] Bazelmans, E., Bleijenberg, G., Voeten, M.J., van der Meer, J.W., & Folgering, H. (2005). Impact of a maximal exercise test on symptoms and activity in chronic fatigue syndrome. *J Psychosom Res*, 59,201–208.

[120] De Becker, P., Roeykens, J., Reynders, M., McGregor, N., & De Meirleir, K. (2000). Exercise capacity in chronic fatigue syndrome. *Arch Intern Med*, 160,3270–3277.

[121] Kadetoff, D., & Kosek, E. (2007). The effects of static muscular contraction on blood pressure, heart rate, pain ratings and pressure pain thresholds in healthy individuals and patients with fibromyalgia. *Eur J Pain*, 11,39–47.

[122] Maquet, D., Croisier, J.L., Renard, C., & Crielaard, J.M. (2002). Muscle performance in patients with fibromyalgia. *Joint Bone Spine*, 69,293–299.

[123] Meeus, M., Nijs, J., & Meirleir, K.D. (2006). Chronic musculoskeletal pain in patients with the chronic fatigue syndrome: a systematic review. *Eur J Pain*, 11,377–386.

[124] Staud, R., Robinson, M.E., & Price, D.D. (2005). Isometric exercise has opposite effects on central pain mechanisms in fibromyalgia patients compared to normal controls. *Pain*, 118,176–184.

[125] Vierck, C.J, Jr., Staud, R., Price, D.D., Cannon, R.L., Mauderli, A.P., & Martin, A.D. (2001). The effect of maximal exercise on temporal summation of second pain (windup) in patients with fibromyalgia syndrome. *J Pain*, 2,334–344.

[126] Whiteside, A,, Hansen, S., & Chaudhuri, A. (2004). Exercise lowers pain threshold in chronic fatigue syndrome. *Pain*, 109,497–499.

[127] Wolfe, F., Hawley, D.J., & Wilson, K. (1996). The prevalence and meaning of fatigue in rheumatic disease. *J Rheumatol*, 23,1407–1417.

[128] Zautra, A.J., Fasman, R., Parish, B.P., & Davis, M.C. (2007). Daily fatigue in women with osteoarthritis, rheumatoid arthritis, and fibromyalgia. *Pain*, 128,128–135.

[129] Yokoyama, T., Lisi, T.L., Moore, S.A., & Sulka, K.A. (2007). Muscle fatigue increases the probability of developing hyperalgesia in mice. *J Pain*, 8,692–699.

[130] Curt, G.A. (2001). Fatigue in cancer. *British Medical Journal*, 322, 1560.

[131] Stone, P., Richardson, A., Ream, E., Smith, A.G., Kerr, D.J., & Kearney, N. (2000). Cancer-related fatigue: Inevitable, unimportant and untreatable? Results of a multi-centre patient survey. Cancer Fatigue Forum. *Annals of Oncology*, 11,971-975.

[132] Vogelzang, N.J., Breitbart, W., Cella, D., Curt, G.A., Groopman, J.E., Horning, S.J., Itri, L.M., Johnson, D.H., Scherr, S.L.,& Portenoy, R.K. (1997). Patient, caregiver, and oncologist perceptions of cancer-related fatigue: Results of a tripart assessment survey. The Fatigue Coalition. *Seminars in Hematology*, 34, 4-12.

[133] Broeckel, J.A., Jacobsen, P.B., Horton, J., Balducci, L., & Lyman, G.H. (1998). Characteristics and correlates of fatigue after adjuvant chemotherapy for breast cancer. *Journal of Clinical Oncology*, 16,1689-1696.

[134] Servaes, P., van der Werf, S., Prins, J., Verhagen, S., & Bleijenberg, G. (2001). Fatigue in disease-free cancer patients compared with fatigue in patients with chronic fatigue syndrome. *Support Care Cancer*, 9,11-17.

[135] Janardhan, V., & Bakshi, R. (2002). Quality of life in patients with multiple sclerosis: the impact of fatigue and depression. *J Neurol Sci*, 205,51-58.

[136] Doward, L.C., Meads, D.M., Fisk, J., Twiss, J., Hagell, P., Oprandi, N.C., Grand'maison, F., Bhan, V., Arbizu, T., Kohlmann, T., Brassat, D., Eckert, B.J., & McKenna, S.P. (2010). International Development of the Unidimensional Fatigue Impact Sale (U-FIS), Value Health, In Press.

[137] National Institutes of Health Consensus Development Panel. (2001). National Institutes of Health Consensus Development Conference statement: Adjuvant therapy for breast cancer; November 1-2, 2000. *Journal of the National Cancer Institute Monographs*, 30,5-15.

[138] Crentsil, V. (2010). Mechanistic contribution of carnitine deficiency to geriatric failty. *Ageing Res Rev*, In Press.

[139] Nozaki, S., Tanaka, M., Mizuno, K., Ataka S., Mizuma, H., Tahara, T., Sugino, T., Shirai, T., Eguchi, A., Okutama K., Yoshida, K., Kajimoto, Y., Kuratsune, H., Kajimoto, O., & Watanabe, Y. (2009). Mental and physical fatigue-related biochemical alternations. *Nutrition*, 25,51-57.

[140] Malaguarnera, M., Gargante, M.P., Colonna, V., Messano, M. Koverech, A., Neri, Sl, Vacante, M., Cammalleri, L., & Motta, M. (2008). Acetyl L-carnitine (ALC) treatment in elderly patients with fatigue. *Arch gerontol Geriatr*, 46,181-190.

[141] Pistone, G., Marino, A., Leotta, C., Dell'Arte, S., Finocchiaro, G., & Malaguarnera, M. (2003). Levocarnitine administration in elderly subjects with rapid muscle fatigue: effect on body composition, lipid profile and fatigue. *Drugs Aging*, 20,761-767.

[142] Malaguarnera, M., Cammaller, L., Gargante, M.P., Vacante, M., Colonna, V., & Motta, M. (2007). L-Carnitine treatment reduces severity of physicual and mental fatigue and increases cognitive functions in centernarians: a randomized and controlled clinnical trial. *Am J Clin Nutr*, 86,1738-1744.

[143] Tejani, A.M., Wasdell, M., Spiwak, R., Rowell, G., & Nathwani, S. (2010). *Cochrane Database Syst Rev*, In Press.

[144] Vucic, S., Burke, D, & Kiernan, M.C. (2010). Fatigue in multiple sclerosis; Mechanisms and Management. *Clin Neurophysiol*, In Press.

[145] Beenakker, E.A., Oparina, T.I., Hartgring, A., Teelken, A., Arutjunyan, A.V., & De Keyser, J. (2001). Cooling garment treatment in MS: clinical improvement and decrease in leukocyte NO production. *Neurology*, 57,892–894.

[146] Schwid, S.R., Petrie, M.D., Murray, R., Leitch, J., Bowen, J., Alquist, A., Pelligrino, R., Roberts, A., Harper-Bennie, J., Milan, M.D., Guisado, R., Luna, B., Montgomery, L., Lamparter, R., Ku, Y.T, Lee, H., Goldwater, D., Cutter, G., Webbon, B.; & NASA/MS Cooling Study Group. (2003). A randomized controlled study of the acute and chronic effects of cooling therapy for MS. *Neurology*, 60,1955–1960.

[147] Burke, D., Mogyoros, I., Vagg, R., & Kiernan, M.C. (1999). Temperature dependence of excitability indices of human cutaneous afferents. *Muscle Nerve*, 22,51–60.

[148] Burke, D., Kiernan, M.C., & Bostock, H. (2001). Excitability of human axons. Clin *Neurophysiol*, 112,1575–1585.

[149] Smith, K., Kapoor, R., & Felts, P. (1999). Demyelination: the role of reactive oxygen and nitrogen species. *Brain Pathol*, 9,69–92.

[150] Bostock, H., Sears, T.A., & Sherratt, R.M. (1981). The effects of 4-aminopyridine and tetraethylammonium ions on normal and demyelinated mammalian nerve fibres. *J Physiol*, 313:301–15.

[151] Bever, C.T. Jr., Young, D., Anderson, P.A., Krumholz, A., Conway, K., Leslie, J., Eddington, N., Plaisance, K.I., Panitch, H.S., Dhib-Jalbut, S., et al. (1994). The effects of 4-aminopyridine in multiple sclerosis patients: results of a randomized, placebo-controlled, double-blind, concentration-controlled, crossover trial. *Neurology*, 44,1054–1059.

[152] Polman, C.H., Bertelsmann, F.W., de Waal, R., van Diemen, H.A., Uitdehaag, B.M., van Loenen, A.C., & Koetsier, J.C. (1994). 4-Aminopyridine is superior to 3,4-diaminopyridine in the treatment of patients with multiple sclerosis. *Arch Neurol*, 51,1136–1139.

[153] Polman, C.H., Bertelsmann, F.W., van Loenen, A.C., & Koetsier, J.C. (1994). 4-Aminopyridine in the treatment of patients with multiple sclerosis. Long-term efficacy and safety. *Arch Neurol*, 51,292–296.

[154] Rossini, P.M., Pasqualetti, P., Pozzilli, C., Grasso, M.G., Millefiorini, E., Graceffa, A., Carlesimo, G.A., Zibellini, G., & Caltagirone, C. (2001). Fatigue in progressive multiple sclerosis: results of a randomized, double-blind, placebo-controlled, crossover trial of oral 4-aminopyridine. *Mult Scler*, 7,354–358.

[155] van Diemen, H.A., Polman, C.H., van Dongen, T.M., van Loenen, A.C., Nauta, J.J., Taphoorn, M.J., van Walbeek, H.K., & Koetsier, J.C.. (1992). The effect of 4-aminopyridine on clinical signs in multiple sclerosis: a randomized, placebo-controlled, double-blind, cross-over study. *Ann Neurol*, 32,123–130.

[156] Bever, Jr., C.T., Anderson, P.A., Leslie, J., Panitch, H.S., Dhib-Jalbut, S., Khan, O.A., Milo, R., Hebel, J.R., Conway, K.L., Katz, E., & Johnson, K.P. (1996). Treatment with oral 3,4-diaminopyridine improves leg strength in multiple sclerosis patients: results of a randomized, double-blind, placebo-controlled, crossover trial. *Neurology*, 47,1457–1462.

[157] Sheean, G.L., Murray, N.M., Rothwell, J.C., Miller, D.H., & Thompson, A.J. (1998), An open-labelled clinical and electrophysiological study of 3,4-diaminopyridine in the treatment of fatigue in multiple sclerosis. *Brain*, 121,967–975.

In: Handbook of Fatigue in Health and Disease
Editor: Howard S. Smith
ISBN 978-1-61761-920-5

Chapter 2

FATIGUE AND CYTOKINES

***Christine Gallati*[1] *and Howard S. Smith*[2]**

[1] Research Assistant
Pharmaceutical Research Institute at Albany College of Pharmacy
106 New Scotland Avenue
Albany, New York 12208, USA
[2] Associate Professor & Academic Director of Pain Management
Albany Medical College
Department of Anesthesiology
47 New Scotland Avenue; MC-131
Albany, New York 12208, USA

ABSTRACT

Fatigue remains an incompletely understood but extremely common symptom that mat be very challenging and difficult to address. One potential class of mediators that may contribute to fatigue, especially in inflammatory states are cytokines. Cytokines are small endogenous hydrophilic proteins and glycoproteins which may be involved in cell-to-cell communication and/or signaling pathways that could contribute to the genesis and/or maintenance of fatigue. It is difficult to find robust evidence for specific cytokines directly resulting in the sensation of fatigue, however it appears that in some circumstances cytokines may be involved in contributing to fatigue. A greater understanding of which cytokines in which medical conditions/states may be involved in contributing to fatigue, may help clinicians to optimally address this potentially debilitating symptom.

[1] Phone: 518-694-7578
Email: gallatc@mai.amc.edu
[2] Phone: 518-262-4461
Fax: 518-262-2671
Email : smithh@mail.amc.edu

INTRODUCTION

Fatigue is that state that follows mental or bodily activity, characterized by lessened capacity for work and reduced efficiency of accomplishment. Fatigue is a subjective sense of weakness, lack of energy, and tiredness [1]. Lee et al. [2] proposed that it can be conceptualized as located on a continuum of exhaustion and tiredness on one end, with energy and vitality at the opposite end of the continuum. Fatigue is usually associated with feelings of weariness, sleepiness, or irritability. Fatigue has historically been overlooked by clinicians and researchers because of its subjective nature and complex etiology. Recently, however, great advances have been made in our understanding of the biological mechanisms responsible for the development of fatigue. We are now beginning to consider that fatigue may not be an inescapable, untreatable condition; as our knowledge of fatigue continues to evolve we can expect new therapeutic tactics to emerge for its treatment.

Fatigue can be characterized as either acute or chronic. Acute fatigue occurs in healthy individuals and is self-limited, relieved by rest, and can be accounted for through identifiable insults. Chronic fatigue, on the other hand, generally accompanies illness, lasts longer than 6 months, is not sufficiently relieved through rest, and has multiple or unknown causes [3]. Chronic fatigue is highly prevalent and can have a significant effect on an individual's quality of life. The incidence of chronic fatigue within the general population, as reported by primary care physicians, is between 10% and 20% [4, 5], and the incidence reported in community-based surveys is between 1% and 3% [6, 7].

Fatigue affects between 70 and 100% of patients with cancer undergoing radio- or chemotherapy and may persist for months or years after treatment [8, 9]. Cancer-related fatigue (CaRF) is a very distressing condition, which has serious impact on the quality of life and is strongly associated with depression [10, 11]; and may be more troublesome to cancer patients than cancer-related pain, nausea or vomiting [12].

Fatigue can have central or peripheral origins. Central fatigue is the result of alterations or abnormalities in neurotransmitter pathways in the central nervous system (CNS) and is often associated with psychological complaints, especially depression and anxiety [2, 13, 14]. Peripheral fatigue, in contrast, arises from neuromuscular dysfunctions outside the CNS. Peripheral fatigue may in part be due to impaired neurotransmission in peripheral nerves and/or defects in muscular contraction. Peripheral fatigue may involve a loss of maximal force, generating capacity that develops during muscular activity (generally within the muscle itself). Lewis and Haller have classified skeletal muscle disorders, which may contribute to peripheral fatigue, into three major groups. One group consists of primary disorders of muscle energy metabolism, including defects in muscle carbohydrate and lipid metabolism, disorders of mitochondrial electron transport, and abnormalities of purine nucleotide metabolism [15]. A second major group of disorders includes patients with decreased muscle mass due to muscle necrosis, atrophy, and replacement of muscle by fat and connective tissue [15]. A third group of disorders includes patients with impaired activation of muscle contraction or relaxation [15]. The distinction between central and peripheral fatigue may be a somewhat arbitrary one; central and peripheral fatigue often coexist in patients and may be brought on by the same underlying conditions.

One underlying cause of chronic fatigue that has received much attention recently is the dysregulation of cytokines, especially pro-inflammatory cytokines. Altered levels of circulating cytokines have been implicated in the pathogenesis of fatigue in a variety of conditions including: Parkinson's disease, fibromyalgia, Crohn's disease, rheumatoid arthritis, atherosclerotic conditions, obesity, multiple sclerosis, cancer, and chronic fatigue syndrome. Altered cytokine levels are believed to contribute to a number of physiological states that can promote fatigue, particularly anemia, dysregulation of the hypothalamo-pituitary-adrenal axis, pathological sleep, serotonin deficits in the central nervous system (CNS), dysfunction of vasoactive neuropeptides, and skeletal muscle dysfunction.

Hansson and Rönnbäck proposed that altered central nervous system (CNS) neuronal-glial signaling may lead to an increase in extracellular glutamate levels in the vicinity of glutamate synapses. The increased extracellular glutamate levels may eventually lead to increased excitability and increased energy requirements. When cellular energy decreases, the CNS glutamate transmission decreases, possibly contributing to mental fatigue [16].

PRO-INFLAMMATORY AND ANTI-INFLAMMATORY CYTOKINE BALANCE IN FATIGUE

Cytokines are small endogenous water-soluble proteins and glycoproteins that are used extensively throughout the body for cell-to-cell communication. There are a wide variety of cytokines produced by a hematopoetic and non-hematopoetic cells. Cytokines can act in autocrine, paracrine, and endocrine fashion to mediate their effects. They bind to specific membrane receptors, often tyrosine kinases, and stimulate signaling cascades in effector cells. Cytokine stimulation can induce a variety of responses in these cells, including: an increase or decrease in the expression of membrane receptors, increased or decreased proliferation, and secretion of effector molecules.

Cytokines are often produced in cascades, i.e. one cytokine can stimulate the production of another cytokine which can in turn stimulate the production of other cytokines. These cascades frequently result in an increase in the levels of a class of cytokines that exhibit redundant activities. Furthermore, cytokines can act in a synergistic or antagonistic fashion with each other. A prime example of this principle is antagonistic relationship between the pro- and anti-inflammatory cytokines.

Pro-inflammatory cytokines are produced mainly by activated macrophages. This group of cytokines includes tumor necrosis factor-α (TNF-α), interleukin-1 (IL-1), interleukin-6 (IL-6), interleukin-11 (IL-11), interferon-α (INF-α), interferon-β (INF-β), and interferon-γ (INF-γ). These cytokines are associated with T_H1 responses which bolster cellular immunity by maximizing the killing efficacy of macrophages and the proliferation of cytotoxic $CD8^+$ T cells. Anti-inflammatory cytokines, on the other hand, are produced primarily by B-cells. This group of cytokines includes interleukin-4 (IL-4), interleukin-5 (IL-5), interleukin-10 (IL-10), and interleukin-13 (IL-13). These cytokines are associated with T_H2 responses that promote the humoral immune system by stimulating B-cell proliferation, inducing B-cell antibody class switching, and increasing antibody production. There is significant cross-regulation between these two groups of cytokines. For instance, INF-γ, which is secreted by the T_H1 subset, inhibits the proliferation of the T_H2. Furthermore, IL-4 and IL-10, secreted by the T_H2 subset, reduce the secretion of IL-12, which is essential for the differentiation of the T_H1 subset [17-19].

The balance between T_H1 and T_H2 subsets and their associated cytokines is dictated by the type of challenge that is presented to the immune system. The balance can also be modulated by other factors such as stress hormones, including glucocorticoids and catecholamines. Recent studies have indicated that glucocorticoids and catecholamines, inhibit the production of proinflammatory cytokines and promote the production of anti-inflammatory cytokines. An excessive inflammatory immune response can trigger the activation of the stress system and release of stress hormones. This negative feedback mechanism can prevent an "overshoot" of the inflammatory response, protecting the body from tissue damage and distress. It is now believed that a breakdown of this negative feedback mechanism, the genesis of a "dysfunctional neuroendocrine-immune interface", may be responsible for the pathological cytokine profile associated with chronic inflammatory diseases [20-22].

Obesity and related atherosclerotic disorders are associated with systemic chronic inflammation. Abdominal fat can be thought of as a secretory organ, preferentially producing proinflammatory cytokines, including: TNF-α, IL-1, and IL-6. The proinflammatory state caused by elevated serum levels of these cytokines promotes the development of the metabolic syndrome (hypertension, hyperglycemia, diyslipidemia, etc.) and atherosclerosis.

In a 2007 study, Kwaijtaal et al found that patients with coronary artery disease who reported exhaustion could be charactertized by hypoactivity of the hypothalamo-pituitary-adrenal axis [23]. If you recall, stimulation of the hypothalamo-pituitary-adrenal axis results in the release of glucocorticoids, which inhibit the production of pro-inflammatory cytokines. Another study found that vital exhaustion in women with coronary artery disease was related to inflammatory activity, which was assessed by IL-6 levels [24].

Immune System-Central Nervous System Communication in Fatigue

There is bidirectional communication between the CNS and the immune system. The CNS can affect immune function through the signaling of target cells via both the autonomic and neuroendocrine pathways. The CNS, thus, has the ability to modulate cytokine production and immune function. Cytokines, in turn, have profound effects on the CNS, modifying neural activity, behaviors, autonomic function, and hormone release. Some experts have found it useful to liken the cells of the immune system to "sensory cells" that relay information to the CNS about peripheral events related to infection. This information is relayed by the action of cytokines through the endocrine route via the blood or by direct neural transmission via the afferent vagus nerve. The CNS responds to this "sensory input" by modifying the behavior of the organism in a way that allows it to cope more effectively with the challenge. These changes in behavior, such as loss of appetite, sleepiness, withdrawal from normal social activities, fever, aching joints, and fatigue, can be referred to as "sickness behavior". The fatigue associated with some chronic inflammatory diseases can therefore be thought of as a result of the body's inability to return to its normal state from the sick state [25, 26]. There appears to be much therapeutic potential in producing appropriate interference in the bidirectional communication of the CNS and the immune system. For example, it was recently demonstrated that inhibition of vagally mediated immune-to-brain signaling by vanadyl sulfate speeds recovery from sickness [27].

Furthermore, an immune-to-brain communication pathway may contribute to the production of a constellation of CNS-mediated phenomena, collectively referred to as 'sickness responses'. These sickness responses are created by immune-to-brain signals activating CNS glia to release glial proinflammatory cytokines [28].

Sickness behavior, (a cluster of symptoms including fatigue, loss of appetite, and disturbed sleep) appears to be triggered by at least in part increased production of the inflammatory cytokines IL-1β, TNF-α, and IL-6. Studies in humans and in animal models have demonstrated the role that these cytokines play in the development of sickness behavior [29-34]. The p38 mitogen activated protein kinase (p38 MAPK) plays a central role in the inflammatory cytokine response to immune challenge and consequently the development of sickness behavior [35]. Pretreatment with a p38 MAPK inhibitor, BIRB796 (Boeringher Ingelheim) blocked p38 MAPK activation in peripheral blood mononuclear cells (PBMC) and the rise in plasma cytokine levels in response to LPS injection [36]. Consequently LPS (lipopolysaccheride)-induced sickness behaviors were attenuated in the BIRB796 pre-treatment group [36].

Animal studies have shown that direct application of IL-1 into the brain leads to a variety of symptoms such as loss of appetite, fever, fatigue, depressed activity, and decreased learning and cognitive functioning [37, 38]. These behavioral manifestations ("sickness behavior") [39], can be partially blocked by IL-1ra (interleukin-1 recetpro antagonist) and may also be triggered by other cytokines such as IL-6 and TNF- α [40]. The parenteral application of high concentrations of recombinant proinflammatory cytokines such as INF, IL-6, IL-12, IL-1β, TNF-α, and interleukin-2 (IL-2) to enhance immune defenses against cancer often leads to a syndrome referred to as the systemic inflammatory response syndrome. One of the major symptoms of this systemic response is intense fatigue, which in many patients calls for dose reduction or even interruption of therapy [38, 41].

Human studies have linked inflammatory cytokines to fatigue in both aging patients and those with such chronic health conditions such as cancer and chronic fatigue syndrome [42-48]. Interestingly, increased levels of proinflammatory cytokines have been linked to an increase in energy expenditure (with increased mortality) and lower functional status in hemodialysis (HD) patients [49-51].

Schubert et al. quantitatively reviewed empirical findings in the literature regarding the association between fatigue and inflammatory marker levels in cancer patients [52]. Analyses of individual inflammatory markers revealed significantly positive correlations between fatigue and IL-6 ($r = 0.12$, $p = 0.004$), fatigue and IL-1ra ($r = 0.24$, $p = 0.0005$), and fatigue and neopterin ($r = 0.22$, $p = 0.0001$) [52].

Motor slowing and its correlation with psychiatric symptoms suggest that altered basal ganglia function may contribute to the pathogenesis of IFN-alpha-induced behavioral changes such as fatigue [53].

Robson-Ansley et al. found that strenuous, prolonged exercise stimulated an increase in soluble IL-6 receptor (sIL-6R) which was associated with CRP and may affect subjective sensations of post-exercise fatigue at rest [54]. Wang and colleagues studied sixty-two patients undergoing chemoradiation therapy (CXRT) for locally advanced non-small cell lung cancer (NSCLC. They evaluated symptoms weekly for 15 weeks via the M. D. Anderson

Symptom Inventory (MDASI) and assessed serum inflammatory cytokines weekly during therapy via enzyme-linked immunosorbent assay [55]. An increase in serum IL-6 was significantly related to increased mean severity for the five most severe symptoms (pain, fatigue, disturbed sleep, lack of appetite, sore throat). These results suggest a role for over-expressed pro-inflammatory cytokines in significant worsening of symptoms in NSCLC patients undergoing CXRT [55]. Bower and colleague studied patients with early-stage breast (n = 28) and prostate cancer (n = 20) who completed questionnaires and provided blood samples for determination of serum levels of interleukin 1beta (IL-1beta) and IL-6 at assessments conducted before, during, and after a course of radiation therapy [56]. There was a significant increase in fatigue during radiation treatment. Changes in serum levels of inflammatory markers C-reactive protein and IL-1 receptor antagonist were positively associated with increases in fatigue symptoms ($Ps < 0.05$), although serum levels of IL-1beta and IL-6 were not associated with fatigue [56]. These effects remained significant in analyses controlling for potential biobehavioral confounding factors, including age, body mass index, hormone therapy, depression, and sleep disturbance [56]. Bower et al. suggested that activation of the proinflammatory cytokine network and associated increases in downstream biomarkers of proinflammatory cytokine activity are associated with fatigue during radiation therapy for breast and prostate cancer [56].

Hypothalamo-Pituitary-Adrenal Axis in Fatigue

The hypothalamo-pituitary-adrenal axis is an important component of the neuroendocrine system that is responsible for regulating metabolism, mood, immune response, and reactions to stress. Dopamine, serotonin, and norepinephrine (noradrenaline) are all important players involved in the regulation of this system. The axis functions by relaying stimulatory and inhibitory messages between the hypothalamus, pituitary gland, and the adrenal gland. One important messenger in the axis is corticotropin releasing hormone (CRH), a polypeptide hormone/ neurotransmitter. CRH is secreted by neuroendocrine cells in the paraventricular nucleus of the hypothalamus and stimulates the secretion of corticotropin (ACTH) by the pituitary into the bloodstream. ACTH acts on the adrenal cortices and stimulates the production of glucocorticoid hormones, which exert a variety of effects on the body and act to inhibit the secretion of CRH and ACTH in a negative feedback loop.

The release of CRH from the hypothalamus is dependent on a number of variables, including: stress, blood cortisol (a glucocorticoid) levels, and the sleep/wake cycle. In humans, cortisol levels peak twice during a normal day, once within 30-45 minutes after waking, and again in the late afternoon. During sleep cortisol levels fall and reach a trough in the middle of the night. Flattened circadian cortisol patterns are associated with chronic fatigue syndrome [57], insomnia [58] and burnout [59]. Due to the fact that pro-inflammatory cytokines are able to stimulate the hypothalamo-pituitary-adrenal axis, it has been hypothesized that perhaps over-stimulation of the axis by these cytokines could result in the loss of the normal circadian cortisol pattern. This hypothesis provides a clear mechanism by which inflammatory disease can promote pathological sleep and, consequently, fatigue. While, this is a clear and elegant explanation of the relationship between cytokines and fatigue, it cannot account for the fatigue associated with all inflammatory conditions, nor can it claim full responsibly for the fatigue in conditions in which it is implicated. Some studies focusing on inflammatory diseases have found no correlation between cortisol levels and fatigue [60].

While there is clear evidence that elevated serum levels of pro-inflammatory cytokines can have role in the pathogenesis of fatigue states in many diseases, in some diseases, such as chronic fatigue syndrome it appears that fatigue symptoms maybe more related to disordered cytokine production by cells within the CNS [61]. This may explains why some studies using serum samples have found no correlation between pro-inflammatory cytokines and fatigue.

Proinflammatory cytokines in the CNS are thought to produce fatigue states through variety of mechanisms. In 2006 Katafuchi et al, using an immunologically induced fatigue model in rats, demonstrated the involvement of brain INF-α and the serotonin transporter in the central mechanisms of fatigue. Compared to control animals, the fatigued rats showed increased expression of INF-α and serotonin transporter, as well as a decrease in serotonin levels in the prefrontal cortex (which can be explained by the increase in serotonin transporter expression) [62].

Serotonin

Depression has historically been associated with fatigue and is often correlated with serotonin deficiencies. There is a body of research that has bolstered the idea that pro-inflammatory cytokines are, to some degree, responsible for depressive behavior/symptoms. Capuron et al. [63] proposed that pro-inflammatory cytokines induce elevated indoleamine 2, 3 dioxygenase (IDO) activity. IDO catalyses the breakdown of tryptophan, the precursor of serotonin. Depressed patients often display decreased plasma levels of tryptophan. Studies in mice have confirmed that immune system is activation is associated with IDO activation [64]. This paradigm is further strengthened by evidence that some antidepressant treatments have immunomodulatory effects, perhaps acting to correct pro- and anti-inflammatory cytokine imbalances [65]. There is strong evidence that fatigue and depression often exist as codependent conditions. Pro-inflammatory cytokines provide one logical mechanistic link between these two complex disease states. Indeed, immunomodulatory treatment regimens may be able to improve both of these disease states in co-morbid patients.

Vasoactive Neuropeptides

Another manner in which fatigue may arise is the dysfunction of endogenous adenylate cyclase (AC)-activating vasoactive neuropeptides (VNs), which include: pituitary adenylate cyclase-activating polypeptide (PACAP), vasoactive intestinal peptide (VIP) and calcitonin gene-related peptide (CGRP). It has been hypothesized that autoimmunity to these neuropetides or their corresponding receptors could be implicated in the pathobiology of some conditions that are associated with fatigue, such as chronic fatigue syndrome, fibromyalgia, and Parkinson's disease [66]. PACAP, VIP, and CGRP belong to the secretin-glucagon super-family and, thus, exert considerable control over carbohydrate and lipid metabolism [67]. Additionally, they play critical roles in vasodilation, neurotropism, nociception, neuroregulation and neurotransmission including thermoregulation, cardio-respiratory control, balance and vestibular function, emotional and intellectual functioning (including memory and concentration), and immunological and hormonal modulation [68]. Many of these effects are exerted through control of the hypothalamo-pituitary-adrenal axis, which we have already identified as a system that is sensitive to inflammatory cytokine imbalance, as well as, a potential site from which fatigue can arise.

VNs function through multiple signaling processes [69] and have complex interactions with a variety of neurotransmitters including cross-talk feedback and control mechanisms. Since a large portion of the CNS is regulated to some degree, through direct, indirect, and cotransmitter functions, by VNs, there are a number of ways that fatigue can be induced through VN dysfunction. Generally speaking, VNs have anti-inflammatory and/or neuroprotective roles in the CNS; dysregulation may lead to inflammation.

VNs and their receptors are thought to be quite susceptible to autoreactive immunological responses. It has been hypothesized that a reduction in VIP by autoantibodies can interfere with the regulation of immune cells, promoting an inflammatory state and exacerbating the autoimmune response [70, 71]. In this paradigm VN dysfunction can result from the stimulation of autoreactivity brought on by minor infection or inflammation. Pro-inflammatory responses in the CNS are associated apoptotic neurodegeneration. PACAP and VIP inhibit the production of inflammatory mediators and, thus, have neuroprotective effects. Dysfunction of PACAP and VIP has been implicated in Parkinson's disease which is characterized by inflammation-mediated degeneration of dopaminergic neurons in the substantia nigra [72]. Along with degeneration of dopaminergic neurons, dopamine levels in individuals suffering from Parkinson's are reduced by high levels of NO, resulting from increased expression of iNOS. This type of sustained high-output NO production is characteristic of a number of acute inflammatory diseases and autoimmune diseases. VIP and PACAP inhibit iNOS expression and activity both in vivo and in vitro through two distinct transduction pathways: (1) a cAMP-dependent pathway that inhibits IFN regulatory factor-1 transactivation and (2) a cAMP-independent pathway that blocks NF-κB binding to the iNOS promoter [73].

Skeletal Muscle Dysfunction

Chronic inflammation can lead to skeletal muscle dysfunction, another condition that can contribute to fatigue. In a 2008 study, Ruiz et al. demonstrated that low-grade inflammation could be negatively associated with muscle strength in adolescents. In the study, 230 boys and 186 girls were categorized as either overweight (including obese) or non-overweight according to body mass index. A number of inflammatory markers were measured in the subjects and muscle strength was determined by recording values for mean had grip and standing broad jump [74].

Recently, research has been conducted which has started to shed some light upon the mechanisms by which inflammation causes skeletal muscle dysfunction. It is well known that individuals with congestive heart failure are susceptible to skeletal muscle fatigue. It is also known that increased circulating concentrations TNF-α and monocyte chemoattractant protein-1(another inflammation-associated cytokine) have the ability to stimulate matrix metalloproteinase activity, which can distort the normal contractile function of skeletal muscle, thereby contributing to increased skeletal muscle fatigue. Schiøtz Thorud et al demonstrated in rats that the development of CHF enhances matrix metalloproteinase activity [75]. Thus, there is a possibility that inflammatory cytokines can contribute to fatigue in some conditions by promoting muscular dysfunction.

POTENTIAL GENETIC INFLUENCES

Smith et al. studied patients with medically unexplained fatigue and examined genetic polymorphisms involved in either HPA axis function or neurotransmitter systems, including: proopiomelanocortin (POMC), nuclear receptor subfamily 3, group C, member 1 (NR3C1), monoamine oxidase A (MAOA), monoamine oxidase B (MAOB), and tryptophan hydroxylase 2 (TPH2) [76]. Smith and colleagues stated that their data suggested that medically unexplained chronic fatigue may be heterogeneous and that genetic mechanisms may underiesome of the putative conditions potentially contributing to fatigue [76].

INFLAMMATORY CYTOKINES AND THERAPEUTICS

NF-κB

NF-κB is a transcription factor that plays a key role in regulating the immune response to infection. NF- κB controls the expression of over 200 genes, including a number of proinflammatory cytokines, such as, IL-6, IL-1, TNF-α, and INFs. Many of these genes are involved in the inflammatory response, including TNF-α. Elevated serum levels of pro-inflammatory cytokines have been correlated with the symptoms of acute sickness behavior in humans, which includes fatigue [30]. Additionally, NF-κB activation has been linked to cancer, autoimmune diseases, and inflammatory diseases.

Tumor Necrosis Factor-α (TNF-α)

TNF-α is considered to be the master inflammatory cytokine. It promotes the expression of other inflammatory cytokines, including IL-1 and IL-6. These cytokines in turn promote further expression of TNF-α, intensifying the inflammatory response. Animal studies have provided support for the hypothesis that the inflammatory response and the expression of pro-inflammatory cytokines are linked to fatigue. In a study performed by Netea et al in 2007, mice deficient for TNF-α were found to demonstrate increased voluntary exercise [77].

Anti-TNF-α therapy has been utilized for several years for the treatment of inflammatory diseases such as rheumatoid arthritis, inflammatory bowel disease, Crohn's disease, psoriasis, and psoriatic arthritis. There are four TNF-alpha antagonist drugs available today: inflixamab, adalimumab, certolizumab, and etanercept. Inflixamab (Remicade) and adalimumab (Humira) are both monoclonal antibodies that bind to TNF-alpha and prevent its interaction with its receptors. Infliximab is a chimeric monoclonal antibody composed of murine variable segments and human Fc domains [78], whereas adalimumab is a fully human monoclonal antibody. Certolizumab pegol (CDP870, Cimzia) is a PEGylated Fab fragment of a humanized TNF-alpha monoclonal antibody that is currently in phase III clinical trials [79]. Etanercept (brand name Enbrel) is a dimeric molecule composed of a soluble form of the human TNF-α receptor linked to the Fc component of human IgG1. The receptor domain of etanercept binds to TNF-α, thereby preventing its activation of TNF-alpha receptors on cell surfaces.

Fatigue related to these disorders appears to be notably improved when patients undergo this type of therapy. In a 6 month, longitudinal, observational study of psoriatic arthritis patients Heiberg et al found that patients receiving a combination of TNF alpha antagonists and methotrexate reported significantly greater reductions in fatigue, as well as global disease activity, in comparison to patients receiving methotrexate monotherapy [80].

Interleukin-1 (IL-1) and Interleukin-6 (IL-6)

IL-1β and IL-6 are proinflammatory cytokines that mediate sickness behavior in humans with acute infection [30]. Both IL-1and IL-6 have stimulatory effects on hematopoesis. IL-1 is secreted by macrophages, monocytes, and dendritic cells. It controls the activities of lymphocytes, including the transmigration of leukocytes via the increased expression of adhesion factors on endothelial cells. There are two known sub types of IL-1, IL-1α and IL-1β. Polymorphisms of these genes have been linked to the development of RA and other inflammatory disorders [81]. There is also evidence that increased levels of IL-1β in the brain contribute to the fatigue associated with muscle-damaging exercise [82].

IL-6 mediates resistance against bacteria and stimulates immune response to trauma. IL-6 is secreted by T cells and macrophages in response to infection, as well as muscle cells, in response to elevated muscle contraction [83]. IL-6 secretion appears to have effects on the circadian cycle in humans and is responsible for the changes of sleep and behavior that accompany infection and inflammatory disorders [83, 84]. IL-6 stimulates hepatocytes to induce acute-phase reactants, including C-reactive protein, serum amyloid A protein, and fibrinogen, and to decrease serum albumin levels [85]. Elevated levels of IL-6 enhance the synthesis of a hepcidin, a peptide that regulates iron recycling, in the liver. Increased hepcidin expression causes hypofferemia, and consequentially anemia, which can act as a source of fatigue [85].

Interferons (IFNS)

INFs are secreted by a variety of cells in response to challenges by viruses, bacteria, parasites, and tumor cells. INFs work against these pathogenic invaders through a number of mechanisms, including: the inhibition viral replication within host cells, the induction of viral resistance in uninfected host cells, activation natural killer cells and macrophages, and by stimulating an increase in antigen presentation to lymphocytes [86]. There are three important types of INFs that are involved inflammatory responses: INF-α, INF-β, and INF-γ. INF therapy has been used as a treatment for hepatitis A and C, and multiple sclerosis, as well as in combination with radio- and chemotherapy for the treatment of cancer.

INF-α therapy has been effectively used in the treatment of chronic hepatitis A and C infections, but is notorious for producing behavioral alterations including: including anxiety, depression, delirium, psychoses, and mania. The adverse neuropsychiatric effects of INF-α have been described as two overlapping syndromes. The first syndrome usually manifests early in the treatment and peaks at 12 weeks. It involves mood/cognitive alterations that can be ameliorated with serotoninergic antidepressants. This syndrome is thought to be the result of the activation of certain neuroendocrine pathways, as well as altered serotonin metabolism. The second syndrome is neurovegetative and occurs early as well, but persists for the duration of the treatment. It is characterized by psychomotor slowing and fatigue and is unresponsive to antidepressant treatment. This second syndrome is thought to be the result of altered dopamine metabolism in the basal ganglia [87-89].

IFN-β therapy has been shown to have beneficial effects on the course of multiple sclerosis (MS). Unfortunately, like INF-α, INF-β therapy has been associated with negative neuropsychiatric effects, including increased fatigue and depression. Although the benefits of this treatment are clear, the side effects may be, in some cases, more debilitating than the disease itself [90].

Conclusion

Fatigue has been identified as an important symptom in a number of chronic inflammatory diseases, including: Parkinson's disease, fibromyalgia, Crohn's disease, rheumatoid arthritis, atherosclerotic conditions, obesity, multiple sclerosis, cancer, and chronic fatigue syndrome. Here we have discussed a variety of mechanisms by which fatigue can be promoted by the over production of pro-inflammatory cytokines.

There is a great deal of evidence that sustained, elevated levels of pro-inflammatory cytokines can lead to the dysregulation of the hypothalamo-pituitary-adrenal axis. This homeostatic system plays a very important role in the maintenance of the sleep-wake cycle and can have profound effects on the quality and quantity of sleep that an individual achieves. Serotonin is a key neurotransmitter, whose proper regulation and expression is essential for restful sleep. There appears to be strong, yet complex and poorly understood connections between depression and fatigue. Elevated levels of pro-inflammatory cytokines can lead to altered tryptophan metabolism and, consequently, serotonin deficits, a well established cause of depressive behavior. Further research on this topic may help to elucidate the mechanistic connection between fatigue and depression.

Our knowledge of VNs' role in the pathogenesis of fatigue is, as of yet, quite incomplete. VNs are a critical class of signaling proteins whose effects are wide-ranging. The involvement of VNs in autoimmune reactions provides what appears to be an interesting rationale for implicating them in a variety of chronic diseases. The interplay between VNs and the immune system deserves further research, as it may provide important insights into the origins and maintenance of fatigue associated with chronic inflammatory conditions.

Fatigue associated with chronic inflammatory diseases has both central and peripheral origins. Alterations in neurotransmitter profiles and dysfunction of the VN regulation and the hypothalamo-pituitary axis are central orgins of fatigue. Phenomena such as anemia and muscular dysfunction represent more peripheral origins of fatigue.

Fatigue is an important symptom associated with inflammatory diseases. Clinicians and researchers are now only beginning its mechanistic and molecular basis. Drugs designed to target pro-inflammatory cytokines are a relativity new development that has shed much light on the importance of understanding and addressing fatigue clinically.

REFERENCES

[1] Stone, P., Richards, M., & Hardy, J. (1998). Fatigue in patients with cancer. *Eur J Cancer*, 34,1670-1676.

[2] Lee, K.A., Hicks, G., & Nino-Murcia, G. (1991). Validity and reliability of a scale to assess fatigue. *Psychiatry Res*, 36,291- 298.

[3] Piper, B.F., Rieger, P.T., Brophy, L., Haeuber, D., Hood, L.E., Lwer, A., & Sharp, E. (1989). Recent advances in the management of biotherapy-related side effects: fatigue. *Oncol Nurs Forum*, 16,27-34.

[4] Bates, D.W., Schmitt, W., Buchwald, D., Ware, N.C., Lee, J., Thoyer, E., Kornish, R.J. & Komaroff, A.L. (1993). Prevalence of fatigue and chronic fatigue syndrome in a primary care practice. *Arch Intern Med*, 153,2759-2765.

[5] Pawlikoska, T., Chalder, T., Hirsch, S.R., Wallace, P., Wright, D.J., & Wessely, S.C. (1994). Population based study of fatigue and psychological distress. *BMJ*, 208,763-766.

[6] Buchwald, D., Umali, P., Umali, J., Kith, P., Pearlman, T., & Komaroff, A.L. (1995). Chronic fatigue and the chronic fatigue syndrome: prevalence in a Pacific Northwest health care system. *Ann Intern Med*, 123,81-88.

[7] Wessely, S., Chalder, T., Hirsch, S., Pawlikowska, T., Wallace, P., & Wright, D.J. (1995). Postinfectious fatigue: prospective cohort study in primary care. *Lancet*, 345,1333-1338.

[8] World Health Organization. (1990). Cancer pain relief and palliative care. Technical report series, 804, Geneva.

[9] Mock, V., Atkinson, A., Barsevick, A., Cella, D., Cimprich, B., Cleeland, C., Donnelly, J., Eisenberger, M.A., Escalante, C., Hinds, P., Jacobsen, P.B., Kaldor, P., Knight, S.J., Peterman, A., Piper, B.F., Rugo, H., Sabbatini, P., Stahl, C.; & National Comprehensive Cancer Network. (2000). NCCN Practice Guidelines for Cancer-Related Fatigue. *Oncology* (Huntingt.), 14,151–161.

[10] Richardson, A. (1995). Fatigue in cancer patients: a review of the literature. *Eur J Cancer Care* (Engl), 4,20–32.

[11] Visser, M.R., & Smets, E.M. (1998). Fatigue, depression and quality of life in cancer patients: how are they related? *Support. Care Cancer*, 6,101–108.

[12] Blohmer, J.U., Dunst, J., Harrison, L., Johnston, P., Khayat, D., Ludwig, H., O'Brien, M. Van Belle, S., & Vaupel, P. (2005). Cancer-related anemia: biological findings, clinical implications and impact on quality of life. *Oncology*, 68,12–21.

[13] Lloyd, A.R. (1998). Chronic fatigue and chronic fatigue syndrome: shifting boundaries and attributions. *Am J Med*, 105,7S-10S.

[14] Aaronson, L.S., Teel, C.S., Cassmeyer, V., Neuberger, G.B., Pallikkathavil, L., Pierce, J., Press, A.N., Williams, P.D., & Wingate, A. (1999). Defining and measuring fatigue. *Image J Nurs Sch*, 31,45-50.

[15] Lewis, S.F., & Haller, R.G. (1989). Skeletal muscle disorders and associated factors that limit exercise performance. *Exerc Sport Sci Rev*, 17,67-113.

[16] Hansson, E., & Rönnbäck, L. (2004). Altered neuronal-glial signaling in glutamatergic transmission as a unifying mechanism in chronic pain and mental fatigue. *Neurochem Res*, 29,989-996.

[17] Abbas, A.K., Murphy, K.M., & Sher, A. (1996). Functional diversity of helper T lymphocytes. *Nature*, 383,787-793.

[18] Rengarajan, J., Szabo, S.J., & Glimcher, L.H. (2000). Transcriptional regulation of Th1/Th2 polarization. *Immunol Today*, 21,479-483.

[19] Szabo, S.J., Kim, S.T., Costa, G.L., Zhang, X., Fathman, C.G., & Glimcher, L.H. (2000). A novel transcription factor, T-bet, directs Th1 lineage commitment. *Cell*, 100,655-669.

[20] Elenkov, I.J., & Chrousos, G.P. (2002). Stress Hormones, Proinflammatory and Anti-inflammatory Cytokines, and Autoimmunity. *Ann NY Acad Sci*, 966,290-303.

[21] Munck, A., Guyre, P.M., & Holbrook, N.J. (1984). Physiological functions of glucocorticoids in stress and their relation to pharmacological actions. *Endocr Rev*, 5,25-44.

[22] Besedovsky, H., del Rey, A., Sorkin, E., & Dinarello, C.A. (1986). Immunoregulatory feedback between interleukin-1 and glucocorticoid hormones. *Science*, 233,652-654.

[23] Kwaijtaal, M., van der Ven, A.J., van Diest, R., Bruggeman, C.A., Bär, F.W., Calandra, T., Appels, A., & Sweep, F.C. (2007). Exhaustion is associated with low macrophage migration inhibitory factor expression in patients with coronary artery disease. *Psychosom Med*, 69,68-73.

[24] Janszky, I., Lekander, M., Blom, M., Georgiades, A., & Ahnve, S. (2005). Self-rated health and vital exhaustion, but not depression, is related to inflammation in women with coronary heart disease. *Brain Behav Immun*, 19,555-563.

[25] Lorton, D., Lubahn, C.L., Estus, C., Millar, B.A., Carter, J.L., Wood, C.A., & Bellinger, D.L.(2006). Bidirectional communication between the brain and the immune system: implications for physiological sleep and disorders with disrupted sleep. *Neuroimmunomodulation*, 13,357-374.

[26] Dantzer, R., & Kelley, K.W. (2007). Twenty years of research on cytokine-induced sickness behavior. *Brain Behav Immun*, 21,153-160.

[27] Johnson, D.R., O'Connor, J.C., Dantzer, R., & Freund, G.G. (2005). Inhibition of vagally mediated immune-to-brain signaling by vanadyl sulfate speeds recovery from sickness. *Proc Natl Acad Sci U S A*, 102,15184-15189.

[28] Watkins, L.R., & Maier, S.F. (2005). Immune regulation of central nervous system functions: from sickness responses to pathological pain. *J Intern Med*, 257,139-155.

[29] Janicki-Deverts, D., Cohen, S., Doyle, W.J., Turner, R.B., & Treanor, J.J. (2007). Infection-induced proinflammatory cytokines are associated with decreases in positive affect, but not increases in negative affect. *Brain Behav Immun*, 21,301–307.

[30] Vollmer-Conna, U., Fazou, C., Cameron, B., Li, H., Brennan, C., Luck, L., Davenport, T., Wakefield, D., Hickie, I., & Lloyd, A. (2004). Production of pro-inflammatory

cytokines correlates with the symptoms of acute sickness behaviour in humans. *Psychol Med*, 34,1289–1297.

[31] Huang,Y., Henry, C.J., Dantzer, R., Johnson, R.W., & Godbout,J.P. (2008). Exaggerated sickness behavior and brain proinflammatory cytokine expression in aged mice in response to intracerebroventricular lipopolysaccharide. *Neurobiol Aging,* 29,1744-1753.

[32] Teeling, J.L., Felton, L.M., Deacon, R.M., Cunningham, C., Rawlins, J.N., & Perry, V.H. (2007). Sub-pyrogenic systemic inflammation impacts on brain and behavior, independent of cytokines. *Brain Behav Immun*, 21,836-850.

[33] Willette, A.A., Lubach, G.R., & Coe, C.L. (2007). Environmental context differentially affects behavioral, leukocyte, cortisol, and interleukin-6 responses to low doses of endotoxin in the rhesus monkey. *Brain Behav Immun*, 21,807-815.

[34] Harden, L.M., du Plessis, I., Poole, S., & Laburn, H.P. (2006). Interleukin-6 and leptin mediate lipopolysaccharide-induced fever and sickness behavior. *Physiol Behav*, 89,146–155.

[35] Elsea, C.R., Roberts, D.A., Druker, B.J., & Wood, L.J. (2008). Inhibition of p38 MAPK Suppresses Inflammaotry Cytokine Induction by Etoposide, 5-Fluorouracil, and Doxorubicin without Affecting Tumoricidal Activity. *PLoS ONE*, 3,e2355.

[36] Branger, J., van den Blink, B., Weijer, S., Madwed, J., Bos, C.L., Gupta, A., Yong, C.L., Polmar, S.H., Olszyna, D.P., Hack, C.E., van Deventer, S.J., Peppelenbosch, M.P., & van der Poll, T. (2002). Anti-inflammatory effects of a p38 mitogen-activated protein kinase inhibitor during human endotoxemia. *J Immunol*, 168,4070–4077.

[37] Larson, S.J., & Dunn, A.J. (2001). Behavioral effects of cytokines. *Brain Behav Immun*, 15,371–387.

[38] Kelley, K.W., Bluthe, R.M., Dantzer, R., Zhou, J.H., Shen, W.H., Johnson, R.W., & Broussard, S.R. (2003). Cytokine-induced sickness behavior. *Brain Behav Immun*, 17,S112–S118.

[39] Kent, S., Bluthe, R.M., Kelley, K.W., & Dantzer, R. (1992). Sickness behavior as a new target for drug development. *Trends Pharmacol Sci*, 13,24–28.

[40] Swiergiel, A.H., Smagin, G.N., Johnson, L.J., & Dunn, A.J. (1997). The role of cytokines in the behavioral responses to endotoxin and influenza virus infection in mice: effects of acute and chronic administration of the interleukin-1-receptor antagonist (IL-1ra). *Brain Res*, 776,96–104.

[41] Pusztai, L., Mendoza, T.R., Reuben, J.M., Martinez, M.M., Willey. J.S., Lara, J., Swed, A., Fritsche, H.A., Bruera, E., Booser, D., Valero, V., Arun, B., Ibrahim, N., Rivera, E., Royce, M. Cleeland, C.S., & Hortobagyi, G.N. (2004). Changes in plasma levels of inflammatory cytokines in response to paclitaxel chemotherapy. *Cytokine*, 25,94–102.

[42] Cesari, M., Penninx, B.W., Pahor, M., Lauretani, F., Corsi, A.M., Rhys Williams, G., Guralnik, J.M., & Ferrucci, L. (2004). Inflammatory markers and physical performance in older persons: The InCHIANTI Study. *J Gerontol A Biol Sci Med Sci*, 59,242-248.

[43] Schubert, C., Hong, S., Natarajan, L., Mills, P.J., & Dimsdale, J.E. (2007). The association between fatigue and inflammatory marker levels in cancer patients:Aquantitative review. *Brain Behav Immun*, 21,413-427.

[44] Collado-Hidalgo, A., Bower, J.E., Ganz, P.A., Cole, S.W., & Irwin, M.R. (2006). Inflammatory biomarkers for persistent fatigue in breast cancer survivors. *Clin Cancer Res*, 12,2759-2766.

[45] Meyers, C.A., Albitar, M., & Estey, E. (2005). Cognitive impairment, fatigue, and cytokine levels in patients with acute myelogenous leukemia or myelodysplastic syndrome. Cancer, 104,788-793.

[46] Buchwald, D., Wener, M.H., Pearlman, T., & Kith, P. (1997). Markers of inflammation and immune activation in chronic fatigue and chronic fatigue syndrome. J Rheumatol, 24,372-376.

[47] Kurzrock, R. (2001). The role of cytokines in cancer-related fatigue. *Cancer*, 92,S1684-S1688.

[48] Seymour, J.F., Talpaz, M., Cabanillas, F., Wetzler, M., & Kurzrock, R. (1995). Serum interleukin-6 levels correlate with prognosis in diffuse large-cell lymphoma. *J Clin Oncol*, 13,575- 582.

[49] Kamimura, M.A., Draibe, S.A., Dalboni, M.A., Cendoroglo, M., Avesani, C.M., Manfredi, S.R., Canziani, M.E., & Cuppari, L. (2007). Serum and cellular interleukin-6 in haemodialysis patients: Relationship with energy expenditure. *Nephrol Dial Transplant*, 22,839-844.

[50] Balakrishnan, V.S., Guo, D., Rao, M., Jaber, B.L., Tighiouart, H., Freeman, R.L., Huang, C., King, A.J., Pereira, B.J.; & HEMO Study Group. (2004). Cytokine gene polymorphisms in hemodialysis patients: Association with comorbidity, functionality, and serum albumin. *Kidney Int*, 65,1449-1460.

[51] Kimme, P.L., Phillips, T.M., Simmens, S.J., Peterson, R.A., Weihs, K.L., Alleyne, S., Cruz, I., Yanovski, J.A., & Veis, J.H. (1998). Immunologic function and survival in hemodialysis patients. *Kidney Int*, 54,236-244.

[52] Schubert, C., Hong, S., Natarajan, L., Mills, P.J., & Dimsdale, J.E (2007). The association between fatigue and inflammatory marker levels in cancer patients. *Brain Behav Immun*, 21,413-427.

[53] Majer, M., Welberg, L.A., Capuron, L., Pagnoni, G., Raison, C.L., & Miller, A.H. (2008). IFN-alpha-induced motor slowing is assoicated with increased depression and fatigue in patients with chronic hepatitis C. *Brain Behav Immun*, 22,870-880.

[54] Robson-Ansley,P., Barwood, M., Canavan, J., Hack, S., Eglin, C., Davey, S., Hewitt, J., Hull, J., & Ansley, L. (2009). The effect of repeated endurance exercise on IL-6 and sIL-6R and their relationship with sensations of fatigue at rest. *Cytokine*, 45,111-116.

[55] Wang, X.S., Shi, Q., Williams, L.A., Mao, L., Cleeland, C.S., Komaki, R.R., Mobley, G.M., & Liao, Z. (2010). Inflammatory cytokines are associated with the development of symptom burden in patients with NSCLC undergoing concurrent chemoradiation therapy. Brain Behav Immun, In Press.

[56] Bower, J.E., Ganz, P.A., Tao, M.L., Hu, W., Belin, T.R., Sepah, S., Cole, S., & Aziz, N. (2009). Inflammatory biomarkers and fatigue during radiation therapy for breast and prostate cancer. *Clin Cancer Res*, 15,5534-5540.

[57] MacHale, S.M., Cavanagh, J.T., Bennie, J., Carroll, S., Goodwin, G.M., & Lawrie, S.M. (1998). Diurnal variation of adrenocortical activity in chronic fatigue syndrome. *Neuropsychobiology*, 38,213-217.

[58] Backhaus, J., Junghanns, K., & Hohagen, F. (2004). Sleep disturbances are correlated with decreased morning awakening salivary cortisol. *Psychoneuroendocrinology*, 29,1184-1191.

[59] Pruessner, J.C., Hellhammer, D.H., & Kirschbaum, C. (1999). Burnout, perceived stress, and cortisol responses to awakening. *Psychosom Med*, 61,197-204.

[60] Minderhoud, I.M., Oldenburg, B., van Dam, P.S., & van Berge Henegouwen, G.P. (2003). High prevalence of fatigue in quiescent inflammatory bowel disease is not related to adrenocortical insufficiency. *Am J Gastroenterol*, 98,1088-1093.

[61] Vollmer-Conna, U., Lloyd, A., Hickie, I., & Wakefield, D. (1998). Chronic fatigue syndrome: an immunological perspective. *Aust N Z J Psychiatry*, 32,523-527.

[62] Katafuchi, T., Kondo, T., Take, S., & Yoshimura, M. (2006). Brain cytokines and the 5-HT system during poly I:C-induced fatigue. *Ann N Y Acad Sci*, 1088, 230-237.

[63] Capuron, L., Neurauter, G., Musselman, D.L., Lawson, D.H., Nemeroff, C.B., Fuchs, D., & Miller, A.H. (2003). Interferon-alpha-induced changes in tryptophan metabolism relationship to depression and paroxetine treatment. *Biol Psychiatry*, 54,906-914.

[64] Moreau, M., Lestage, J., Verrier, D., Mormede, C., Kelley, K.W., Dantzer, R., & Castanon, N. (2005). Bacille Calmette-Guerin inoculation induces chronic activation of peripheral and brain indoleamine 2,3-dioxygenase in mice. *J Infect Dis*, 192,537–544.

[65] Sutcigi, L., Oktenli, C., Musabak, U., Bozkurt, A., Cansever, A., Uzun, O., Sanisoglu, S.Y., Yesilova, Z., Ozmenler, N., Ozsahin, A., & Sengul, A. (2007). Pro- and anti-inflammatory cytokine balance in major depression: effect of sertraline therapy. *Clin Dev Immunol*, 2007,76396.

[66] Staines, D.R. (2004). Overview of an autoimmune theory of endogenous vasoactive neuropeptides in the aetiology of certain conditions. *Med Hypotheses*, 62,643-645.

[67] Sherwood, N.M., Krueckl, S.L., & McRory, J.E. (2000). The origin and function of the pituitary adenylate cyclase-activating polypeptide (PACAP)/glucagon superfamily. *Endocr Rev*, 21,619-670.

[68] Staines, D.R. (2006). Postulated vasoactive neurpetide autoimmunity in fatigue-related conditions: a brief review and hypothesis. *Clin Dev immunol*, 13, 25-39.

[69] Zhou, C.J., Shioda, S., Yada, T., Inagaki, N., Pleasure, S.J., & Kikuyama, S. (2002). PACAP and its receptors exert pleiotropic effects in the nervous system by activating multiple signaling pathways. *Curr Protein Pept Sci*, 3,423-439.

[70] Bangale, Y., Cavill, D., Gordon, T., Planque, S., Taguchi, H., Bhatia, G., Nishuyama, Y., Arnett, F., & Paul, S. (2002). Vasoactive intestinal peptide binding autoantibodies in autoimmune humans and mice. *Peptides*, 23,2251-2257.

[71] Johnson, M.C., McCormack, R.J., Delgado, M., Martinex, C., & Ganea, D. (1996). Lymphocytes express vasoactive intestinal peptide receptor 1 (VIP-R1) mRNA. *J Neuroimmunol*, 68,109-119.

[72] Staines, D.R. (2007). Is Parkinson's disease an autoimmune disorder of endogenous vasoactive neuropeptides? *Med Hypotheses*, 69,1208-1211.

[73] Delgado, M., Munoz-Elias, E.J., Gomariz, R.P., & Ganea, D. (1999). Vasoactive intestinal peptide and pituitary adenylate cyclase-activating polypeptide prevent inducible nitric oxide synthase transcription in macrophages by inhibiting NF-kappa B and IFN regulatory factor 1 activation. *J Immunol*, 162,4685-4696.

[74] Ruiz, J.R., Ortega, F.B., Wärnberg, J., Moreno, L.A., Carrero, J.J., Gonzalez-Gross, M., Marcos, A., Gutierrez, A., & Sjöström, M. (2008). Inflammatory proteins and muscle strength in adolescents: the Avena study. *Arch Pediatr Adolesc Med*, 162,462-468.

[75] Schiøtz Thorud, H.M., Stranda, A., Birkeland, J.A., Lunde, P.K., Siaastad, I., Kolset, S.O., Sejersted, O.M. & Iversen, P.O. (2005). Enhanced matrix metalloproteinase activity in skeletal muscles of rats with congestive heart failure. *Am J Physiol Regul Integr Comp Physiol*, 289,R389-R394.

[76] Smith, A.K., White, P.D., Aslakson, E., Vollmer-Conna, U., & Rejeevan, M.S. (2006). Polymorphisms in genes regulating the HPA axis associated with empirically delineated classes of unexplained chronic fatigue. *Pharmacogenomics*, 7,387-394.

[77] Netea, M.G., Kullberg, B.J., Vonk, A.G., Verschueren, I., Joosten, L.A., & van der Meer, J.W. (2007). Increased voluntary exercise in mice deficient for tumour necrosis factor-alpha and lymphotoxin-alpha. *Eur J Clin Invest*, 37,737-741.

[78] Knight, D.M., Trinh, H., Le, J., Siegel, S., Shealy, D., McDonough, M., Scallon, B., Moore, M.A., Vilcek. J., Daddona, P., & et al. (1993). Construction and initial characterization of a mouse-human chimeric anti-TNF antibody. *Mol Immunol*, 30,1443-1453.

[79] Kaushik, V.V., & Moots, R.J. (2005). CDP-870 (certolizumab) in rheumatoid arthritis. *Expert Opin Biol Ther*, 5,601-606.

[80] Heiberg, M.S., Kaufmann, C., Rødevand, E., Mikkelsen, K., Koldingsnes, W., Mowinckel, P., & Kvien, T.K. (2007). The comparative effectiveness of anti-TNF therapy and methotrexate in patients with psoriatic arthritis: 6 month results from a longitudinal, observational, multicentre study. Ann Rheum Dis, 66,1038-1042.

[81] Arman, A., Yilmaz, B., Coker, A., Inanc, N., & Direskeneli, H. (2006). Interleukin-1 receptor antagonist (IL-1RN) and interleukin-1B gene polymorphisms in Turkish patients with rheumatoid arthritis. *Clin Exp Rheumatol*, 24,643-648.

[82] Carmichael, M.D., Davis, J.M., Murphy, E.A., Brown, A.S., Carson, J.A., Mayer, E.P., & Ghaffar, A. (2006). Role of brain IL-1beta on fatigue after exercise-induced muscle damage. *Am J Physiol Regul Integr Comp Physiol*, 291, R1344-R1348.

[83] Vgontzas, A.N., Bixler, E.O., Lin, H.M., Prolo, P., Trakada, G., & Chrousos, G.P.(2005). IL-6 and its circadian secretion in humans. *Neuroimmunomodulation*, 12,131-140.

[84] Späth-Schwalbe. E., Hansen. K., Schmidt, F., Schrezenmeir, H., Marshall, L., Burger, K., Fehm, H.L., & Born, J. (1998). Acute effects of recombinant human interleukin-6 on endocrine and central nervous sleep functions in healthy men._J Clin Endocrinol Metab, 83,1573-1579.

[85] Ohsugi, Y. (2007). Recent advances in immunopathophysiology of interleukin-6: an innovative therapeutic drug, tocilizumab (recombinant humanized anti-human interleukin-6 receptor antibody), unveils the mysterious etiology of immune-mediated inflammatory diseases. *Biol Pharm Bull*, 30,2001-2006.

[86] Watanabe, Y. (2004). Fifty years of interference. Nat Immunol, 5,1193.

[87] Capuron, L., & Miller, A.H. (2004). Cytokines and psychopathology: lessons from interferon-alpha. *Biol Psychiatry*, 56,819-824.

[88] Martin, K.A., Krahn, L.E., Balan, V., & Rosati, M.J. (2007). Modafinil's use in combating interferon-induced fatigue. *Dig Dis Sci*, 52,893-896.

[89] Sleijfer, S., Bannink, M., Van Gool, A.R., Kruit, W.H., & Stoter G. (2005). Side effects of interferon-alpha therapy. *Pharm World Sci*, 27,423-431.

[90] Simone, I.L., Ceccarelli, A., Tortorella, C., Bellacosa, A., Pellegrini, F., Plasmati, I., De Caro, M.F., Lopez, M., Girolamo, F., & Livrea, P. (2006). Influence of Interferon beta treatment on quality of life in multiple sclerosis patients. *Health Qual Life Outcomes*, 4,96.

In: Handbook of Fatigue in Health and Disease
Editor: Howard S. Smith
ISBN 978-1-61761-920-5

Chapter 3

BARRIERS TO FATIGUE COMMUNICATION

***Steven D. Passik*[1] *and Kenneth L. Kirsh*[2]**

[1] Memorial Sloan-Kettering Cancer Center
Department of Psychiatry and Behavioral Sciences
641 Lexington Ave.
New York, NY 10022
[2] Assistant Professor
Pharmacy Practice and Science
University of Kentucky
725 Rose Street, 401C
Lexington, KY 40536-0082, USA

ABSTRACT

Fatigue is a highly prevalent multidimensional and distressing symptom which is difficult to define and quantify. Often fatigue is not fully assessed in terms of its intensity, associated distress, impact, or patients beliefs regarding it. Barriers to the communication of fatigue may include: patient-related barriers, provider-related barriers, and system-related barriers. Patient-related barriers to communicating about fatigue may include: concerns that fatigue is a sign that my illness is getting worse, concerns regarding taking away focus from the major illness, concerns that if I talk about fatigue, my doctor will have less time for other more important things, concerns that my doctor will think that I am a "complainer", and/or having the impression that everyone has fatigue and I should just "suck it up" and continue my usual routine. More research and

[1] Phone: (646) 888-0022
Fax: (212) 888-2356
Email: passiks@mskcc.org
[2] Phone: (859) 552-5011
Email: doctorken@windstream.net

perhaps the use of novel instruments may help patients to better report their experiences regarding this potentially devastating and treatable symptom.

INTRODUCTION

Fatigue is a highly prevalent and distressing symptom of cancer and its treatment. Unfortunately, it has proven to be difficult to define and quantify in a consistent way and can be extremely distressing for the patient [1]. Despite these issues, it is highly treatable through a variety of treatment modalities. Complicating matters, however, is that cancer patients often fail to communicate with their oncologists about fatigue.

Fatigue is the most common symptom reported by cancer patients [2-5]. Past studies report prevalence rates ranging from 61% to 90% for fatigue in various oncology samples [5-7]. Cancer-related fatigue (CRF) is associated with significant impairment. A study by Ashbury and colleagues (1998) found that cancer patients with CRF were more likely to have impairment in performing normal daily activities and to more frequently use healthcare services than their non-fatigued counterparts [8]. To date, the mechanisms of CRF are not fully understood, nor is there consensus on how to best identify clinically relevant fatigue [9].

Perhaps the best way to characterize fatigue is to view it as a multidimensional problem involving chronic exhaustion and diminished capacity for physical activity that is not alleviated by rest [2, 10]. This is not to say that fatigue is solely a physical entity, however. The etiology may be physical, psychological, pathological, or a combination of any of these [2, 11, 12]. In addition, fatigue level may be influenced by a variety of factors including treatment, changes in sleeping patterns, symptom distress, mood disturbance, low hemoglobin levels, or poor performance status [6, 7, 13, 14]. Bower and colleagues (2002) report correlations between fatigue level and economic status, as well as, fatigue level and relationship status, in women suffering or recovering from breast cancer. The results show that women with increased fatigue are more likely to be single or have lower incomes [15]. One can speculate that the single cancer population may lack a significant other to attend oncology visits with them to help communicate about fatigue and its impact to the physician. Additionally, cancer patients with lower income may encounter some very specific communication barriers where fatigue is concerned, such as language barriers and lack of translators. However, there have not been any specific studies that focus on marital and economic status as factors affecting fatigue communication. In another study, assessing fatigue and women with breast cancer, the time between surgery and first chemotherapy treatment proved to be a significant factor in severity of fatigue. De Jong and colleagues (2004) found that, following surgery, the longer the patient had to wait for their initial treatment, the more intensely they reported their level of fatigue [16]. It is not clear what this delay may do to communication about fatigue; one might speculate that the patient's haste in wanting to start a delayed treatment may push quality of life matters "off of the agenda" so that the focus might be exclusively on treatment issues. Or, alternatively, perhaps the fatigue arises from certain medical complications that, in fact, cause such delays, again tending to skew communication in the direction of medical issues rather than quality of life concerns.

In a survey of nearly 200 oncologists [5], 80% reported that fatigue is either neglected or under-treated in cancer patients. In addition, the survey found that most patients (74%)

believed fatigue to be an untreatable symptom that one had to endure as a normal part of cancer and its accompanying treatment. However, a large number of potential treatments are available to combat fatigue. For instance, self-care activities and education for the patient and family can be useful [17]. Further, several studies [18-23] have shown that aerobic exercise can help to improve the physical performance of cancer patients. Finally, recombinant human erythropoietin (r-HuEPO, epoetin alfa) has been shown to increase hemoglobin levels and to subsequently reduce fatigue in cancer patients [24-27]. Epoetin alfa improved patients' perceived energy levels, functional status, and overall quality of life.

Patient-related barriers to communicating about fatigue have not been well studied, but similar barriers have been described in cancer pain and AIDS pain [28, 29]. Ward and colleagues (1993) found that patient concerns were fairly universal with regard to treatment of cancer pain. Fears of addiction, tolerance, side effects, and distracting physicians were reported as barriers by over 70% of patients [28]. Endorsement of these barriers was related to the under-medication of the patient's pain. Breitbart and colleagues (1998) reported similar findings with regard to barriers endorsed by people with AID [29]. In addition, these investigations added concerns specific to AIDS patients. They observed that patients often showed a preference for "natural" or alternative interventions and a desire to limit their overall use of medications.

It is clear that it is an important undertaking to understand specific barriers to fatigue communication commonly endorsed by cancer patients. When better understood, knowledge of the prominent barriers can lead to tailored educational efforts to facilitate such communication. As prior research suggests [30], successful interventions for fatigue should be patient-specific, and several points must be kept in mind when attempting such a task.

First, it is important to explore the relationship between self-efficacy and communication about fatigue as cited by patients. It is important to explore whether individual levels of self-efficacy have an impact on this construct. It has been suggested that increased levels of self-efficacy are associated with greater levels of treatment adherence and increased self-care behavior [31], so it is an important area to consider. It may well be that patients with higher levels of self-efficacy are more apt to communicate or endorse different barriers compared to patients with low self-efficacy. Ultimately, this could lead to a more tailored approach to the treatment of fatigue.

Second, there is a likely relationship between depression and fatigue that needs to be addressed in any attempt to explore fatigue communication. In fact, our work [32] has shown that a single-item taken from a depression scale can be utilized as a triage-like screen for more detailed follow-up for cancer-related fatigue, indicating some level of overlap. Indeed, some researchers [33] have shown significant correlations between fatigue and depression. However, this is not to indicate that depression causes fatigue or vice versa. Past research [34] has suggested that there is little evidence for such a cause-and-effect relationship and that depression and fatigue run different temporal courses in cancer patients. This issue of what role depression plays is important because such patients might have different reasons for not communicating (i.e., are more fatalistic).

Third, it is important to understand whether an urban versus rural location creates any differences in fatigue communication. While research has shown that geographical location was unlikely to affect cancer mortality rates [35], differences between these locations do exist. Specifically, rural patients are more likely to be unstaged at diagnosis and to have more advanced disease when diagnosed compared to urban patients [36, 37]. Further, one survey found that rural patients had lower expectations about health care and had to overcome more obstacles before reaching the care of a specialist [38]. In addition, it might be expected that stoicism would play a larger role for the rural patient, again leading to potential differences in style of communication and therefore different potential barriers to discussing fatigue.

Barriers to Fatigue Communication in Rural Populations

We performed a study [39] that attempted to identify the patient-related barriers to communication about fatigue as cited by patients from both rural and urban settings. Two hundred patients (100 rural, 100 urban) were sampled across a community cancer network in Indiana using the Cancer Behavior Inventory-Brief scale (CBI-B) [40], the Zung Self-Rating Depression Scale (ZSDS) [41-44], the Functional Assessment of Cancer Inventory-Anemia scale (FACT-An) [45-47], the Fatigue Management Barriers Questionnaire (FMBQ) (See Table 1), and a checklist of possible interventions communicated by the healthcare staff (See Table 2). The FMBQ questionnaire was devised by experts in the field of cancer-related fatigue and also upon the NCCN guidelines [48].

The average age of the sample was 59.62 years (SD = 13.62) and was comprised of 114 women (57%) and 86 men (43%). The majority (41%, n = 82) had a high school education, followed by those with some college (18%, n = 36) or some high school (16%, n = 16). The vast majority were married (69.5%, n = 139) and the sample was predominantly white (89%, n = 178). The most common employment status was retired (37%, n = 74), followed by disabled (23%, n = 46), or currently working full time (15.5%, n = 31). The type of tumor varied among the population, with lung (23%, n = 45), breast (19.9%, n = 39), and colon (13.8%, n = 27) cancer being most common followed by lymphoma (10.2%, n = 20).

There were no statistically significant correlations between the demographic variables and any of the assessment instruments. In addition, a series of one-way ANOVAs showed no differences amongst the FACT-An, ZSDS, BZSDS, CBI-B, or FMBQ based on whether the patient was in a rural or urban site. We found it surprising that scores on the instruments did not differ significantly based on whether the patient was from a rural or urban site. Only two individual items from the FMBQ showed any differences between the two groups. Of the 28 FMBQ items, only item 18 "I try to be strong by not complaining about fatigue to my doctor" and item 21 "I'm afraid to tell doctor how fatigued I am because he won't continue treatment" were significantly different based on the rural versus urban split. The urban patients had a mean of 2.60 (SD = 1.05) on item 18 and 2.02 (SD = .72) on item 21. Rural patients had a mean of 2.27 (SD = 1.01) on item 18 and 1.77 (SD = .66) on item 21. This indicates that urban patients were more likely to agree with these statements, possibly indicating greater stoicism or fear in the urban sample.

For the total sample, 132 patients (66%) reported that they had never spoken to their doctor about fatigue. The most frequently reported reasons for this lack of patient communication about fatigue included the doctor's failure to offer interventions (47%), patients' lack of awareness of effective treatments for fatigue (43%), a desire on the patient's part to treat fatigue without medications (40%), and not wanting to complain to the doctor (28%). Patients reported that medical staff offered a mean of 11.63 recommendations for dealing with fatigue. The FMBQ was found to correlate with self-efficacy (CBI-B, $r = -.20$, $p<.01$) and weakly with the number of recommendations made ($r = -.15$, $p<.05$). The FMBQ was noted to have acceptable internal consistency ($\alpha = 0.88$) and validity and may prove to be a useful instrument for understanding why patients do not communicate about fatigue. Multiple barriers contribute to why cancer patients do not comment about fatigue but may be overcome if physicians screen and assess for fatigue.

The separation of respondents from the sample that scored at the extremes of the depression and self-efficacy spectrum offer some interesting insights into the beliefs about fatigue. The depressed patients were more likely than their non-depressed counterparts to have heard about potential interventions from their doctors, want medications for the treatment of fatigue but yet claim that they were unaware of any effective treatments. It may be that the depressed group received more global attention because of their depressed mood but still retained a hopeless outlook even when attention and possible treatment options are offered. Similarly, the low self-efficacy group was more apt than their high self-efficacy counterparts to want medication interventions while also believing that there were no effective fatigue interventions.

This study has important implications for patient education. Barriers endorsed regarding fatigue are unlike those in the pain literature in that they are not as universal as patient-related barriers to pain treatment and are more numerous. Even the most commonly endorsed barriers identified herein aren't nearly as universal as those seen in pain management. The use of the FMBQ to identify fatalistic attitudes and other barriers might be a reasonable start as we continue to figure out ways to enhance patient reporting of symptoms. This study raises interesting questions that should be explored through further research that does not rely on cross-sectional data alone. It may well turn out that clinicians will experience better patient outcome by making a stronger effort to individualize patient education and tailor measures regarding fatigue definitions based on whether or not the patient is depressed.

Conclusion

Fatigue is a highly prevalent, multidimensional problem for cancer patients. It is distressing for the patient, but our clinical experience, as well as the work of others [12], suggests that it is highly treatable through a variety of treatment modalities. However, to treat this symptom, we must first be able to adequately identify fatigue in cancer patients. To accomplish this, it is necessary to understand the barriers to communication about fatigue, so we can help patients to better report their experiences.

References

[1] Jacobsen, P.B. (2004). Assessment of fatigue in cancer patients. *J Natl Cancer Inst Monogr*, 32,93-97.

[2] Cella, D., Peterman, A., Passik, S.D., Jacobsen, P., & Breitbart, W. (1998). Progress toward guidelines for the management of fatigue. *Oncology*, 12,369-377.

[3] Curt, G.A., Breitbart, W., Cella, D., Groopman, J.E., Horning, S.J., Itri, L.M., Johnson, D.H., Miaskowski, C., & Scherr, S.L. (2000). Impact of cancer-related fatigue on the lives of patients: new findings from the Fatigue Coalition. *Oncologist*, 5,353-360.

[4] Glaus, A., Crow, R., & Hammond, S. (1996). A qualitative study to explore the concept of fatigue/tiredness in cancer patients and in healthy individuals. *Support Care Cancer*, 4,82-96.

[5] Vogelzang, N.J., Breitbart, W., Cella, D., Curt, G.A., Groopman, J.E., Horning, S.J., Itri, L.M., Johnson, D.H., Scherr, S.L., & Portenoy, R.K. (1997). Patient, caregiver, and oncologist perceptions of cancer-related fatigue: results of a tripart assessment survey. *Semin Hematol*, 34,4-12.

[6] Irvine, D., Vincent, L., Graydon, J., Bubela, N, & Thompson, L. (1994). The prevalence and correlates of fatigue in patients receiving treatment with chemotherapy and radiotherapy. A comparison with the fatigue experienced by healthy individuals. *Cancer Nurs*, 17,367-378.

[7] Richardson, A., & Ream, E. (1996). The experience of fatigue and other symptoms in patients receiving chemotherapy. *Eur J Cancer Care*, 5,24-30.

[8] Ashbury, F.D., Findlay, H., Reynolds, B., & McKerracher, K. (1998). A canadian survey of cancer patients' experiences: are their needs being met? *J Pain Symptom Manage*, 16,298-306.

[9] Richardson, A., Ream, E., & Wilson-Barnett, J. (1998). Fatigue in patients receiving chemotherapy: patterns of change. *Cancer Nurs*, 21,17-30.

[10] Smets, E.M., Garssen, B., Schuster-Uitterhoeve, A.L., de Haes, J.C. (1993). Fatigue in cancer patients. *Br J Cancer*, 68,220-224.

[11] Kirk, J., Douglass, R., Nelson, E., Jaffe, J., Lopez, A., Ohler, J., Blanchard, C., Chapman, R., McHugo, G., & Stone, K. (1990). Chief complaint of fatigue: a prospective study. *J Fam Pract*, 30,33-39.

[12] Portenoy, R.K., & Itri, L.M. (1999). Cancer-related fatigue: guidelines for evaluation and management. *Oncologist*, 4,1-10.

[13] Cella, D. (1998). Factors influencing quality of life in cancer patients: anemia and fatigue. *Semin Oncol*, 25,43-46.

[14] Pater, J.L., Zee, B., Palmer, M., Johnston, D., & Osoba, D. (1997). Fatigue in patients with cancer: results with National Cancer Institute of Canada Clinical Trials Group studies employing the EORTC QLQ-30. *Support Care Cancer*, 5,410-413.

[15] Bower, J., Ganz, P., Aziz, N., & Fahey, J. (2002). Fatigue and proinflammatory cytokine activity in breast cancer survivors. *Psychosomatic Medicine*, 64,604-611.

[16] de Jong, N., Candel, M.J.J.M., Schouten, H.C., Abu-Saad, H.H., & Courtens, A.M. (2004). Prevalence and course of fatigue in breast cancer patients receiving adjuvant chemotherapy. *Annals of Oncology*, 15,896-905.

[17] Yarbro, C.H. (1996). Interventions for fatigue. *Eur J Cancer Care*, 5,35-38.

[18] Dimeo, F.C. (2001). Effects of exercise on cancer-related fatigue. *Cancer*, 92,1689-1693.

[19] Dimeo, F.C., Rumberger, B.G., & Keul ,J. (1998). Aerobic exercise as therapy for cancer fatigue. *Med Sci Sports Exerc*, 30,475-478.

[20] Dimeo, F.C., Tilmann, M.H., Bertz, H., Kanz, L., Mertelsmann, R., & Keul, J. (1997). Aerobic exercise of cancer patients after high dose chemotherapy and autologous peripheral stem cell transplantation. *Cancer*, 79,1717-1722.

[21] MacVicar, M.G., Winningham, M.L., & Nickel, J.L. (1989). Effects of aerobic interval training on cancer patient's functional capacity. *Nursing Research*, 38,348-351.

[22] Mock, V., Ropka, M.E., Rhodes, V.A,, Pickett, M., Grimm, P.M., McDaniel, R., Lin, E.M., Allocca, P., Dienemann, J.A., Haisfield-Wolfe, M.E., Stewart, K.J., & McCorkle, R. (1998). Establishing mechanisms to conduct multi-institutional research-fatigue in patients with cancer: and exercise intervention. *Oncology Nursing Forum*, 25,1391-1397.

[23] Schwartz, A.L., Mori, M., Gao, R., Nail, L.M., & King, M.E. (2001). Exercise reduces daily fatigue in women with breast cancer receiving chemotherapy. *Med Sci Sports Exercise*, 33,718-723.

[24] Demetri, G.D., Kris, M., Wade, J., Degos, L., & Cella, D. (1998). Quality of life benefit in chemotherapy patients treated with epoetin alfa is independent of disease response or tumor type: results from a prospective community oncology study. *J Clin Oncol*, 16,3412-3425.

[25] Gabrilove, J., Cleeland, C., Livingston, R., Sarokhan, B., Winer, E., & Einhorn, L.H. (2001). Clinical evaluation of once-weekly dosing of epoetin alfa in chemotherapy patients: improvements in hemoglobin and quality of life similar to three-times-weekly dosing. *J Clin Oncol*, 19,2875-2882.

[26] Glaspy, J. (1997). The impact of epoetin alfa on quality of life during cancer chemotherapy: a fresh look at an old problem. *Semin Hematol*, 34,20-26.

[27] Glaspy, J., Bukowski, R., Steinberg, D., Taylor, C., Tchekmedyian, S., & Vadhan-Raj, S. (1997). Impact of therapy with epoetin alfa on chemical outcomes in patients with nonmyeloid malignancies during cancer chemotherapy in community oncology practice. Procrit study group. *J Clin Oncol*, 15,1218-1234.

[28] Ward, S.E., Goldberg, N., Miller-McCauley, V., Mueller, C., Nolam, A., Pawlik-Plank, D. Robbins, A., Stormoen, D., & Weissman, D.E. (1993). Patient-related barriers to management of cancer pain. *Pain*, 52,319-324

[29] Breitbart,W., Passik, S.D., McDonald, M.V., Rosenfeld, B., Smith, M., Kaim, M., & Funesti-Esch, J. (1998). Patient-related barriers to pain management in ambulatory AIDS patients. *Pain*, 76,9-16.

[30] Valentine, A.D., & Myers, C.A. (2001). Cognitive and mood disturbance as causes and symptoms of fatigue in cancer patients. *Cancer*, 92,1694-1698.

[31] Lev, E.L. (1997). Bandura's theory of self-efficacy: applications to oncology. *Schol Inq Nurs Pract*, 11,21-37.

[32] Kirsh, K.L., Passik, S.D., Holtsclaw, E., Donaghy, K., & Theobald, D. (2001). I get tired for no reason: A single item screening for cancer-related fatigue. *J Pain Symptom Manage*, 22,931-937.

[33] Redeker, N.S., Lev, E.L., & Ruggiero, J. (2000). Insomnia, fatigue, anxiety, depression, and quality of life of cancer patients undergoing chemotherapy. *Schol Inquiry Nurs Pract*, 14,275-290.

[34] Visser, M.R., & Smets, E.M. (1998). Fatigue, depression and quality of life in cancer patients: how are they related? *Supportive Care Cancer*, 6,101-108.

[35] Horner, R.D., & Chirikos, T.N. (1987). Survivorship differences in geographical comparisons of cancer mortality: an urban-rural analysis. *Int J Epidemiology*, 16,184-189.

[36] Liff ,J.M., Chow, W.H., & Greenberg, R.S. (1991). Rural-urban differences in stage at diagnosis. Possible relationship to cancer screening. *Cancer*, 67,1454-1459.

[37] Monroe, A.C., Ricketts T.C., & Savitz, L.A. (1992). Cancer in rural versus urban populations: a review. *J Rural Health*, 8,212-220.

[38] Bain, N.S., & Campbell, N.C. (2000). Treating patients with colorectal cancer in rural and urban areas: a qualitative study of the patients' perspective. *Family Practice*, 17,475-479.

[39] Passik, S.D., Kirsh, K.L., Donaghy, K., Holtsclaw, E., Theobald, D., Cella, D., Breitbart, W.; & Fatigue Coalition. (2002). Patient-related barriers to fatigue communication: initial validation of the fatigue management barriers questionnaire. *Journal of Pain and Symptom Management*, 24,481-493.

[40] Merluzzi, T., & Sanchez, M. (1997). Assessment of self-efficacy and coping with cancer: Development and validation of the cancer behavior inventory. *Health Psychology*, 16,163-170.

[41] Dugan, W., McDonald, M,, Passik, S., Rosenfeld, B.D., Theobald, D., & Edgerton, S. (1998). Use of the zung self-rating depression scale in cancer patients: Feasibility as a screening tool. *Psycho-Oncology*, 7,483-493.

[42] Tate, D.G., Forchheimer, M., Maynard, F., Tate, Maynard, F., Davidoff, G., Dijkers, M. (1993). Comparing two measures of depression in spinal cord injury. Rehabilitation Psychology, 38,53-61.

[43] Zung, W. (1967). Depression in the normal aged. *Psychosomatics*, 7,287-292.

[44] Zung, W. (1967). Factors influencing the self-rating depression scale. *Arch Gen Psych*, 16,543-547.

[45] Cella, D.F., Tulsky, D.S., Gray, G.G., Sarafian, B., Linn, E., Bonomi, A., Silberman, M., Yellen, S.B., Winicour, P., Brannon, J., Eckberg, K., Lloyd, S., Purl, S., Blendowski, C., Goodman, M., Barnicle, M., Stewart, I., McHale, M., Bonomi, P., Kaplan, E., Taylor IV, S., Thomas, C.R. Jr., & Harris, J. (1993). The functional assessment of cancer therapy scale: Development and validation. *J Clin Oncol*, 11,570-579.

[46] Winstead-Fry, P., & Schultz, A. (1997). Psychometric analysis of the functional assessment of cancer therapy-general (FACT-G) scale in a rural sample. *Cancer*, 79,2446-2452.

[47] Yellen, S., Cella, D., Webster, K., Blendowski, C., & Kaplan, E. (1997). Measuring fatigue and other anemia-related symptoms with the functional assessment of cancer therapy (FACT-G) measurement system. *J Pain Symp Manage*, 13,63-74.

[48] Mock, V., Atkinson, A., Barsevick, A., Cella, D., Cimprich, B., Cleeland, C., Donnelly, J., Eisenberger, M.A., Escalante, C., Hinds, P., Jacobsen, P.B., Kaldor, P., Knight, S.J., Peterman, A., Piper, B.F., Rugo, H., Sabbatini, P., Stahl, C.; & National Comprehensive Cancer Network. (2000). NCCN practice guidelines for cancer-related fatigue. *Oncology*, 14,151-161.

In: Handbook of Fatigue in Health and Disease
Editor: Howard S. Smith

ISBN 978-1-61761-920-5

Chapter 4

EVALUATION TOOLS IN FATIGUE

Howard S. Smith*

Associate Professor & Academic Director of Pain Management
Albany Medical College
Department of Anesthesiology
47 New Scotland Avenue; MC-131
Albany, New York 12208, USA

ABSTRACT

In efforts to fully understand and assess any symptom, its impact on an individual subject, and the distress and suffering that it may produce in multiple domains, clinicians need among other things a clinically helpful symptom definition and a practical and useful method of assessing symptom characteristics (e.g. quality, intensity, distress) as well as its impact on quality of life in multiple domains. Fatigue has been referred to as a vague symptom. Over the past two decades, a number of novel instruments have been developed to aid in the assessment of fatigue. Some of these tools are specific to a particular medical condition.

INTRODUCTION

In order to appropriately approach the treatment of fatigue effectively and to appreciate case-specific contributing factors to fatigue, each case needs to be carefully evaluated including a comprehensive history and physical with appropriate ancillary testing. Furthermore, fatigue needs an appropriate assessment in order to optimally approach potential

* Phone: 518-262-4461
Fax: 518-262-2671
Email: smithh@mail.amc.edu

therapeutic strategies. Treatment strategies for fatigue may involve: pharmacologic approaches, physical medicine approaches, and/or behavioral medicine approaches and perhaps in the future neuromodulation approaches. Fatigue is a universal and daily phenomenon and is ranked third on the list of most reported problems in the general practitioner's surgery [1].

Despite the high incidence of fatigue and its negative impact on quality of life as well as productivity; there remain few studies evaluating therapeutic approaches to prevention and/or palliation of this symptom. Furthermore, this parallels the relative lack of attention which clinicians tend to devote to fatigue. All too often, complaints of fatigue are completely ignored, not taken seriously, or saved for last, even if this is the patient's chief complaint. Additionally, there is no uniform consensus of a particular tool or instrument which should be used to assess fatigue and for the majority of medical care provided; it appears that there is no assessment of fatigue documented at all.

In the basic sciences, especially physiology, fatigue has been defined as a time-related phenomenon of decline in the maximal force-generation capacity [2-4]. Usually, this is expressed by a deterioration in maximal voluntary contraction (MVC). Medical literature usually defines fatigue in the sense of 'experienced fatigue' as an overwhelming sense of tiredness, lack of energy and feeling of exhaustion [5-8]. A problem arises when one wishes to discriminate fatigue levels between patients. Everyone knows feelings of fatigue, but do we always mean the same thing [9]. To allow between-patient comparisons, the self-perceived fatigue needs to be quantified. For physicians this has practical relevance. Fatigue is a concept determined by two dimensions, psychological and physiological (i.e. bodily phenomena contributing to the perception of fatigue). Psychological factors such as well-being, concentration problems, attributions, physical activity and social functioning may all affect the way the fatigue is experienced [10]. "Physiologic Fatigue" has been categorized into peripheral and central fatigue. Although not commonly utilized in clinical practice, various objectives as tools will be presented to help assess peripheral and central fatigue longitudinally.

Peripheral Fatigue

The most direct measure of peripheral fatigue is the change in force response to electrical stimulation during rest following exercise relative to the pre-stimulation force, which will reveal any loss of force in the muscle tissue after constant activation [9]. It also shows the change in contractile characteristics like a fatigue-induced dominant slowing of the relaxation phase [11, 12].

Changes in sarcolemma can be studied noninvasively by means of Surface EMG (sEMG), which allows various variables to be monitored online, among which are the amplitude (e.g. integrated EMG (iEMG) or rectified EMG), frequency content of the signal and muscle-fibre conduction velocity (MFCV [9]).

The amplitude of the sEMG signal (often expressed by iEMG recordings over a specified time, i.e. the area under the full-wave rectified signal within a time interval) is a measure of the voluntary drive to the muscle. During submaximal contractions the iEMG usually increases considerably due to the recruitment of extra motor units and an increase in firing frequency [9]. Both are mechanisms to cope with the declining force output during a sustained contraction of the motor units. Contrariwise, during high and maximal contractions the amplitude usually declines, concomitant with a change of the muscle-fibre action potentials and possibly a drop in firing frequencies [13-16]. Multichannel surface electrodes allow MFCV to be conveniently assessed [17, 18], at least in several muscles. Changes in the frequency spectrum and MFCV during fatigue are well-known phenomena and mainly due to changes in the metabolic environment (and in the muscle membrane) [19, 20].

Central Fatigue

A muscle receiving suboptimal input from the CNS will not be able to develop its maximal force capacity. In the case of submaximal central activation, central activation failure (CAF) is said to be present [9]. An increase of CAF during exercise is called central fatigue.

Twitch Interpolation

Submaximal voluntary drive may have several causes, e.g. a lack of motivation or exhaustion of the cortical neurons in the motor cortex [9]. Usually, CAF can be confirmed with a version of the so-called twitch-interpolation technique [9, 21]. Subjects are instructed to make an MVC with a specific muscle, during which electrical stimulation is applied to the motor nerve or motor endplate. If the muscle's voluntary central drive is optimal, this will not lead to additional force production [9]. However, if the voluntary activation is submaximal, the electrical stimulation will result in an increased exertion of force, demonstrating CAF [9]. With this technique, CAF can be quantified and its change over time (central fatigue) studied, although it cannot discriminate between the different causes of CAF at the central level (e.g. whether the impaired drive has a spinal or a cortical origin) [22] have shown that even in the course of a sustained contraction, the technique allows the peripheral and central contributions to the force reduction to be calculated [9].

Motor Cortex Stimulation

Magnetic and electrical stimulation of the motor cortex have been used to study correlates of fatigue higher up in the nervous system [21, 23, 24]. The stimulation of the motor cortex artificially activates the CNS and the response is measured at the output site by recording the force or the electrical muscle response. Numerous studies have reported diminished output by the motor cortex following magnetic stimulation after a fatiguing contraction [25]. Todd and colleagues suggest that magnetic stimulation may capture voluntary output at force levels of 50–100% [26, 27].

Readiness Potential

Freude and Ullsperger (1987) introduced readiness potentials (RPs) for the study of fatigue [28]. This negative movement-related cortical EEG potential appears over the human scalp about 1 s before a self-paced motor act [29]. It is mainly generated by the supplementary motor area and the primary motor cortex [30]. Although it cannot be used during sustained contractions, RP recordings are a prominent tool to study central changes during more natural repetitive contractions [9].

Fatigue assessment tools should allow for detection of temporal changes in the level of distress caused by fatigue. Similar to pain and many other symptoms, there exists general agreement that the approach to the assessment of the sensation of fatigue should be based on self-report [31-33]. Any tool which attempts to evaluate fatigue should be clear, concise, dynamic, and reactive. If the instrument is too cumbersome, efforts to complete it may represent too much of a burden for the fatigues respondent. Also, fatigue assessment tools should attempt to truly measure fatigue and not potentially associates issues, such as worsening medical/neurological conditions, muscle weakness, diminished functional status, depression, insomnia, or diminished cardiopulmonary status. Ideally, the tool should be able to be used repeatedly to follow treatment response specific for fatigue (e.g. testosterone dose-dependently increases maximal voluntary strength and leg power, but does not affect fatigability or specific tension [34]).

Perhaps the "easiest" assessment of fatigue is to apply reasonable well known tools, used to assess other symptoms (e.g. pain) such as the numerical rating scale-11 (NRS-11) where patients circle the number (0 through ten) which best related to their fatigue, or the visual analog scale (VAS) where the respondent puts a mark along a 10-cm line (anchored on one end with no fatigue and on the other end with worst fatigue imaginable) which best relates to their fatigue. These unidimensional tools assess fatigue intensity but do not give any information regarding how the fatigue interferes with the patient's life, any associated distress related to the fatigue, or any other domains affected by fatigue.

Assessment tools for fatigue remain suboptimal. The Piper Fatigue Scale (Piper) was an early multidimensional tool attempting to subdivide the experience of pain into several distinct domains, but it seems to be too cumbersome to be used in clinical practice. The Schwartz Cancer Fatigue Scale which has four subscales (physical, emotional, cognitive, and temporal) was developed specifically for the cancer patient [35].

Van Belle et al. attempted to validate the use of the proposed International Statistical Classification of Diseases and Related Health Problems (10th version) (ICD-10) criteria for fatigue (P-ICD10) through comparison with the Functional Assessment of Cancer Therapy Fatigue (FACT-F) subscale and three visual analogue scale (VAS) qualities in 834 cancer patients through to be fatigued at three clinical centers in Belgium, using P-ICD10, FACT-F, and VAS to assess: level of energy (VAS1), quality of life (VAS2), and ability to perform daily activities (VAS3) [36].

A logistic regression model between P-ICD10 criteria diagnosis and FACT-F (VAS1) identified a score of 34 (61) on the FACT-F scale as a proposed cut-off point for the diagnosis of fatigue [36]. The ICD-10 criteria can be recommended as a diagnostic tool, whereas the FACT-F scale and the level of energy 100-mm VAS, assess the intensity of fatigue, and are more suitable for follow-up cancer-related fatigue [36].

A self-rating scale was developed to measure the severity of fatigue. Two-hundred and seventy-four new registrations on a general practice list completed a multi-item fatigue scale with Likert scoring [37]. The scale was found to be both reliable and valid. There was a high degree of internal consistency, and the principal components analysis supported the notion of a two-factor solution (physical and mental fatigue). The validation coefficients for the fatigue scale, using an arbitrary cut off score of ¾ and the item on the CIS-R were sensitivity 75.5 and specificity 74.5 [37]. This has become known as the Chalder Fatigue Scale [37].

This scale [37] also called the Fatigue Questionnaire (FQ) or the Bidimensional Fatigue Scale (BFS) has been used to measure fatigue in large community [38, 39] and primary care [40] studies. The scale consists of 11 items, 7 of which form a physical fatigue subscale (BFS-P) and 4 of which form a mental fatigue subscale (BFS-M). A combined score for the total scale can also be constructed (BFS-T) [41]. Each of the 11 items can be scored on a four-point (0–3) scale, thus the BFS-T can range between 0 (minimum fatigue) and 33 (maximum fatigue) [41]. The "Shortened fatigue questionnaire' (SFQ) is a short, reliable and easily used instrument to determine the intensity of the patient's bodily fatigue. It consists of four questions which the patient answers by checking an item at a 7-point scale ('I feel tired', 'I tire easily', 'I feel fit' and' I feel physically exhausted' [42].

An instrument has been developed to assess the current health status of women with the fibromyalgia syndrome. The Fibromyalgia Impact Questionnaire (FIQ) is a brief 10-item, self-administered instrument that measures physical functioning, work status, morning tiredness, depression, anxiety, sleep, pain, stiffness, fatigue (ability to do the job, number of workdays missed), and well being (number of days the subject felt good) [43].

Fibromyalgia (FM) and chronic fatigue syndrome (CFS) are both chronic clinical conditions characterized by a variety of nonspecific symptoms, including prominent fatigue, myalgia and sleep disturbances. Despite different diagnostic criteria, FM and CFS have many demographic and clinical similarities with few differences in the domains of symptoms [44, 45]. Observer's rating scales are also considered quite important in addition to self-rating scales. For this reason, FibroFatigue Scale (FFS) was designed as a new observer's rating scale aimed at the assessment of core symptoms and treatment outcome in FM and CFS [46]. Due to substantial overlap in symptomatology between both conditions, it was decided to develop a scale suitable for FM and CFS.

The FibroFatigue scale (FFS) is a 12-item observer's rating instrument derived from the Comprehensive Psychopathological Rating Scale [47, 48], which measures pain, muscular tension, fatigue, concentration difficulties, failing memory, irritability, sadness, sleep disturbances, autonomic disturbances, irritable bowel symptoms, headache and subjective experience of infection [46]. The third item [fatigue] from the FFS is assessed as follows:

Fatigue is frequently found in chronic pain patients (CPPs) and may be etiologically related to the presence of pain. Fishbain et al. have demonstrated that chronic low back pain (LBP) and chronic neck pain patients are more fatigued than controls [49]. Fishbain and colleagues set out to determine whether chronic LBP- and chronic neck pain-associated fatigue responded to multidisciplinary multimodal treatment not specifically targeted to the treatment of fatigue.

FATIGUE EVALUTION

Representing the experience of debilitating fatigue and lack of energy and the experience of tiring more easily than usual.

0	Ordinary staying power; not easily fatigued
1	Tires easily but does not have to take a break more often than usual
2	Considerable fatigue and lack of energy; easily wearied; frequently forced to pause or rest
3	Exhaustion interrupts almost all activities or even makes them impossible [46]

Fishbain and colleagues studied a total of 85 chronic LBP and 33 chronic neck pain patients who completed the Multidimensional Fatigue Inventory (MFI), Neuropathic Pain Scale (NPS), and Beck Depression Inventory on admission to a multidisciplinary pain treatment facility. At completion of the multidisciplinary multimodal treatment, each CPP again completed the MFI. Student's *t*-test was utilized to test for statistical changes on the MFI five scales from pre- to post-treatment. Pearson and point-biserial correlations were utilized to determine which variables significantly correlated with MFI change scores. Variables found significant at less than or equal to 0.01 were utilized in a stepwise aggression analysis to find variables predictive of change in MFI scores.

Multidisciplinary multimodal treatment significantly improved CPP fatigue as measured by the MFI. The available variables utilized to predict fatigue best explained only a small percentage (28.9%) of the variance. Improvement in fatigue was related to NPS-10 scale scores (neuropathic pain) and a previous diagnosis of fibromyalgia [49]. Fishbain et al. concluded that multidisciplinary multimodal pain facility treatment improves chronic LBP- and neck pain-associated fatigue [49].

Various empirical studies link persistent failure to recover from acute fatigue to the evolution of chronic fatigue. However, existing fatigue measurement scales do not tend to distinguish between acute and chronic fatigue elements as well, and none include a measure of effective recovery from fatigue [50]. The 15 item Occupational Fatigue Exhaustion Recovery (OFER) scale has been developed and validated in three study populations specifically to measure work-related fatigue [50]. The OFER scale possesses robust, gender-bias free psychometric characteristics. Its three subscales identify and distinguish between chronic work-related fatigue traits, acute end-of-shift states and effective fatigue recovery between shifts [50].

Gentile et al. described the validation step of the French version of the 'Multidimensional Fatigue Inventory' (MFI) and presented the psychometric properties of this instrument [51]. A sample of 225 patients was divided into three groups 'Tired' (82 subjects), 'Moderately tired' (36) and 'Not tired' (107). The analysis of the structure validity found four dimensions: 'General Fatigue', 'Mental Fatigue', 'Reduced Activities' and 'Motivation' [51]. The convergent validity showed highly significant correlation ($P < 0.001$) with a visual analogue scale. The French MFI has been able to distinguish patients with different fatigue levels. Cronbach's alpha measurement of the scale and the subscales are good, (cronbach alpha > 0.70). The reproducibility and sensitivity to change in patients who were followed up one month later show satisfactory results [51].

The Motivation and Energy Inventory (MEI) was developed to facilitate the evaluation of vitality [52]. Consistent with the measurement model of the MEI, the psychometric results confirm that the instrument has three factors generally addressing physical energy, mental energy, and social motivation. Furthermore, these results provide evidence for the internal consistency; construct validity, and responsiveness of all three MEI subscales [52].

Tiesinga et al. analyzed patients with chronic heart failure (n = 138) was to develop and test both the Dutch Fatigue Scale (DUFS) and the Dutch Exertion Fatigue Scale (DEFS) [53]. Psychometric testing of these scales included measurement of internal consistency, construct validity and criterion-related validity. Statistical analyses of both scales showed sufficient reliability and validity. The DUFS (scale coefficient H = 0.48; Rho = 0.80; KR-20 = 0.79) is suitable as a measurement instrument for the diagnosis of fatigue and makes it possible to compare results of fatigue on the level of groups of patients. The DEFS (scale coefficient H = 0.61; Rho = 0.91; Cronbach's alpha = 0.91) can be used in clinical practice for the measurement of patients' exertion fatigue [53].

All three visual analog scales (VAS) [the Fatigue Severity Scale (FSS) (range 7-63), the Modified Fatigue Impact Scale (MFIS) (range 0-84), and the Guy's Neurological Disability Scale (GNDS) (range 0-5)] were able to discriminate between subjects with multiple sclerosis (MS) and controls [54]. The three visual analog scales are seen below:

VAS_1	How much influence does fatigue have on your daily life (the everyday life at home and at work) and on your relationships? no influence at all -------------------------------- a lot of influence*
VAS_2	How much influence does fatigue have on daily activities, like grooming and dressing ,etc.? no influence at all -------------------------------- a lot of influence*
VAS_3	How much influence does fatigue have on household or occupational activities? no influence at all -------------------------------- a lot of influence*

* Lines are 100 mm
Reproduced from [Kos, 2006 Ref 54].

Twenty five subjects with MS had a Fatigue Severity Scale score of 36 or more and were classified into the "fatigue" group [54]. ROC analysis showed that VAS_1 is most useful to classify subjects in the "fatigue" group. A cut-off value of VAS_1 of 59 displayed 76% sensitivity and 72% specificity. When using the MFIS, a score of 40 or more to classify the groups, VAS_1 remained the strongest tool, with 81% sensitivity and 77% specificity at a cut-off value of 59 [54]. Kos et al. concluded that the VAS for the impact of fatigue on daily life (VAS_1) is a moderately reliable, though valid and useful tool to screen rapidly for fatigue impact in multiple sclerosis. A cut-off value of 59 satisfactorily classifies individuals having severe fatigue with a high impact on daily life [54].

van Nes et al. removed two items from the original 9-item Fatigue Severity scale (FSS) and collapsed the original 7-point Likert options to 4-point response categories for the remaining items, theerby constructing a 7-item Rasch-built scale that fulfilled all requirements of unidimensionality, linearity, and rating scale model. Good reliability and validity were also obtained for the modified FSS scale. In conclusion, a 7-item linearly weighted Rasch-built modified FSS is presented for better assessment of fatigue in future studies in patients with immune-mediated neuropathies [55].

Fatigue Assessment for Specific Conditions

Immune Disorder – Related Fatigue

Chronic fatigue is a prominent symptom of many autoimmune rheumatic diseases, including Sjögren's Syndrome (SS) [56] and Rheumatoid Arthritis (RA) [57].

Smets et al. (1995) developed the Multidimensional Fatigue Inventory (MFI) to assess five facets of fatigue that they noted in the existing literature on illness [58]. Evidence in support of its validity was provided following completion by patients with cancer or chronic fatigue syndrome, and by students, junior physicians and army personnel. Smets and colleagues (1995) reported that the MFI can distinguish five facets of fatigue (which they referred to as 'dimensions'), which they created based on previous questionnaire studies [58]. These facets were labeled General Fatigue (GF), Physical Fatigue (PF), Reduced Activity (RAct), Reduced Motivation (RM) and Mental Fatigue (MF). Certain items of the MFI, such as 'Physically I feel I am in bad condition', could be confounded by inflammatory symptoms of both Sjögren's Syndrome (SS) and Rheumatoid Arthritis (RA) [59].

In order to increase the content validity of quantitative assessment of fatigue in patients with SS, Bowman et al. [60, 61] utilized the qualitative technique of allowing patients with SS to provide their own accounts of variations in fatigue and other clinical features of the disease as the sole basis of the wording of the items in a new questionnaire tool. The resulting Profile of Fatigue and Discomfort contained six facets of fatigue that can be employed as a stand-alone Profile of Fatigue (ProF). These six facets of fatigue formed two overarching 'domains': the domain of Somatic Fatigue (SF) contained the facets Need Rest (NR), Poor Starting (PS), Low Stamina (LS) and Weak Muscles (WM), while the facets of Poor Concentration (PC) and Poor Memory (PM) formed the domain of Mental Fatigue (MF) [61].

Neuromuscular Disorders – Related Fatigue

Fatigue is a symptoms very frequently reported by patients with neuromuscular disorders. Fatigue is mainly evaluated by strength loss after an exercise, by change in electromyographic activity during a given exercise and by questionnaires that takes into account the subjective (psychological) part of fatigue [62]. Due to the large diversity of motor disorders, there are multiple clinical expressions of fatigue that differ in their presentation, consequences and therapeutic approach [62].

Many neuromuscular disorders are associated with significant and profound fatigue. Although specific disease state fatigue assessment tools exist, such as the MS-specific Fatigue Severity Scale (MFSS) [63] and the Würzburger Fatigue Inventory for Multiple Sclerosis (WEIMuS) [64] for multiple sclerosis, other fatigue assessment tools such as the D-FIS may be utilized for non-neuromuscular disorders such as multiple sclerosis [65] or Parkinson's disease [66].

Fatigue was assessed in 158 MS patients by four published quantitative scales: the Fatigue Severity Scale (FSS), Modified Fatigue Impact Scale (MFIS), MS-specific Fatigue Severity Scale (MFSS), and Visual Analogue Scale. From these a new fatigue scale, the Würzburger Fatigue Inventory for Multiple Sclerosis (WEIMuS), was assembled [64]. It contains 17 items with values from 0 to 4 [64]. The WEIMuS scale was validated in a subgroup of 67 patients and a control group of 68 patients. The MFIS and FSS but not the MFSS showed high internal consistency and split-half reliability. After applying factor analysis within the scales, fairly reliable and valid items originally found in the MFIS and FSS were selected to contrast the final 17-item WEIMuS scale, which showed a high degree of reliability. In the validation study, varimax rotated factor analysis extracted two main factors corresponding to both cognitive and physical fatigue [64]. The new, two-dimensional WEIMuS showed good psychometric properties, is easy to use, and may therefore be a useful tool for the assessment of MS-associated fatigue [64]. Multiple sclerosis patients suffer from different types of fatigue which could be attributed to cognitive and physical fatigue [64]. Thus, MS-associated fatigue is different from common tiredness [64].

The fatigue impact scale (FIS) was developed previously as a symptom-specific profile measure of health-related quality of life (HRQoL) for use in medical conditions in which fatigue is a prominent chronic symptom. Thus, it was not developed to be a responsive measure of daily changes in fatigue. This 8-item D-FIS demonstrated good relations to flu symptom rating and to other general health rating. It also proved to be a responsive measure of change in reported fatigue impact for subjects who were followed longitudinally. This initial validation study indicates that the D-FIS has considerable promise as a valid measure of the subjective daily experience of fatigue [67].

The Fatigue Impact Scale for Daily Use (D-FIS) is an eight-item instrument designed to measure subjective daily experience of fatigue [67]. Benito-León et al. studied the metric properties of the D-FIS in multiple sclerosis patients [65].

The MFI-20 consists of five subscales of fatigue" General Fatigue (GF), Physical Fatigue (PF), Reduced Motivation (RM), Reduced Activity (RA) and Mental Fatigue (MF) [68]. Patients with fatigue completed the Fatigue Descriptive Scale, [a Visual Analog Scale for Fatigue (VAS-F)], the Multidimensional Fatigue Inventory (MFI), and a Global Perception of Fatigure Scale (GPF) [65]. There is a strong association between health-related quality of life (HRQoL) (FAMS) and D-FIS (rS=0.07) [65]. Benito-León et al. concluded that D-FIS is a feasible and valid instrument for measuring MS related fatigue, a frequent symptom associated with deterioration of patients' HRQoL [65].

The Daily Fatigue Impact Scale

Fatigue is a feeling of physical tiredness and lack of energy that many people experience from time to time. In certain medical conditions, feelings of fatigue can be more frequent and more of a problem than usual. The FIS questionnaire was designed to aid in understanding the patient's experience of fatigue and how it has affected their life (e.g. the impact of fatigue). Patients rate 8 statements choosing one of the 5 responses (No problem [0], Small problem

[1], Moderate problem [2], Big problem [3], Extreme problem [4]). Statements include: 1.) Because of fatigue, I feel less alert, 2.) Because of fatigue, I have to reduce my workload or responsibilities, 3) Because of fatigue, I am less motivated to do anything that requires physical effort, 4.) Because of fatigue, I have trouble maintaining physical effort for long periods, 5.) Because of fatigue, I find it difficult to make decisions, 6) Because of fatigue, I am less able to finish tasks that require thinking, 7. Because of fatigue, I feel slowed down in my thinking, and 8.) Because of fatigue, I have to limit my physical activities. [67].

Cancer-Related Fatigue

Fatigue is a commonly reported symptom by individuals suffering from various diseases, including multiple sclerosis, rheumatoid arthritis, and cancer. Fatigue is the most frequently reported symptom of cancer patients [69]. Because of its prevalence, it is often reported as the symptom that is the most distressing and causes the greatest amount of interference with daily life [70].

The FACT-F [71] was designed to measure the fatigue symptoms of cancer patients with anemia. It consists of the 28 items of the FACT-General (FACT-G) to assess health-related quality of life and an additional 13 items to assess fatigue. Examples of these fatigue items are "feel weak all over," "have energy," and "I am frustrated by being too tired to do the things I want to do." Each item was rated on a five-point Likert scale ranging from "0" (not at all) to "4" (very much so).

Other scales were designed to portray more than one dimension of fatigue, including the Piper Fatigue Self-Report Scale (PFS) [72], the MFI [58], and the MFSI [73]. Many of these scales have been developed carefully from a theoretical standpoint, taking into account the multifactorial nature of fatigue, and meet accepted standards of validity and reliability. However, their length makes them difficult for cancer patients to complete, especially for those who are very tired [74].

Mendoza et al. developed a new fatigue measure, the Brief Fatigue Inventory (BFI), to address some of the concerns with existing instruments. The BFI was based on the Brief Pain Inventory (BPI) [75], which has been used successfully to assess the severity and impact of cancer pain in the United States [76] and in European [77] and Asian countries [78]. The simple wording of the BPI makes it easy to understand for educationally disadvantaged patients as well as easy to translate. The BPI measures the severity of pain and interference caused by pain using 0-10 scales. In addition, the level of pain assessed by the BPI can be divided into categories of "mild" (1-4), "moderate" (5-6), and "severe" (7-10) pain based on the amount of pain-related interference with function [79].

Cancer-related fatigue (CRF) is a significant clinical symptom. Effective assessment of CRF attributes from the patients' perspective is essential. Wu and colleagues tested the psychometric properties of the Wu Cancer Fatigue Scale (WCFS) [80]. A total of 172 outpatients with breast cancer, who were at various stages and on various chemotherapy regimens, and were undergoing treatment at one of three cancer clinics in a Midwest metropolitan area, participated in this study. The participants were instructed to complete four instruments in the following order: the 16-item WCFS, Schwartz Cancer Fatigue Scale

(SCFS), Geriatric Depression Scale (GDS), and Cancer-Related Fatigue Distress Scale (CRFDS).

Internal consistency reliability was $\alpha = 0.91$ for the nine-item scale. The revised WCFS is a reliable and valid instrument that aims to measure the subjective characteristics of CRF from the patients' perspective [80].

The Brief Fatigue Inventory (BFI) has been validated as a short and comprehensive instrument to assess severity of fatigue and fatigue-related impairment in cancer patients. Radbruch and colleagues validated the German version of the BFI in patients with chronic cancer-related pain treatment in a tertiary pain center [81].

Glaus and Müller described the development of a new fatigue measurement instrument in the German language, the Fatigue Assessment Questionnaire and used it to compare different populations of cancer patients and healthy patients [82].

A difference was found in physical tiredness for patients with different types of cancer ($p = 0.008$) but this was not the case for affective and cognitive tiredness. More fatigue feelings were experienced by cancer patients with advanced disease than by patients in remission and this was true for physical fatigue ($p = 0.0001$), affective fatigue ($p = 0.01$), cognitive fatigue ($p = 0.02$) as well as for fatigue intensity ($p = 0.0001$) and distress ($p = 0.0001$). This group of patients also experiences significantly higher levels of depression and anxiety ($p = 0.0001$). The Fatigue Assessment Questionnaire, developed in the German speaking part of Switzerland, can be used for further activities in the field of quality of life and nursing care in oncology [82]. The 'Shortened fatigue questionnaire' (SFQ) or abbreviated fatigue questionnaire is a short reliable and easily used instrument to determine the intensity of the patient's bodily fatigue. It consists of four questions which the patient answers by checking an item at a 7-point scale ('I feel tired', 'I tire easily', 'I feel fit', and 'I feel physically exhausted') [42]. The Checklist Individual Strength (CIS) which includes an eight-item fatigue subscale and a fatigue-severity subscale [10, 83]. The CIS is used both for scientific research and for patient care.

The 28-item Schwartz Cancer Fatigue Scale (SCFS) has demonstrated reliability and content and construct validity. Factor analysis supports the four subscales (physical, emotional, cognitive, and temporal). Preliminary construct validity has been demonstrated by difference in fatigue between those people who are currently receiving treatment and those who have completed treatment and by scores on a visual analogue scale of fatigue [35].

The Cancer-Related Fatigue Distress Scale (CRFDS) was developed from 23 in-depth audiotaped interviews with patients experiencing CRF [84]. The CRFDS has strong content validity, high reliability, and very good construct validity. The CRFDS is a clinically useful and psychometrically sound tool for the measurement of CRF distress. This tool is clinically useful because of its brevity (20 items), clear instructions that required no training to use, and a readability score at the third-grade level [84]. Meek et al. evaluated four different instruments for their assessment of cancer-related fatigue, examining their reliability, ease of use, construct validity, and responsiveness to change in cancer patients receiving treatment [85]. The instruments selected were the Profile of Mood States short form fatigue subscale (F_POMS-sf), Multidimensional Assessment of Fatigue (MAF), Lee Fatigue Scale (LFS), and Multidimensional Fatigue Inventory (MFI).

The F_POMS-sf has been well studied for CRF and in many other chronic medical conditions [86-88]. The POMS is an adjective checklist that has been reduced via factor analysis to a short form (POMS-sf) containing 30 items [89] with 6 subscales (Tension-

Anxiety, Depression-Dejection, Anger-Hostility, Vigor-Activity, Confusion-Bewilderment, and Fatigue-Inertia). Scoring is on a 5-point Likert-type scale from 0=not at all – to 4=extremely, with F_POMS-sf calculated by adding together the responses to five items.

The MAF initially utilized with arthritis patients has also been used in chronic pulmonary disease [90-92]. The severity, distress, and interference items are scaled from 0 to 10, with ends anchored by "not at all" to "a great deal" respectively. Each frequency item is a categorical scale (0-4) with descriptors for each choice. A global fatigue score is calculated by adding together the severity and distress items, adding the item mean for the interference items and adding the product of the categorical score on frequency multiplied by a constant (2.5). If fatigue severity is zero, then there is no need to complete any other items and total score is zero. Also, if there is anything other than fatigue which interfering in an activity, the item would not be able to be included in the total score. The LFS (scored as a visual analog scale) was originally developed to be used for subjects with sleep disorders but it has been utilized in chronic illness [93].

The MFI was initially developed in the Netherlands for use in cancer and has been studied in Europe [58, 94]. It originally had a mixture of positively and negatively phrased questions, thus some MFI users changed certain items. The responses are on a five-point Likert-type scale and scored so that the higher the score, the less the fatigue experienced.

Meek et al. published a series of recommendations about using each of these instruments to measure CRF is appropriate [85]. First, the F_POMS-sf scale performed well in internal consistency stability, factor analysis, interinstrument correlations, and responsiveness. It was the strongest performer in this study. The F_POMS-sf could be used in clinical situations to evaluate programs aimed at minimizing the impact of treatment on fatigue or simply to assess the levels of fatigue seen in a particular population [85].

In general, the MAF was recommended for use as a measure of CRF, because it may require great effort to obtain completed scales and may not detect small changes [85]. Testing of the LFS in this study indicated that the LFS is relatively easy to use with good reliability, having strong internal consistency, but slightly low stability, potentially because of the instrument's sensitivity to morning and evening changes [85]. Overall, the LFS showed good performance and could be recommended for use with CRF during treatment if administration controlled for time of day effects [85]. The MFI, which was developed in a very rigorous psychometric manner and included cancer patients in the original sample, produced confusing findings [85]. The MFI was not recommended for used in a clinical setting unless it is being used in combination with other instruments and subjected to additional psychometric analysis [85].

The BFS and FACT-F cutoff scores can be used to identify breast cancer survivors at higher risk of clinically significant ongoing post treatment fatigue. Neither scale can be used as a diagnostic instrument for CRFS [95]. In order to rigorously define the clinical phenotype of CRF, Cella and colleagues [96] proposed a set of diagnostic criteria modeled on the International Classification of Diseases manual. The criteria are a set of symptoms which relate to fatigue, its functional impact, and duration [95]. To fulfill these diagnostic criteria, the subject must have experienced six of 11 fatigue related symptoms on most days or every day for 2 weeks in the previous month [95]. At least one of these symptoms must have been "significant fatigue, lack of energy, or an increased need to rest." The fatigue needs to be sufficiently severe to have had an impact on daily life [95]. There must be evidence from the history, physical examination, or laboratory findings that the symptoms are a consequence of cancer or cancer therapy, and not as a consequence of any psychiatric disorders [95].

Minton and Stone performed a systematic review methodology to identify scales that have been validated to measure CRF [97]. Unidimensional scales are the easiest to administer and have been most widely used. The authors recommend the use of the EORTC QLQ C30 fatigue subscale or the FACT F. The FQ gives a multidimensional assessment and has also been widely used [97].

HIV-Related Fatigue

Bormann et al. evaluated the psychometric properties of the Global Fatigue Index (GFI) in a community-based sample of 209 patients with HIV/AIDS. The GFI is a measure that quantifies five dimensions of fatigue from the Multidimensional Assessment of Fatigue instrument into one score [98]. The GFI was found to be easily self-administered, reliable, and a valid measure of overall fatigue burden in an HIV population. This instrument may be used by clinicians and researchers for assessing fatigue [98].

The HIV-Related Fatigue Scale (HRFS) was developed to address the specific aspects of fatigue experienced by people who are HIV-positive and are not measured in any commonly used fatigue scale [99]. The HRFS has 56 items, most of which as on a 1-to-10 scale, drawn from five existing fatigue scales and the data from this qualitative study. The items were deemed content valid, easy to understand, and not fatiguing to complete by people with HIV-related fatigue [99].

Pediatric Fatigue

The PedsQLtrade mark (Pediatric Quality of Life Inventorytrade mark) is a modular instrument designed to measure health-related quality of life (HRQOL) and disease-specific symptoms in children and adolescents ages 2-18 [100].

Conclusion

Multiple tools have been developed to assess reasonable reliability and validity of the perception of fatigue. Despite the numerous instruments which exist to assess fatigue; it appears that documentation of the assessment of fatigue only occurs in a minority of patients' medical records. Choosing the most appropriate tool to assess fatigue should be left to individual clinicians, and multiple factors may play a role in making this choice including: specific medical conditions, specific clinical needs, specific therapeutic approaches and the need to follow tends and responses to treatments, as well as the need for the patient to perform various activities. Especially with respect to advanced chronic kidney disease, the F_POMS-sf appears to be a particularly good instrument. It is hoped that future efforts will improve the documentation of fatigue, at least in medical conditions known to have a reasonable high incidence of fatigue (e.g. multiple sclerosis, cancer, advanced heart failure, advanced chronic pulmonary disease, advanced chronic kidney disease).

References

[1] Lamberts, H. In het huis van de huisarts. Verslag van het Transitieproject. Meditekst, 1991.

[2] Gandevia, S.C., Enoka, R.M., McComas, A.J., Stuart, D.G., & Thomas, C.K. Fatigue, neural and muscular mechanisms. New York: Plenum Press; 1995.

[3] Hill, A.V. (1913). The heat production in prolonged contractions of an isolated frog's muscle. *J Physiol*, 47,305–324.

[4] Vøllestad, N.K. (1997). Measurement of human muscle fatigue. *J Neurosci Methods*, 27,219–227.

[5] Bleijenberg, G. De ene vermoeidheid is de andere niet. Nijmegen, 2003. Available from: http://webdoc.ubn.kun.nl/mono/b/bleijenberg_g/ene_veisd.pdf. (accessed May 2008).

[6] Friedman, J., & Friedman, H. (1993). Fatigue in Parkinson's disease. *Neurology*, 43,2016–2018.

[7] Karlsen, K., Larsen, J.P., Tandberg, E., & Jorgensen, K. (1999). Fatigue in patients with Parkinson's disease. *Mov Disord*, 14,237–241.

[8] Krupp, L.B. Fatigue. Philadelphia: Butterworth Heinemann; 2003.

[9] Zwarts, M.J., Bleijenberg, G., & van Engelen, B.G.M. (2008). Clinical neurophysiology of fatigue. *Clin Neurophysiology*, 119,2-10.

[10] Vercoulen, J.H., Swanink, C.M., Fennis, J.F., Galama, J.M., van der Meer, J.W., & Bleijenberg, G. (1994). Dimensional assessment of chronic fatigue syndrome. *J Psychosom Res*, 38,383–392.

[11] De Ruiter,C.J., Jones, D.A., Sargeant, A.J., & De Haan, A. (1999). The measurement of force/velocity relationships of fresh and fatigued human adductor pollicis muscle. *Eur J Appl Physiol Occup Physiol*, 80,386–393.

[12] Fitts, R.H. (1994). Cellular mechanisms of muscle fatigue. *Physiol Rev*, 74,49–94.

[13] Behm, D.G. (2004). Force maintenance with submaximal fatiguing contractions. *Can J Appl Physiol*, 29,274–290.

[14] Houtman, C.J., Stegeman, D.F., Van Dijk, J.P., & Zwarts, M.J. (2003). Changes in muscle fiber conduction velocity indicate recruitment of distinct motor unit populations. *J Appl Physiol*, 95,1045–1054.

[15] Kuchinad, R.A., Ivanova, T.D., & Garland, S.J. (2004). Modulation of motor unit discharge rate and H-reflex amplitude during submaximal fatigue of the human soleus muscle. *Exp Brain Res*, 158,345–355.

[16] Zijdewind, I., Zwarts, N.J., & Kernell, D. (1999). Fatigue-associated changes in the electromyogram of the human first dorsal interosseus muscle. *Muscle Nerve*, 22,1432–1436.

[17] Zwarts, M.J., Drost, G., & Stegeman, D.F. (2000). Recent progress in the diagnostic use of surface EMG for neurological diseases. *J Electromyogr Kinesiol*, 10,287–291.

[18] Zwarts, M.J., & Stegeman, D.F. (2003). Multichannel surface EMG: basic aspects and clinical utility. Muscle Nerve, 28,1–17.

[19] Lindström, L., Magnusson, R., & Peterson, I. (1970). Muscular fatigue and action potential conduction velocity changes studied with frequency analysis of EMG signals. *Electromyography*, 4,341–356.

[20] Zwarts, M.J., & Arendt-Nielsen, L. (1988). The influence of force and circulation on average muscle fibre conduction velocity during local muscle fatigue. *Eur J Appl Physiol Occup Physiol*, 58,278–283.

[21] Gandevia, S.C. (1998). Neural control in human muscle fatigue: changes in muscle afferents, motoneurones and motor cortical drive. *Acta Physiol Scand*, 162,275–283.

[22] Schillings, M.L., Stegeman, D.F., & Zwarts, M.J. (2005). Determining central activation failure and peripheral fatigue in the course of sustained maximal voluntary contractions – a model based approach. *J Appl Physiol*, 98,2292–2297.

[23] Di Lazzaro, V., Oliviero, A., Tonali, P.A., Mazzone, P., Insola, A., Pilato, F., Saturno, E., Dileone, M., & Rothwell, J.C. (2003). Direct demonstration of reduction of the output of the human motor cortex induced by a fatiguing muscle contraction. *Exp Brain Res*, 149,535–538.

[24] Taylor, J.L., Butler, J.E., & Gandevia, S.C. (2000). Changes in muscle afferents, motoneurons and motor drive during muscle fatigue. *Eur J Appl Physiol*, 83,106–115.

[25] Gandevia, S.C. (2001). Spinal and supraspinal factors in human muscle fatigue. *Physiol Rev*, 81,1725–1789.

[26] Todd, G., Taylor, J.L., & Gandevia, S.C. (2003). Measurement of voluntary activation of fresh and fatigued human muscles using transcranial magnetic stimulation, J Physiol, 551, 661–671.

[27] Todd, G., Taylor, J.L., & Gandevia, S.C. (2004). Reproducible measurement of voluntary activation of human elbow flexors with motor cortical stimulation. *J Appl Physiol*, 97, 236–242.

[28] Freude, G., & Ullsperger, P. (1987). Changes in Bereitschaftspotential during fatiguing and non-fatiguing hand movements. *Eur J Appl Physiol Occup Physiol*, 56,105–108.

[29] Shibasaki, H., & Hallett, M. (2006). What is the Bereitschaftspotential? *Clin Neurophysiol*, 117,2341–2356.

[30] Deecke, L. (1996). Planning, preparation, execution, and imagery of volitional action. *Brain Res Cogn Brain Res*, 3,59–64.

[31] Pearce, S., & Richardson, A. (1996). Fatigue in cancer; a phenomenological perspective. *Eur J Cancer Care*, 5,111-115.

[32] Ferrell, B.R., Grant, M., Funk, B., Garcia, N., Otis-Green, S., & Schaffner, M.L. (1996). Quality of life in breast cancer. *Cancer Pract*, 4,331-340.

[33] Ream, E., & Richardson, A. (1996). Fatigue: a concept analysis. *Int J Nurs Stud*, 5,519-529.

[34] Storer, T.W., Magliano, L., Woodhouse, L., Lee, M.L., Dzekov, C., Dzekov, J., Casaburi, R., & Bhasin, S. (2003). Testosterone dose-dependently increases maximal voluntary strength and leg power, but does not affect fatigability or specific tension. *J Clin Endocrinol Metab*, 88,1478-1485,

[35] Schwartz, A. (1998). The Schwartz Cancer Fatigue Scale: testing reliability and validity. Oncol Nurs Forum, 25,711-717.

[36] Van Belle, S., Paridaens, R., Evers, G., Kerger, J., Bron, D., Foubert, J., Ponnet, G., Vander Steichel, D., Heremans, C., & Rosillon, D. (2005). Comparison of proposed diagnostic critieria with FACT-F and VAS for cancer-related fatigue: proposal for use as a screening tool. *Support Care Cancer*, 13,246-254.

[37] Chalder, T., Berelowitz, G., Pawlikowska, T., Watts, L., Wesseky, S., Wright, D., & Wallace, E.P. (1993). Development of a fatigue scale. *J Psychosom Res*, 37,147-153.

[38] Pawlikowska, T., Chalder, T., Hirsch, S., Wallace, P., Wright, D.J., & Wessely, S.C. (1994). A population based study of fatigue and psychological distress. *BMJ*, 308,763-766.

[39] Lawrie, S., & Pelosi, A. (1995). Chronic fatigue syndrome in the community: prevalence and associations. Br J Psychiat, 166,793–797.

[40] David, A., Pelosi, A., McDonald, E., Stephens, D., Ledger, D., Rathbone, R., & Mann, A. (1990). Tired, weak, or in need of rest: fatigue among general practice attenders. *BMJ*, 301,1199–1202.

[41] Stone, P., Richards, M., A'Hern, R., & Hardy, J. (2001). Fatigue in patients with cancers of the breast or prostate undergoing radical radiotherapy. *J Pain Symptom Manage*, 22,1007-1015.

[42] Alberts, M., Smets, E.M., Vercoulen J.H., Garssen, B., & Bleijenberg, G. (1997). 'Abbreviated fatigue questionnaire': a practical tool in the classification of fatigue. Ned Tijdschr Geneeskd, 141,1526-1530.

[43] Burckhardt, C.S., Clark, S.R., & Bennett, R.M. (1991). The fibromyalgia impact questionnaire: development and validation. *J Rheumatol*,18, 728-733.

[44] Buchwald, D., & Garrity, D. (1994). Comparison of patients with chronic fatigue syndrome, fibromyalgia, and multiple chemical sensitivities. Arch Intern Med, 15,2049-2053.

[45] Buchwald, D. (1996). Fibromyalgia and chronic fatigue syndrome: similarities and differences. *Rheum Dis Clin North Am*,22, 219-243.

[46] Zachrisson, O., Regland, B., Jahreskog, M., Kron, M., & Gottfries, C.G. (2002). A rating scale for fibromyalgia and chronic fatigue syndrome (the FibroFatigue scale). *J Psychosome Res*, 52,501-509.

[47] Asberg, M., Montgomery, S.A., Perris, C., Schalling, D., & Sedvall, G. (1978). A comprehensive psychopathological rating scale. Acta Psychiatr Scand, 271,5-27.

[48] Asberg, M., & Schalling, D. (1979). Construction of a new psychiatric rating instrument, the Comprehensive Psychopathological Rating Scale (CRPS). *Prog Neuropsychopharmacol*, 3,405-412.

[49] Fishbain, D.A., Lewis, J., Cole, B., Cutler, B., Smets, E., Rosomoff, H., & Rosomoff, R.S. (2005). Multidisciplinary pain facility treatment outcome for pain-associated fatigue. *Pain Med*, 6,299-304

[50] Winwood, P.C., Winefield, A.H., Dawson, D., & Lushington, K. (2005). Development and validation of a scale to measure work-related fatigue and recovery: the Occupational Fatigue Exhaustion/Recovery Scale (OFER). *J Occup Environ Med*, 47,594-606.

[51] Gentile, S., Delarozière, J.C., Favre, F., Sambuc, R., San Marco, J.L. (2003). Validation of the French 'multidimensional fatigue inventory' (MFI 20). *Eur J Cancer Care*, 12,58-64.

[52] Fehnel, S.E., Bann, C.M., Hogue, S.L., Kwong, W.J., & Mahajan, S,S. (2004). The development and psychometric evaluation of the Motivation and Energy Inventory (MEI). *Qual Life Res*, 13,1321-1336.

[53] Tiesinga, L.J., Dassen, T.W., & Halfens, R.J. (1998). DUFS and DEFS development, reliability and validity of the Dutch Fatigue Scale and the Dutch Exertion Fatigue Scale. Int J Nurs Stud, 35,115-123.

[54] Kos, D., Nagels, G., D'Hooghe, M.B., Duportail, M., & Kerckhofs, E. (2006). A rapid screening tool for fatigue impact in multiple sclerosis. *BMC Neurol*, 6,27.

[55] van Nes, S.I., Vanhoutte, E.K., Faber, C.G., Garssen, M., van Doorn, P.A., Merkies, I.S.; & PeriNomS Study Group. (2009). Improving fatigue assessment in immune-mediated neuropathies: the modified Rasch-built fatigue severity scale. *J Peripher Nerv Syst*, 14,268-278.

[56] Godaert, G.L.R., Hartkamp, A., Geenen, R., Garssen, A., Kruize, A.A., Bijlsma, J.W., & Derksen, R.H. (2002). Fatigue in daily life in patients with primary Sjögren's syndrome and systematic lupus erythematosus. *Annals of the New York Academy of Sciences*, 966,320–326.

[57] Pollard, L.C., Choy, E.H., Gonzalez, J., Khoshaba, B., & Scott, D.L. (2006). Fatigue in rheumatoid arthritis reflects pain, not disease activity. *Rheumatology*, 45,885–889.

[58] Smets, E.M., Garssen, B., Bronke, B., & De Haes, J.C. (1995). The Multidimensional Fatigue Inventory (MFI): Psychometric qualities of an instrument to assess fatigue. *Journal of Psychosomatic Research*, 39,315–325.

[59] Goodchild, C.E., Treharne, G.J., Booth, D.A., Kitas, G.D., & Bowman, S.J. (2008). Measuring fatigue among women with Sjögren's syndrome or rheumatoid arthritis: A comparison of the Profile of Fatigue (ProF) and the Multidimensional Fatigue Inventory (MFI). Musculoskeletal Care, 6,31-48.

[60] Bowman, S.J., Booth, D.A., Platts, R.G., Field, A., Rostron, J.; & UK Sjögren's Interest Group. (2003). Validation of the Sicca Symptoms Inventory for clinical studies of Sjögren's syndrome. *Journal of Rheumatology*, 30,1259–1266.

[61] Bowman, S.J., Booth, D.A., Platts, R.G., & UK Sjögren's Interest Group. (2004). Measurement of fatigue and discomfort in primary Sjögren's syndrome using a new questionnaire tool. *Rheumatology*, 43,758–764.

[62] Féasson, L., Camdessanché, J.P., El Mandhi, L., Calmels, P., & Millet, G.Y. (2006). Fatigue and neuromuscular diseases. *Ann Readapt Med Phys*, 49,289-300.

[63] Bakshi, R., Shaikh, Z.A., Miletich, R.S., Czarnecki, D., Dmochowski, J., Henschel, K., Janardhan, V., Dubey, N., & Kinkel, P.R. (2000). Fatigue in multiple sclerosis and its relationship to depression and neurologic disability. *Mult Scler*, 6,181-185.

[64] Flachenecker, P., Müller, G., König, H., Meissner, H., Toyka, K.V., & Rieckmann, P. (2006). "Fatigue" in multiple sclerosis. Development and validation of the "Würzburger Fatigue Inventory for MS". Nervenarzt, 77,165-166.

[65] Benito-León, J., Marinez-Martin, P., Frades, B., Martínez-Ginés, M.L., de Andrés, C., Meca-Lallana, J.E., Antiqüedad, A.R., Huete-Antón, B., Rodríquez-García, E., & Ruiz-Martínez, J. (2007). Impact of fatigue in multiple sclerosis: the Fatigue Impact Scale for Daily Use (D-FIS). *Mult Scler*, 13,645-651.

[66] Martinez-Martin, P., Catalan, M.J., Benito-Leon, J., Moreno, A.O., Zamarbide, I., Cubo, E., van Blercon, N., Arillo, V.C., Pondal, M., Linazasoro, G., Alonso, F., Ruiz,

P.G., & Frades, B. (2006). Impact of fatigue in Parkinson's disease: the Fatigue Impact Scale for Daily Use (D-FIS). Qual Life Res, 15,597-606.

[67] Fisk, J.D., & Doble, S.E. (2002). Construction and validation of a fatigue impact scale for daily administration. *Qual Life Res*, 11,263-272.

[68] Hagelin, C.L., Wengström, Y., Runesdotter, S., & Fürst, C.J.. (2007). The psychometric properties of the Swedish Multidimensional Fatigue Inventory MF1-20 in four different populations. *Acta Oncol*, 46, 97-104.

[69] Glaus, A., Crow, R., & Hammond, S. (1996). A qualitative study to explore the concept of fatigue/tiredness in cancer patients and in healthy individuals. *Support Care Cancer*, 4,82–96.

[70] Richardson, A. (1995). Fatigue in cancer patients: a review of the literature. *Eur J Cancer Care*, 4,20 –32.

[71] Yellen, S.B., Cella, D.F., Webster, K., Blendowski, C., & Kaplan E. (1997). Measuring fatigue and other anemia-related symptoms with the Functional Assessment of Cancer Therapy (FACT) measurement system. *J Pain Symptom Manage*, 13,63–74.

[72] Piper, B.F., Lindsey, A.M., Dodd, M.J., Ferketich, S., Paul, S. & Weller, S. The development of an instrument to measure the subjective dimension of fatigue. In: Funk, S., Tornquist, E., Champagne, M., Archer, C.L., & Wiese, R., editors. Key aspects of comfort: management of pain, fatigue and nausea. New York: Springer; 1989; 199–208.

[73] Stein, K.D., Martin, S.C., Hann, D.M., & Jacobsen, P.B. (1998). A multidimensional measure of fatigue for use with cancer patients. *Cancer Practice*, 6,143–152.

[74] Mendoza, T.R., Wang, X.S., Cleeland, C.S., Morrissey, M., Johnson, B.A., Wendt, J.K., & Huber, S.L. (1999). The Rapid Assessment of Fatigue Severity in Cancer Patients. *Cancer*, 85,1186-1196.

[75] Cleeland, C.S. Measurement of pain by subjective report. In: Chapman, C.R., & Loeser, J.D., editors. Issues in pain measurement. Vol. 12 of advances in pain research and therapy. New York: Raven Press; 1989; 391–403.

[76] Cleeland, C.S., Gonin, R., Hatfield, A.K., Edmonson, J.H., Blum, R.H., Stewart, J.A., & Pandya, K.J. (1994). Pain and its treatment in outpatients with metastatic cancer. *New Engl J Med*, 330,592–596.

[77] Larue, F., Colleau, S.M., Brasseur, L., & Cleeland, C.S. (1995). Multicentre study of pain and its treatment in France BMJ, 310,1034–1037.

[78] Wang, X.S., Mendoza, T.R., Gao, S.Z., & Cleeland, C.S. (1996). The Chinese version of the Brief Pain Inventory (BPI-C): its development and use in a study of cancer pain. *Pain*, 61,407–416.

[79] Serlin, R.C., Mendoza, T.R., Nakamura, Y., Edwards, K.R., & Cleeland, C.S. (1995). When is cancer pain mild, moderate or severe? Grading pain severity by its interference with function. Pain, 61,277–284.

[80] Wu, H.S., Wyrwich, K.W., & McSweeney, M. (2006). Assessing fatigue in persons with cancer: further validation of the Wu Cancer Fatigue Scale. *J Pain Symptom Manage*, 32,255-265.

[81] Radbruch, L., Sabatowski, R., Elsner, F., Everts, J., Mendoza, T., & Cleeland, C. (2003). Validation of the German version of the brief fatigue inventory. *J Pain Symptom Manage*, 25,449-458.

[82] Glaus, A., & Müller, S. (2001). Measuring fatigue of cancer patients in the German-speaking region: development of the Fatigue Assessment Questionnaire. Pfleg, 14,161-170.

[83] Dittner, A.J., Wessely, S.C., & Brown, R.G. (2004). The assessment of fatigue. A practical guide for clinicians and researchers. *J Psychosom Res*, 56(2),157–170.

[84] Holley, S.K. (2000). Evaluating patient distress from cancer-related fatigue: an instrument development study. *Oncol Nurs Forum*, 27,1425-1431.

[85] Meek, P.M., Nail, L.M., Barsevick, A., Schwartz, A.L., Stephen, S., Whitmer, K., Beck, S.L., Jones, L.S., & Walker, B.L. (2000). Psychometric testing of fatigue instruments for use with cancer patients. *Nurs Res*, 49,181-190.

[86] Larson, P.J., Vuiele, C.S., Coleman, S., Dibble, S.L., & Cebulski, C. (1993). Comparison of perceived symptoms of patients undergoing bone marrow transplant and the nurses caring for them. *Oncology Nursing Forum*, 20,81-87.

[87] Holland, J.C., Korzun, A.H., Tross, S., Silberfarb, P., Perry, M., Comis, R., & Oster, M. (1986). Comparative psychological disturbance in patients with pancreatic and gastric cancer. *American Journal of Psychiatry*, 143,982-986.

[88] McCorkle, R., & Quint-Benoliel, J. (1983). Symptom distress, current concerns and mood disturbance after diagnosis of life-threatening disease. Social Science Medicine, 17,431-438.

[89] McNair, D.M., Lorr, M., & Droppleman, L.F. Profile of mood states manual (2nd ed). San Diego, CA: Educational & Industrial Testing Service, 1991.

[90] Belza, B.L. (1995). Comparison of self-reported fatigue in rheumatoid arthritis and controls. *J Rhematology*, 22,639-643.

[91] Belza, B.L., Henke, C.J., Yelin, E.H., Epstein, W.V., & Gilliss, C.L. (1993). Correlates of fatigue in older adults with rheumatoid arthritis. *Nursing Research*, 42:93-99

[92] Tack, B. Dimensions and correlates of fatigue in older adults with rheumatoid arthritis. Unpublished doctoral dissertation. University of California San Francisco, School of Nursing, 1991.

[93] Lee, K.A., Hicks, G., & Nino-Murcia, G. (1991). Validity and reliability of a scale to assess fatigue. *Psychiatry Research*, 36,291-298.

[94] Smets, E.M., Garssen, B., Cull, A., & de Haes, J.C. (1996). Application of the Multidimensional Fatigue Inventory (MFI-20) in cancer patients receiving radiotherapy. *British Journal of Cancer*, 73,241-245.

[95] Alexander, S., Minton, O., & Stone, P.C. (2009). Evaluation of screening instruments for cancer-related fatigue syndrome in breast cancer survivors. *J Clin Oncol*, 27,1197-1201.

[96] Cella,D., Peterman, A., Passik, S., Jacobsen, P., & Breitbart, W. (1998). Progress toward guidelines for the management of fatigue. Oncology (Huntington),12,369-377.

[97] Minton, O., & Stone, P. (2009). A systemative review of the scales used for the measurement of cancer-related fatigue (CRF). *Ann Oncol*, 20,17-25.

[98] Bormann, J., Shively, M., Smith, T.L., & Gifford, A.L. (2001). Measurement of fatigue in HIV-positive adults: reliability and validity of the Global Fatigue Index. *J Assoc Nurses AIDS Care*, 12,75-83.

[99] Barroso, J., & Lynn, M.R. (2002). Psychometric properties of the HIV-Related Fatigue Scale. *J Assoc Nurses AIDS Care*, 13,66-75.

[100] Varni, J.W., & Limbers, C.A. (2008). The PedsQLtrade mark Multidimensional Fatigue Scale in young adults: feasibility, reliability and validity in a University student population. *Qual Life Res*, 17,105-114.

In: Handbook of Fatigue in Health and Disease
Editor: Howard S. Smith
ISBN 978-1-61761-920-5

Chapter 5

IS THERE A RELATIONSHIP BETWEEN CANCER-RELATED CACHEXIA AND FATIGUE?

Sheryl L. Ziegler[1] and Jamie H. Von Roenn[2*]

[1] Medical Oncologist, Hematologist Oncology Hematology Associates of Southwest Indiana, Newburgh, Indiana, USA

[2] Professor of Medicine, Department of Medicine, Division of Hematology/Oncology Feinberg School of Medicine, Northwestern University and the Robert H. Lurie Comprehensive Cancer Center of Northwestern University, USA

Medical Director, Palliative Care and Home Hospice Program Northwestern Memorial Hospital Chicago, Illinois, USA

ABSTRACT

Cancer cachexia is a complex metabolic syndrome characterized by severe chronic unintentional and progressive weight loss, reduced muscle mass usually associated with diminished muscle strength, as well as fatigue, anorexia, and/or early satiation. It is intimately associated with severe fatigue impacting physical function and quality of life.

* Address correspondence to:
Jamie H. Von Roenn, MD
Professor of Medicine
Feinberg School of Medicine
Northwestern University
676 North St. Clair Street
Suite 850
Chicago, Illinois 60611
Phone: (312) 695-4542
Fax: (312) 695-6189
Email: j-vonroenn@northwestern.edu

The precise pathophysiologic mechanisms leading to cancer cachexia remain elusive, but inflammatory mediators likely contribute. Pharmacologic treatment includes orexigenic agents anti-inflammatory modulators, and anabolic agents. Targeting anti-inflammatory cytokines as well as other inflammatory mediators and their downstream signaling pathways may have potential utility in the future.

INTRODUCTION

Cancer- and treatment-related symptoms are highly prevalent throughout the course of cancer and its therapy. Symptom burden diminishes quality of life and has only recently become a primary focus of care. Cancer cachexia reduces patient response to anti-neoplastic treatments, increases the risk of postoperative complications and accounts for > 20% of cancer-related deaths [1]. Fatigue, pain, nausea, and cachexia are commonly reported symptoms, particularly by patients with advanced disease. While pain, nausea, and emesis are effectively controlled for most patients, fatigue and cachexia remain poorly understood. In advanced disease, these symptoms frequently occur together and have a profound impact on quality of life [2]. With our incomplete understanding of the pathogenesis of these symptoms, treatment options remain limited and often ineffective. This chapter will explore the relationship between cancer-related fatigue and cachexia.

The cancer anorexia-cachexia syndrome is characterized by accelerated loss of skeletal muscle, loss of appetite, decreased food intake, increasing debility, and fatigue [3, 4]. In patients with advanced cancer, fatigue and weight loss are highly prevalent, occurring in more than 75% of patients [5]. In spite of their high prevalence, both fatigue and cachexia are under-evaluated and under-treated [6, 7]. Interestingly, in one study, only 52% of patients ever reported fatigue to their physician [8]. This may in part be from patients' own beliefs that no effective therapy is available. Only 22% of patients who experience fatigue felt that something could be done to relieve or control it [8]. Similar beliefs are held by patients regarding cachexia, feeling that the wasting is an expected sequelae of advanced cancer.

The progressive weakness, fatigue, and debilitation that complicate weight loss raises the question as to whether a common mechanism results in the severe wasting and fatigue of advanced cancer. Fatigue and cachexia each result in decreased physical activity and increasing amounts of time in bed. Bed rest, lack of activity, and/or passive stretching of muscle results in a predictable decrease in functional capacity and degradation of contractile protein [9]. Stuart and colleagues demonstrated that seven days of absolute bed rest for healthy volunteers resulted in muscle volume loss of 1%-4%, as quantified by magnetic resonance imaging, in the back and lower extremities [10]. Bed rest decreases glucose tolerance, increases peripheral insulin resistance, abolishes the synthetic response to IGF-1, and dramatically increases the sensitivity of protein catabolism to cortisol [11].

CANCER-RELATED CACHEXIA-DEFINITIONS AND ASSESSMENT

Strasser has proposed that muscle strength should be measured directly in cancer cachexia and be included in diagnostic criteria [12]. Cachexia seems a dominant cause for decreased muscle strength. Most cachectic patients lose muscle strength, usually together with reduced muscle mass [12].

Fatigue is – in advanced cancer – a multifactorial phenomenon with insecure independent diagnostic value for cachexia, but representing an important 'global outcome' of cachexia [12].

The mechanism of muscle strength decline in cachexia is both a decreased protein synthesis and increased muscle proteolysis [12]. Measurement of body and skeletal muscle protein turnover in cachectic patients in contrast with control patients showed that the skeletal muscle protein turnover (nmol/100 ml/min.) is significantly reduced in cachectic compared with control patients (P¼004), whereas whole body turnover (g/kg/day) is not [12, 13].

Lasheen and Walsh analyzed date from 484 consecutive patients with complete data who were referred to palliative medicine and completed a 38-symptom questionnaire [14]. The data of Lasheen and Walsh suggests that CACS is a subtype of cachexia and not a different syndrome [14]. Just like insulin- and noninsulin-dependent diabetes; they are both subtypes of diabetes, yet essentially distinct. Cachexia has been classified [15] into (1) primary cachexia or CACS and (2) secondary cachexia.

Cachexia has been variously defined as weight loss of:

1) >10% of pre-illness weight [16, 17]
2) >10% in the past 6 months [18]
3) >5% of pre-illness weight [19]
4) >5% in the previous 6 months [15]
5) >5% in the previous 6 weeks [20]
6) >5 lb in the last 2 months [14, 21]. .

Experts at a consensus conference [22] proposed a new cachexia definition: weight loss of at least 5% of body weight over at most the past 12 months and at least three of the following:

1) Decreased muscle strength
2) Fatigue
3) Anorexia
4) Low fat-free mass index or
5) Abnormal biochemistry: as increased inflammatory markers (CRP and IL-6), anemia, or low serum albumin.

Bozzetti et al. used a database of an ongoing multicenter prospective investigation on the screening of the nutrition risk of 1307 oncology (the SCRINIO working group) outpatients from different university or scientific institutes or hospitals [23].

The patients were divided into 4 classes based on combinations of body weight loss (<10%, precachexia; ≥10%, cachexia) and the presence/absence of at least 1 symptom of anorexia, fatigue, or early satiation [Class 1-Asymptomatic precachexia; Class 2-Symptomatic precachexia; Class 3-Asymptomatic cachexia; Class 4-Symptomatic cachexia] [23] (See Figure 1).

	Asymptomatic	**Symptomatic (Anorexia, Fatigue, or Early Satiation)**
Precachexia (< 10% Body Weight Loss)	Class I (Asymptomatic Precachexia)	Class II (Symptomatic Precachexia)
Cachexia (≥ 10% Body Weight Loss)	Class III (Asymptomatic Cachexia)	Class IV (Symptomatic Cachexia)

Figure 1. Classes of Cancer Related-Cachexia.

As patients progress from "asymptomatic precachexia" (class 1) to "symptomatic cachexia" (class 4), there were statistically significant trends ($P < .0001$) in the percentage of gastrointestinal vs nongastrointestinal tumors, severity of cancer stage, percentage of weight loss, number of symptoms per patient, Eastern Cooperative Oncology Group (ECOG) performance status, and nutritional risk score [23].

The European Society for Clinical Nutrition and Metabolism on Parenteral Nutrition in Oncology in 2006 proposed a qualitative definition of cancer cachexia which can be shortened to the following: "cachexia is a complex syndrome characterized by a severe, chronic, unintentional and progressive weight loss, which is poorly responsive to the usual nutritional support, and may be associated with anorexia, asthenia and early satiation" [23].

Also in 2006, a Committee of Experts approved the following definition (J. E. Morley, W. Evans, S. Anker, unpublished data): "Cachexia is a complex metabolic syndrome associated with underlying illness and characterised by loss of muscle with or without loss of fat mass. The prominent clinical feature of cachexia is weight loss in adults and growth failure in children. Anorexia, inflammation, insulin resistance and increased muscle breakdown are frequently associated with cachexia. Cachexia is distinct from starvation, agerelated loss of muscle mass, primary depression, malabsorption and primary hyperthyroidism and is associated with increased morbidity" [23].

PATHOGENESIS

The pathogenesis of both cancer-related fatigue and cachexia is poorly understood, a result of complex interactions between treatment and tumor-related factors. Cachexia, in its simplest definition, is a catabolic syndrome characterized by progressive loss of muscle and body fat. Cachexia is distinguished from starvation in that repletion of normal body composition is not amenable to the simple provision of adequate protein and calories [3, 4]. While anorexia is a frequent symptom associated with cancer-related weight loss, it alone does not explain the clinical findings. The negative nitrogen balance in patients with cancer cachexia results from an imbalance between protein synthesis (anabolism) and protein degradation (catabolism). This imbalance results from decreased intake, hormonal abnormalities, and tumor- (e.g., proteolysis-inducing factor) and host-related factors (e.g., cytokines) that lead to metabolic abnormalities. Cytokine-mediated metabolic alterations are thought to be the basis, at least in part, of the observed disproportionate loss of muscle mass and may play an etiologic role in cancer-associated fatigue as well.

Proinflammatory cytokines likely play a pathogenetic role in multiple symptoms, including fever, anorexia, fatigue, cachexia, and night sweats [24]. Weight loss and a reduced lean body mass in patients with lung cancer are associated with an elevated acute-phase response. IL-6 levels in newly diagnosed patients with lung cancer have independent prognostic value and are related to the degree of wasting, disease progression, impairment of performance status, acute phase response, and to shorter survival [25]. It has been hypothesized that the demand for amino acids to produce the acute-phase proteins is met at the expense of skeletal muscle.

Elevated inflammatory cytokine levels are characteristic of both fatigue and cachexia [26]. Furthermore, fatigue and cachexia are recognized toxicities of cytokines used therapeutically in humans (e.g., TNF). Higher concentrations of cytokines are identified in many cancer patients compared to healthy controls [26, 27]. Peripheral blood mononuclear cell cytokine concentrations, especially TNF-α and IL-6, are particularly increased among weight-losing patients with cancer [25-28]. In weight-losing patients with both non-small cell lung cancer and pancreatic cancer, a systemic inflammatory response has been observed, characterized by high concentrations of TNF-α and IL-6 in peripheral blood mononuclear cells, increased plasma concentrations of soluble TNF receptor 55, as well as other adhesion molecules [28, 29]. The wasting effect of these proinflammatory cytokines appears to be targeted against the myosin heavy chain of skeletal muscle, leading to the severe skeletal muscle wasting characteristic of cachexia [30-32]. In patients with advanced pancreatic cancer, the presence of an acute-phase response (a marker of elevated proinflammatory cytokines) is associated with accelerated weight loss, hypermetabolism, anorexia, and shortened survival [29]. In patients with advanced colon cancer, elevated levels of tumor necrosis factor-alpha and interleukin-6 have been associated with both fatigue and anorexia [26].

Elevated resting energy expenditure, a frequent finding in patients with advanced lung cancer, hematologic malignancies, and sarcomas, may further contribute to patient wasting and fatigue [33, 34]. Hypermetabolism may occur secondary to tumor growth, increase in the Cori cycle, the acute phase protein response, gluconeogenesis, and increased protein turnover [33-35]. To balance energy output to the frequently reduced intake in patients with advanced disease, conservation of energy may be achieved via decreased physical activity, an adaptation that results in decreased functional status [36]. This only leads to further loss of skeletal muscle, mobility, and independence. The loss of lean muscle mass leads to decreased quality of life and poor outcomes overall.

Basic research targeting skeletal muscle is ongoing with respect to future agents which may beneficial to patients with cancer cachexia. Although human data is lacking for future agents which may be taking an interest in include: inhibitors of mediators (cytokines, tumor-derived substances) or their receptors (TNFR, androgen receptors), inhibitors of the proteolytic pathways [calpains (e.g. calpetin) and ubiquitin-proteasome (e.g. Dipeptidic boronic acids)], inhibitors of intracellular signaling pathways [NF-κB (e.g. Resveratrol), AP-1 (e.g. TAM67 protein), FOXO (e.g RNA oligonucleotides), PKR activation (e.g. leucine), and inhibitors of negative modulators of muscle growth/hypertrophy (myostatin (e.g. JA16 antibody-an antibody against myostatin), and GSK3-β (e.g. SB415286) [37].

In physiological conditions, overall rates of protein synthesis and degradation in tissue is delicately balanced [37]. In a normal 70-kg adult, about 280 grams of protein are synthesized and degraded each day, the majority of these proteins being intracellular. Small decreases in synthesis or increases in degradation may result in significant losses of lean body mass [37]. Four major proteolytic systems exist in the skeletal muscle; the endosome-lysosome system that relies on the activity of acidic proteases, the caspases, the calpains, and the ubiquitin-proteasome system [38, 39].

The observed anabolic effect of etanercept in patients with rheumatoid arthritis [40, 41] authorizes investigators to replicate clinical investigation with etanercept or other TNF-α antagonists in other cachectic conditions such as cancer cachexia [37].

Two agents that inhibit the IL-6 synthesis at the tumor level through the inhibition of NF-κB have been shown to attenuate the development of cachexia in vivo [dehydroxymethylepoxyquinomicin (DHMEQ) [42], pyrrolidine dithiocarbamate [43]].

Fujiki et al. evaluated the effects of gene transfer of Interleukin-10 (IL-10), a cytokine potentially capable of inhibiting the production of pro-inflammatory cytokines including IL-6, on the development of cachexia in mice injected with a colon adenocarcinoma cell line. Mice inoculated with IL-10-transfectant cells did not exhibit progressive weight loss, a reduction in food intake, or severe hypoglysemia, which was observed in mice, inoculated with parental or control vector-transfectant cells [44]. Similarly, IL-15 administration has been shown to inhibit skeletal muscle wasting [45].

This relationship between body composition, nutritional state, and fatigue has been demonstrated in multiple disease states. For example, total body protein and lean body index in patients with severe emphysema correlates with nutritional status; lean body mass and nutritional status correlate with muscle strength. Muscle protein metabolism is highly sensitive to indicators of nutritional status. Decreased oral intake and decreased insulin levels stimulate a catabolic response—protein mobilization.

Alterations in nutrient metabolism are associated with cancer cachexia. Frequently observed metabolic alterations include hypoglycemia with relative insulin resistance, hypertriglyceridemia, and excessive protein breakdown [46, 47]. Recently, research has focused on the ubiquitin proteasome pathway as a potential mediator of cachexia-associated muscle wasting. This pathway is responsible for the bulk of basal proteolysis in skeletal muscle [3]. Animal models and human investigations demonstrate increases in ubiquitin mRNA levels in skeletal muscle in the face of cachexia [30, 31]. This pathway, which appears regulated at least in part by proinflammatory cytokines, is down regulated by anticytokine treatment in animal models [48].

Alterations in the hypothalamic-pituitary-gonadal axis in patients with advanced cancer also may contribute to both fatigue and muscle wasting. In patients with advanced lung cancer, for example, a hypogonadal state is often present [25]. Fatigue and muscle wasting are well recognized consequences of subnormal gonadotropin levels from any cause. In men with prostate cancer undergoing hormonal ablative therapy, gonadotropin function correlates with fatigue [49]. The incidence of fatigue more than doubled after only three months of treatment in one study [49]. Conversely, in hypogonadal men, testosterone therapy increases lean body mass and energy, improves mood, and may improve quality of life.

Treatment

What is the clinical data to support a relationship between cachexia and fatigue? What therapeutic interventions favorably impact both symptoms? Pharmacologic treatment for cachexia includes orexigenic agents, anti-inflammatory/ cytokine modulating interventions, and anabolic agents.

Orexigenic Agents

Corticosteroids

Corticosteroids, potent anti-inflammatory agents, are frequently recommended to patients with advanced cancer to reduce fatigue and improve appetite. Multiple randomized, placebo-controlled trials demonstrate a short term (6-8 weeks) improvement in appetite with steroids and, frequently, an improved "sense of well-being" [36, 46-55]. The catabolic effect of chronic corticosteroids (muscle wasting, glucose intolerance, etc.) underscore the ineffectiveness of these agents, however, for prevention or chronic treatment of fatigue or cachexia.

Progestational Agents

Megestrol acetate and medroxyprogesterone acetate are the most effective appetite stimulants available [56]. The mechanism of action of progestational agents is unclear and probably multifactorial. Megestrol acetate may stimulate appetite via inhibition of proinflammatory cytokines (e.g., IL-1, IL-6, TNF-α) or through modulation of calcium channels in the satiety center of the ventromedial hypothalamus [57-61]. Decreased levels of TNF-α and IL-6 have been observed in both animal models and clinical trials of megestrol acetate in patients with cancer cachexia [57-59]. Lower circulating levels of soluble cytokines (IL-1α, IL-1β, TNF-α) were measured in one trial of patients with head and neck carcinoma after treatment with megestrol acetate [57].

The clinical efficacy of progesterones for the improvement of appetite and reversal of cancer-related weight loss has been demonstrated in more than 15 randomized, placebo-controlled trials [56]. While appetite was uniformly increased with megestrol acetate compared with placebo, weight gain and the degree of weight change varied with the dose and the population studied. A number of trials assessed the impact of treatment on changes in performance status [56]. Only one study prospectively evaluated the effect of megestrol acetate on fatigue [62]. A total of 84 patients with advanced, non-hormone responsive stolid tumors and weight loss were randomized to receive 10 days of megestrol acetate 480 mg daily or placebo. After a two-day washout period, participants were crossed over to the other treatment. In addition to significant improvement in appetite (p=0.005), megestrol acetate-treated patients reported improvement in activity (p=0.007) and general sense of well-being (p=0.03). Utilizing the Piper Fatigue Scale, there was a significant improvement in two of the three factors measured by the scale and in the overall fatigue score for the megestrol acetate-treated patients.

Trials currently in development will specifically evaluate the impact of megestrol acetate on fatigue. While these data are intriguing, it is likely that progesterones will be most useful as a single agent for patients with anorexia as a major feature of their weight loss or given in combination with an anabolic stimulus. The latter is of particular importance in view of the fact that increased fat mass is the primary component of megestrol acetate-induced weight gain and the agent causes reversible hypogonadism.

Anti-Inflammatory Cytokine-Modulating Therapy

Cytokines

Tumors or host immune cells responding to the tumuor release several pro-inflammatory cytokines including TNF-α [63], IL-6 [63] and IFN-γ [28], which have been implicated in cancer cachexia. In vitro studies have shown that TNF-α and IFN-γ may induce cachexia by activating the nuclear transcription factor, NF-κB, to suppress transcription of the myogenic regulatory factor, MyoD [64].

Tumors may also release proteolysis-inducing factor (PIF), a catabolic protein identified in the sera of cachexic patients which enhances protein degradation and reduces protein synthesis in isolated murine skeletal muscle [1, 65-67]. In the future, inhibitors may be helpful [37].

Expression of myostatin, a negative regulator of muscle mass [68], is increased in experimental cancer cachexia [1]. This may be due to elevated systematic levels of TNF-α the increase in myostatin can be blocked with the TNF-α inhibator, pentoxifylline [69]. Myostatin inhibits protein synthesis by suppressing the transcription of MyoD and another myogenic regulatory factor, myogenic [70], and inhibits the Akt/mTOR sihnalling pathway that leads to skeletal muscle hypertrophy [1, 71]. Furthermore, myostatin activates the forkhead box O signaling pathway, leading to increased expression of MuRF-1 and another ubiquitin E3 ligase, Atrogin-1 (MAFbx) [1, 72].

Because both genetic deletion of the melanocortin-4 receptor and administration of AgRP via intracerebroventrivular injection in mice enhances appetite and induced weight gain [73], investigations have focused on the therapeutic potential of melanocortin-4 receptor antagonism for cancer cachexia. Treatment of Lewis lung carcinoma (LLC) tumour-bearing mice with the melanocortin-4 receptor antagonists, ML00253764, increased food intake and attenuated the loss of lean body mass compared with vehicle-treated controls [74].

Ghrelin, a 28-amino acid peptide, is an endogenous ligand for the growth hormone secretagogue receptor (GHSR). In addition to stimulating growth hormone (GH) release, ghrelin has potent stimulatory effects on gut motility [75].

Compounds AKL-0707, AEZS-130, TZP-101, Anamorelin hydrochloride, and SUN-11031 include ghrelin analogues peptides and GH secretagogue peptidomimetrics [1].

However, a clinical trial investigating the efficacy of infliximab for cancer cachexia yielded negative results [76]. Eighty-nine pancreatic cancer patients receiving the chemotherapeutic agent, gemcitabine, also received placebo or infliximab at a dose of 3 or 5 mg/kg for 24 weeks [76]. No differences between groups were reported for lean body mass, overall survival and quality of life, indicating that infliximab lacks efficacy for treating cancer cachexia.

Inhibition of IL-6 has typically involved the production of IL-6 neutralizing antibodies, such as CNTO-328, a high-affinity human-mouse anti-IL-6 monoclonal antibody.

In a Phase I study investigating the safety and efficacy of ALD-158 and another humanized anti-IL-6 antibody, nine patients with advanced cancer were assigned to one of three escalating doses of ALD-158 which were administered as a single intravenous infusion [77]. Patients were followed up at 4 weeks (9/9) and 12 weeks (5/9). ALD-518 was safe and well tolerated, improved levels of haemoglobin and albumin, and there was a trend for improvements in handgrip strength [77].

Eicosapentaenoic Acid

Eicosanoids are inflammatory mediators produced by some tumors and by the host that have been implicated in the pathogenesis of cancer cachexia. Eicosapentaenoic acid is a polyunsaturated fatty acid, a component of fish oil, which has demonstrated inhibition of lipolysis and muscle protein degradation in animal models of cachexia [78]. A three-month, open-label study of a supplement of fish oil capsules, in pancreatic cancer patients, observed minimal body weight gain, a reduction in acute-phase protein, and an improvement in patient-reported levels of fatigue [79]. A second phase II study, also in patients with pancreatic cancer, reported a significant weight gain after administration of a fish oil-enriched nutritional supplement [80]. Unfortunately, fatigue was not evaluated. Multiple randomized, placebo-controlled trials have now been reported, with overall negative results [81, 82]. A North Central Cancer Treatment Group trial of EPA versus megestrol acetate versus the combination of both agents compared the effects of treatment on appetite, weight, and body composition in patients with advanced cancer anorexia or weight loss [82]. There was no improvement with the combination therapy over megestrol acetate alone. EPA did not appear to significantly improve study outcomes. Unfortunately, fatigue was not specifically addressed in this trial.

Thalidomide

Thalidomide, a TNF-α inhibitor, has been evaluated for its impact on weight and lean body mass. Two small, randomized, placebo-controlled trials showed improvement in appetite, weight, and lean body mass with thalidomide in patients with AIDS-related cachexia [83, 84]. An open-label trial in patients with metastatic breast cancer suggested improvement in appetite and overall sense of well-being with thalidomide, but no major impact on weight [19]. While the anti-inflammatory effect of thalidomide may be anticipated to impact both fatigue and cachexia, its mechanism of action may be too specific to adequately address the multifactorial symptoms of fatigue and cachexia for the majority of patients.

Nonsteroidal Anti-Inflammatory Drugs

Nonsteroidal anti-inflammatory drugs have been shown to reduce levels of IL-6 and cortisol in cachectic colorectal cancer patient [85]. These alterations in cytokine levels are associated with normalization of whole body protein kinetics to at least some extent [86]. In addition, several small clinical trials in patients with gastrointestinal malignancies and weight loss demonstrated modest weight gain with the use of ibuprofen, presumably due to its anti-inflammatory effects. While it appears that the proinflammatory cytokines have a multi-pronged effect on cachexia and fatigue, the impact of anti-cytokine and anti-inflammatory agents tested to date have had a limited impact.

Wigmore and colleagues studied patients with irresectable pancreatic cancer (n = 16) treated with either ibuprofen (1200 mg day-1 for 7 days (n = 10) or placebo (n = 6) [87]. Following treatment the mean REE of the ibuprofen group fell significantly (1386 +/- 89 kcal) compared with pretreatment values (1468 +/- 99 kcal) ($P < 0.02$), whereas no change was observed in the placebo group. Serum CRP concentration was also reduced in the ibuprofen-treated group (pre-ibuprofen, 51 mg l-1; post-ibuprofen, 29 mg l-1; $P < 0.05$). These results suggest that ibuprofen may have a role in abrogating the catabolic processes which contribute to weight loss in patients with pancreatic cancer [87].

McMillan and colleagues comparde the combination of megestrol acetate and placebo with megestrol acetate and ibuprofen in the treatment of weight loss in patients with gastrointestinal cancer [88]. After 12 weeks, there was a decrease in weight (median 2.8 kg) in the megestrol acetate/placebo group compared with an increase (median 2.3 kg) in the megestrol acetate/ibuprofen group ($P<0.001$). There was also an improvement in the EuroQol-EQ-5D quality of life scores of the latter group ($P<0.05$). The combination of megestrol acetate/ibuprofen appeared to reverse weight loss and appeared to improve quality of life in patients with advanced gastrointestinal cancer [88].

Mantovani and colleagues carried out a small prospective phase II clinical trial of 24 patients to test the safety and effectiveness of an intervention with the COX-2 inhibitor celecoxib (300 mg/day for 4 months) on key variables of cachexia (lean body mass, resting energy expenditure (REE), serum levels of proinflammatory cytokines, and fatigue) in patients with advanced cancer at different sites [89].

A significant increase of lean body mass and a significant decrease of TNF-α were observed. Moreover, an improvement of grip strength, quality of life, performance status, and Glasgow prognostic score was shown [89].

REE and fatigue did not change significantly, although, both of them showed a trend toward a decrease (p=0.07 for REE and p=0.09 for MFSI-SF score) [89].

Anabolic Agents

Anabolic agents have the potential to improve body weight, especially lean body mass, leading to improved exercise functional capacity and potentially decreased fatigue. Anabolic agents maintain working muscle mass and strength. As a result, these agents have the potential to improve both cancer-related fatigue and cachexia. The anabolic effect of androgens have long been recognized and utilized by athletes to improve muscle mass and strength. In hypogonadal states, whether HIV related or secondary to advanced illness such as cancer, hypogonadism is frequently present [12, 90, 91]. Testosterone replacement in hypogonadal men has been associated with increase in fat-free mass, muscle size, strength, and improvement in fatigue [91. 92]. In advanced cancer patients with wasting and fatigue, testosterone levels are rarely evaluated, and testosterone replacement has not been adequately evaluated in this population. In patients with HIV infection and acquired hypogonadism, androgen administration increases lean body mass as well as quality of life [92]. A meta-analysis of testosterone therapy for men with HIV wasting syndrome concluded that testosterone increased lean body mass more than placebo, with the increase greater if therapy was given intramuscularly [93]. A small positive effect also was noted from testosterone therapy on total body weight. In some series, fatigue also has been reported improved with testosterone treatment.

Synthetic testosterone analogs have been developed with reported greater anabolic versus androgenic activity compared with testosterone. Nandrolone decanoate has been evaluated in two small studies in HIV-infected patients with wasting, both in women and men [94, 95]. Intramuscular therapy weekly for 12 weeks led to increased weight and lean body mass in both studies, though the impact of therapy on fatigue was not evaluated. A single, small, randomized, prospective trial in patients with lung cancer evaluated the impact of nandrolone IM weekly for one month in patients receiving chemotherapy for newly diagnosed lung cancer [96]. No significant difference between the groups was identified in terms of the percentage of patients losing weight, though fewer patients on nandrolone had progressive weight loss compared to those receiving placebo.

Oxymetholone is an oral anabolic steroid evaluated in the setting of HIV-related wasting. A double-blind, randomized, placebo-controlled trial in eugonadal men and women with significant weight loss reported an increase in weight and lean body mass with oxymetholone [97]. Fifty-eight percent of the patients in the oxymetholone group reported decreased weakness and fatigue, compared to no change in the placebo-treated patients. The primary toxicity of this therapy, as in previous evaluations of oxymetholone, was liver-related side effects leading to interruption of therapy for 19% of patients. This agent has not yet been evaluated for cancer-related fatigue or cachexia.

Oxandrolone is an oral anabolic agent indicated for adjunctive therapy to promote weight gain after weight loss following extensive surgery, chronic infection, or trauma or for patients without definite pathophysiologic reasons for unexplained weight loss. A recently completed study of 131 patients with advanced cancer and weight loss, treated with nutritional counseling, a recommendation for exercise, and oxandrolone 10 mg orally twice daily, observed a significant weight gain ($p=0.0002$), averaging 9 to 14 lbs. in four months and increase in body cell mass ($p=0.001$) [98]. Body composition assessment, evaluated by bioelectric impedance analysis, demonstrated an increase in lean tissue in patients who gained, maintained, or lost weight. Specifically, for patients who gained weight, the gain was predominantly as lean tissue rather than as fat. In the patients who were weight stable, lean tissue was gained while fat was lost. Finally, in patients who lost weight, the loss was disproportionately loss of fat as compared to muscle. Furthermore, the increase in muscle mass correlated with improvements in quality of life, performance status, and function.

The significant improvement in quality of life at two months ($p<0.001$) and four months ($p=0.0306$), in addition to the significant improvement in performance status for those patients who gained lean tissue, suggests a potential favorable impact on fatigue as well. Of note, improved performance status also was associated with an increase in the number of subjects who walked at least 3-5 days per week compared to baseline. The association between improvement in lean muscle mass and improved quality of life underscores the potential impact of improved lean tissue on other symptoms of advanced cancer, such as fatigue. A trial is currently in development to specifically analyze this effect.

Future research may lead to the development of useful non-steroidal tissue-selective androgen receptor modulators (SARMs) that retain the beneficial properties of natural androgens and exhibit better therapeutic indices [99-103]. SARMs, unlike testosterone, do not undergo aromatization or 5-α-reduction, and act as agonists in muscle and bone and as partial agonists in prostate and seminal vesicles without significant androgenic activity [37].

Mantovani et al. conducted a 4 month phase III, randomized study to establish the most effective and safest pharmacologic treatment to improve the primary endpoints of cancer cachexia-lean body mass (LBM), resting energy expenditure (REE), and fatigue-and relevant secondary endpoints: appetite, quality of life, grip strength, Glasgow Prognostic Score (GPS) and proinflammatory cytokines [104]. Three hundred thirty-two assessable patients with cancer-related anorexia/cachexia syndrome were randomly assigned to one of five treatment arms: arm 1, medroxyprogesterone (500 mg/day) or megestrol acetate (320 mg/day); arm 2, oral supplementation with eicosapentaenoic acid; arm 3, L-carnitine (4 g/day); arm 4, thalidomide (200 mg/day); and arm 5, a combination of the above [104]).

Toxicity was quite negligible, and was comparable between arms. The most effective treatment in terms of all three primary efficacy endpoints and the secondary endpoints appetite, IL-6, GPS, and ECOG PS score was the combination regimen that included all agents (e.g. medroxy progesterone or megestrol acetate, oral eicosapentaenoic acid, L-carnitine, and thalidomide) [104].

Exercise

Physical activity is essential for the maintenance of skeletal muscle mass and may also decrease fatigue possibly by modifying cytokine levels [105]. Though few randomized, placebo-controlled trials are available, physical activity, in particular cardiovascular training with a combination of cardiovascular and resistance training and resistance training alone, has been recommended to decrease fatigue and improve muscle strength [106]. In addition, exercise, in particular resistance training, is a potent anabolic stimulus, resulting in improvement in lean body mass in multiple clinical settings, including HIV-related wasting, sarcopenia of the elderly, and in patients with cancer [106-110]. Endurance training attenuates muscle atrophy associated with tumor growth in animals as well [111].

A recent review of exercise in cancer patients identified improvement in fatigue and/or lean body mass with relatively short duration, overall low intensity, exercise programs [106]. It is noteworthy that in none of the studies were patients with cachexia evaluated, in spite of the fact that exercise in the frail elderly and in patients with HIV-related wasting have resulted in significant improvement in muscle strength and performance [108, 112]. A progressive resistance exercise program in HIV-infected patients led to an increase in lean body mass on average of 0.5 kg/week [108]. This increase in muscle mass was directly correlated with increased strength. Sequential studies by Mock et al. examined the effect of a home-based walking exercise intervention in patients with cancer [113, 114]. In both studies, 10-30 minutes of a progressive walking program 5-6 days/week improved physical performance and reduced fatigue. Similar findings were reported by Schwartz et al. in a group of women with breast cancer [115]. Subjects participated in an eight-week, home-based walking program with self-paced intensity measured by an accelerometer and noted improvement in physical performance as well as decreased fatigue compared with subjects who did not adopt the training program.

It is noteworthy that, to date, there are no published investigations evaluating the impact of exercise, particularly resistance training, on patients with cancer-related weight loss. The clear relationship between muscle mass and function, and the recognized disproportionate loss of muscle mass in cachexia, suggests a need for these investigations.

Conclusion

The pathogenesis of both cancer-related fatigue and cachexia is multifactorial. Within a given patient with a particular tumor, the pathogenesis of these symptoms varies. While patients with lung cancer generally have increased resting energy expenditure, this is not true for malignancies such as breast cancer. Furthermore, elevations in cytokine levels vary by malignancy, as do other tumor-host interactions. Maintenance of lean body mass appears an essential component of patient strength, performance, and energy. As loss of muscle mass is dependent on adequate nutrients, protein synthesis, and control of proteolysis, a multi-pronged approach is likely necessary. Adequate nutrition in combination with an anabolic stimulus and an anti-catabolic intervention are likely to have the greatest impact on the symptoms of cachexia and fatigue. We await future studies that will evaluate combinations of both pharmacologic and non-pharmacologic interventions.

REFERENCES

[1] Murphy., K.T., & Lunch, G.S. (2009). Update on emerging drugs for cancer cachexia. *Expert Opion Emerg Drugs*, 14,619-632.

[2] Portenoy, R.K., Thalen, H.T., Kornblith, A.B., Lepore, J.M., Friedlander-Klar, H., Coyle, N., Smart-Curley, T., Kemeny, N., Norton, L., Hoskins, W., & Scher, H. (1994). Symptom prevalence, characteristics and distress in a cancer population. *Qual Life Res*, 3,183-189.

[3] MacDonald, N., Easson, A.M., Mazurak, C.V., Dunn, G.P. Baracos, V.E. (2003). Understanding and managing cancer cachexia. *J Am Coll Surg*, 197,143-161.

[4] Inui, A. (2002). Cancer anorexia-cachexia syndrome: current issues in research and management. *CA Cancer J Clin*, 52, 72-91.

[5] Miaskowski, C., & Portenoy, R. (1998). Update on the assessment and management of cancer-related fatigue. *Supportive Oncol*, 1,1-10.

[6] Wolfe, J., Grier, H.E., Klar, N., Levin, S.B., Ellenbogen, J.M., Salem-Schatz, S., Emanuel, E.J., & Weeks, J.C. (2000). Symptoms and suffering at the end of life in children with cancer. *N Engl J Med*, 342,326-333.

[7] Langer, C.J., Hoffman, J.P., & Ottery, F.D. (2001). Clinical significance of weight loss in cancer patients: rationale for the use of anabolic agents in the treatment of cancer-related cachexia. *Nutrition*, 17,S1-S20.

[8] Stone, P., Richardson, A., Ream, E., Smith, A.G., Kerr, D.J., & Kearney, N. (2000). Cancer-related fatigue: inevitable, unimportant and untreatable? Results of a multi-centre patient survey. *Ann Oncol*, 11,971-975.

[9] Baracos, V.E. (2001). Management of muscle wasting in cancer-associated cachexia: Understanding gained from experimental studies. *Cancer*, 92,1669-1677.

[10] Stuart, C.A., Shangraw, R.E., Prince, M.J., Peters, E.J., & Wolfe, R.R. (1988). Bed rest induced insulin resistance occurs primarily in muscle. *Metabolism*, 37,802-806.

[11] Shangraw, R.E., Stuart, C.A., Prince, M.E., Peters, E.J., & Wolfe, R.R (1988). Insulin responsiveness of protein metabolism in vivo following bed rest in humans. *Am J Physiol*, 255,E548-E558.

[12] Strasser, F. (2008) Diagnostic criteria of cachexia and their assessment: decreased muscle strength and fatigue. *Curr Opin Clin Nutr Metab Care*, 11,:417-421.

[13] Dworzak, F., Ferrari, P., Gavazzi, C., Maiorana, C., & Bozzetti, F. (1998). Effects of cachexia due to cancer on whole body and skeletal muscle protein turnover. *Cancer*, 82,42–48.

[14] Lasheen, W., & Walsh, D. (2010). The cancer anorexia-cachexia syndrome: myth or reality? *Support Care Cancer*, 18,265-272.

[15] Strasser, F., & Bruera, E. (2002) Cancer anorexia cachexia syndrome: epidemiology, pathogenesis and assessment. In: Ripamonti C, Bruera E (eds) Gastrointestinal symptoms in advanced cancer. Oxford University, New York, pp 39–80.

[16] Giacosa, A., Frascio, F., Sukkar, S.G., et al (1997). Changes of nutritional and psychological status after megestrol acetate treatment of cancer cachexia. Rivista Italian di Nutrizione Parenterale ed Enterale, 15,20–23.

[17] Feliu, J., González Barón, M., Berrocal, A., Artal, A., Ordóñez, A., Garrido, P., Zamora, P., García de Paredes, M.L., & Montero, J.M. (1992). Usefulness of megestrol

acetate in cancer cachexia and anorexia. A placebo controlled study. *Am J Clin Oncol*, 15,436–440.

[18] Fietkau, R., Riepl, M., Kettner, H., Hinke, A., & Sauer, R. (1997). Supportive use of megestrol acetate in patients with head and neck cancer during radio (chemo)therapy. *Eur J Cancer*, 33,75–79.

[19] Bruera, E., Neumann, C.M., Pituskin, E., Calder, K., Ball, G., & Hanson, J. (1999). Thalidomide in patients with cachexia due to terminal cancer: preliminary report. *Ann Oncol*, 10,857–859.

[20] Rowland, K.M. Jr, Loprinzi, C.L., Shaw, E.G., Maksymiuk, A.W., Kuross, S.A., Jung, S.H., Kugler, J.W., Tschetter, L.K., Ghosh, C., Schaefer, P.L., Owen, D., Washburn, J.H. Jr, Webb, T.A., Mailliard, J.A., & Jett, J.R. (1996). Randomized double blind placebo controlled trial of cisplatin and etoposide plus megestrol acetate/placebo in extensive stage small cell lung cancer: A North Central Cancer Treatment Group Study. *J Clin Oncol*, 14,135–141.

[21] Loprinzi, C.L., Bernath, A.M., Schaid, D.J., Malliard, J.A., Athmann, L.M., Michalak, J.C., Tschetter, L.K., Hatfield, A.K., & Morton, R.F. (1994). Phase III evaluation of 4 doses of megestrol acetate for patients with cancer anorexia and/or cachexia. *Oncology*, 51,2–7.

[22] Evans, W.J., Morley, J.E., Argilés, J., Bales, C., Baracos, V., Guttridge, D., Jatoi, A., Kalantar-Zadeh, K., Lochs, H., Mantovani, G., Marks, D., Mitch, W.E., Muscaritoli, M., Najand, A., Ponikowski, P., Rossi Fanelli, F, Schambelan, M., Schols, A., Schuster, M., Thomas, D., Wolfe, R,, & Anker, S.D. (2008). Cachexia: a new definition. *Clin Nutr*. 27,793–799.

[23] Bozzetti, F., & Mariani, L. (2009). Defining and classifying cancer cachexia: a proposal by the SCRINIO Working Group. *JPEN J Parenter Enteral Nutr*, 33,361-367.

[24] Kurzrock, R. (2001). The role of cytokines in cancer-related fatigue. *Cancer*, 92,1684-1688.

[25] Simons, J.P., Schols, A.M., Buurman, W.A., & Wouters, E.F. (1999). Weight loss and low body cell mass in males with lung cancer: relationship with systemic inflammation, acute-phase response, resting energy expenditure, and catabolic and anabolic hormones. *Clin Sci*, 97,215-223.

[26] Rich, T.A., Innominato, P., Mormont, M.C., Boerner, J., Iacobelli, S., Jasmin, C., Boran, B., & Levi, F. (2004). Performance status, global quality of life, fatigue, and appetite loss are correlated with serum TGFa and IL-6 in patients with metastatic colorectal cancer (MCC). J Clin Oncol, ASCO Meeting Abstracts, 2004,8024.

[27] Illman, J., Corringham, R., Robinson, D. Jr., Davis, H.M., Rossi, J.F., Cella, D., & Trikha, M. (2005). Are inflammatory cytokines the common link between cancer-associated cachexia and depression? *J Supp Oncol*, 3,37-57.

[28] Martin, F., Santolaria, F., Batista, N., Milena, A., González-Reimers, E., Brito, M.J., & Oramas, J. (1999). Cytokine levels (IL-6 and IFN-gamma), acute phase response and nutritional status as prognostic factors in lung cancer. *Cytokine*, 11,80-86.

[29] Fearon, K.C., Barber, M.D., Falconer, J.S., McMillan, D.C., Ross, J.A., & Preston, T. (1999). Pancreatic cancer as a model: inflammatory mediators, acute-phase response, and cancer cachexia. *World J Surg*, 23,584-588.

[30] Lazarus, D.D., Destree, A.T., Mazzola, L.M., McCormack, T.A., Dick, L.R., Xu, B., Huang, J.Q., Pierce, J.W., Readm M.A., Coggins, M.B., Solomon, V., Goldberg, A.L.,

Brand, S.J., & Elliott, P.J. (1999). A new model of cancer cachexia: contribution of the ubiquitin-proteasome pathway. *Am J Physiol*, 277,E332-E341.

[31] Bossola, M., Muscaritoli, M., Costelli, P., Bellantone, R., Pacelli, F., Busquets, S., Argilès, J., Lopez-Soriano, F.J., Civello, I.M., Baccino, F.M., Rossi Fanelli, F., & Doglietto, G.B. (2001). Increased muscle ubiquitin mRNA levels in gastric cancer patients. *Am J Physiol*, 280,R1518-R1523.

[32] Acharyya, S., Ladner, K.J., Nelsen, L.L., Damrauer, J., Reiser, P.J., Swoap, S., & Guttridge, D.C. (2004). Cancer cachexia is regulated by selective targeting of skeletal muscle gene products. *J Clin Invest*, 114, 370-378.

[33] Bosaeus, I., Daneryd, P.,& Lundholm, K. (2002). Dietary intake, resting energy expenditure, weight loss and survival in cancer patients. *J Nutr*, 132,3465S-3466S.

[34] Fredrix, E.W.H.M., Soeters, P.B., Wouters, E.F.M., Deerenberg, I.M., von Meyenfeldt, M.F., & Saris, W.H.. (1991). Effect of different tumor types of resting energy expenditure. *Cancer Res*, 51,6138-6141.

[35] Harvie, M.N., & Campbell, I.T. (2000). Energy balance, cancer, and the sympathetic nervous system. Eur J Cancer, 36,289-292.

[36] Stasi, R., Abriani, L., Beccaglia, P., Terzoli, E., & Amadori, S. (2003). Cancer-related fatigue. *Cancer*, 98,1786-1801.

[37] Bossola, M., Pacelli, F., Tortorelli, A., Rosa, F., & Doglietto, G.B. (2008). Skeletal muscle in cancer cachexia: the ideal target of drug therapy. *Curr Cancer Drug Targets.*, 8,285-298.

[38] Camps, C., Iranzo, V., Bremnes, R.M., & Sirera, R. (2006). Anorexia-Cachexia syndrome in cancer : implications of the ubiquitin-proteasome pathway. *Support Care Cancer*, 14,1173-1183.

[39] Costelli, P., & Baccino, F.M. (2003). Mechanisms of skeletal muscle depletion in wasting syndromes: role of ATP-ubiquitin-dependent proteolysis. *Curr Opin Clin Nutr Metab Care*, 6,407-412.

[40] Briot, K., Garnero, P., Le Henanff, A., Dougados, M., & Roux, C. (2005). Body weight, body composition, and bone turnover changes in patients with spondyloarthropathy receiving anti-tumour necrosis factor [alpha] treatment. *Ann Rheum Dis*, 64,1137-1140.

[41] Marcora, S., Chester, K.R., Mittal, G., Lemmey, A.B., & Maddison, P.J. (2006). Randomized phase 2 trial of anti-tumor necrosis factor therapy for cachexia in patients with early rheumatoid arthritis. *Am J Clin Nutr*, 84,1463-1472.

[42] Kuroda, K., Horiguchi, Y, Nakashima, J., Kikuchi, E., Kanao, K., Miyajima, A., Ohigashi, T., Umezawa, K., Murai, M. (2005). Prevention of cancer cachexia by a novel nuclear factor kB inhibitor in prostate cancer. *Clin Cancer Res*, 11,5590-5594.

[43] Nai, Y.J., Jiang, Z.W., Wang, Z.M., Li, N., Li, J.S. (2007). Prevention of cancer cachexia by pyrrolidine dithiocarbamate (PDTC) in colon 26 tumor-bearing mice. JPEN J Parenter Enteral Nutr, 31,18-25.

[44] Fujiki, K., Mukaida, N., Hirose, K., Ishida, H., Harada, A., Ohno, S., Bkuethmann, H., Kawakami, M., Akiyama, H., Sone, S., & Matsushima, K. (1997). Prevention of adenocarcinoma colon 26-induced cachexia by interleukin 10 gene transfer. *Cancer Res*, 57,94-99.

[45] Carbo, N., Lopez-Soriano, J., Costelli, P., Busquets, S., Alvarez, B., Baccino, F.M., Quinn, L.S., Lopez-Soriano, F.J., & Argilés, J.M. (2000). Interleukin-15 antagonizes muscle protein waste in tumour-bearing rats. *Br J Cancer*, 83,526-531.

[46] Argilés, J.M., Moore-Carrasco, R., Fuster, G., Busquets, S., & López-Soriano, F.J. (2003). Cancer cachexia: the molecular mechanisms. *Int J Biochem Cell Biol*, 35,405-409.

[47] Argilés, J.M., Moore-Carrasco, R., Busquets, S., & López-Soriano, F.J. (2003). Catabolic mediators as targets for cancer cachexia. *Drugs Discov Today*, 8,838-844.

[48] Costelli, P., Bossola, M., Muscaritoli, M., Grieco, G., Bonelli, G., Bellantone, R., Doglietto, G.B., Baccino, F.M., & Rossi Fanelli, F. (2002). Anticytokine treatment prevents the increase in the activity to ATP-ubiquitin and Ca2+-dependent proteolytic systems in the muscle of tumor-bearing rats. *Cytokine*, 19,1-5.

[49] Stone, P., Hardy, J., Huddart, R., A'Hern, R., & Richards, M. (2000). Fatigue in patients with prostate cancer receiving hormone therapy. *Eur J Cancer*, 36,1134-1141.

[50] Moertel, C., Schutt, A.J., Reitemeier, R.J., & Hahn, R.G. (1974). Corticosteroid therapy of preterminal gastrointestinal cancer. *Cancer*, 33, 1607-1609.

[51] Pommatau, E., Revillard, J., & Gignous, M. (1962). Interet de methyl-6-prednisolone hemisuccinate de sodium (Solumedrol) dans les traitements des tumeurs malignes. *Lyon Med*, 49,1179-1198.

[52] Popiela, T., Lucchi, R., & Giongo, F. (1989). Methylprednisolone as palliative therapy for female terminal cancer patients. *Eur J Cancer Clin Oncol*, 25,1823-1829.

[53] Robustelli Della Cuna, G., Pellegrini, A., & Piazzi, M. (1989). Effect of methylprednisolone sodium succinate on quality of life in pre-terminal cancer patients: a placebo controlled, multi-center study. *Eur J Cancer Clin Oncol*, 25,1817-1821.

[54] Schell, H. (1972). Adrenal corticosteroid therapy in far-advanced cancer. *Geriatrics*, 27,131-141.

[55] Bruera, E., Roca, E., Cedaro, L., Carraro, S., & Chacon, R. (1985). Action of oral methylprednisolone in terminal cancer patients: a prospective randomized double-blind study. *Cancer Treat Rep*, 69,751-754.

[56] Maltoni, M., Nanni, O., Scarpi, E., Rossi, D., Serra, P., & Amadori, D. (2001). High-dose progestins for the treatment of cancer anorexia-cachexia syndrome: a systematic review of randomised clinical trials. *Ann Oncol*, 12,289-300.

[57] Mantovani, G., Maccio, A., Bianchi, A., Curreli, L., Ghiani, M., Santona, M.C., & Del Giacco, G.S. (1995). Megestrol acetate in neoplastic anorexia/cachexia: clinical evaluation and comparison with cytokine levels in patients with head and neck carcinoma treated with neoadjuvant chemotherapy. *Int J Clin Lab Res*, 25,135-141.

[58] Yamashita, J-I., & Ogawa, M. (2000). Medroxyprogesterone acetate and cancer cachexia: interleukin-6 involvement. *Breast Cancer*, 7,130-135.

[59] Mantovani, A., Maccio, A., Esu, S., Lai, P., Santona, M.C., Massa, E., Dessì, D., Melis, G.B., & Del Giacco, G.S. (1997). Medroxyprogesterone acetate reduces the in vitro production of cytokines and serotonin involved in anorexia/cachexia and emesis by peripheral blood mononuclear cells of cancer patients. *Eur J Cancer*, 33,602-607.

[60] Kalra, S.P., Dube, M.G., Pu, S., Xu, B., Horvath, T.L., & Kalra, P.S. (1999). Interacting appetite-regulating pathways in the hypothalamic regulation of body weight. *Endocr Rev*, 20,68-100.

[61] Plata-Salaman, C.R. (2000). Central nervous system mechanisms contributing to the cachexia-anorexia syndrome. *Nutrition*, 16,1009-1012.

[62] Bruera, E., Ernst, S., Hagen, N., Spachynski, K., Belzile, M., Hanson, J., Summers, N., Brown, B., Dulude, H., & Gallant, G. (1998). Effectiveness of megestrol acetate in

patients with advanced cancer: a randomized, double-blind, crossover study. *Cancer Prev Control*, 2,74-78.

[63] Mantovani, G., Maccio, A., Mura, L., Massa, E., Mudu, M.C., Mulas, C., Lusso, M.R., Madeddu, C., & Dessì, A. (2000). Serum levels of leptin and proinflammatory cytokines in patients with advanced-stage cancer at different sites. *J Mol Med*, 78,554-561.

[64] Guttridge, D.C., Mayo, M.W., Madrid, L.V., Wang, C.Y., & Baldwin, A.S., Jr. (2000). NF-κB-induced loss of MyoD messenger RNAs possible role in muscle decay and cachexia. *Science*, 289,2363-2366.

[65] Lorite, M.J., Cariuk, P., & Tisdale, M.J. (1997). Induction of muscle protein degradation by a tumour factor. *Br J Cancer*, 76,1035-1040.

[66] Emery, P.W., Edwards, R.H., Rennie, M.J., Souhami, R.L., & Halliday, D. (1984). Protein synthesis in muscle measured in vivo in cachextic patients with cancer. *Br Med J*. (Clin Res Ed), 289,584-586.

[67] Emery, P.W., Lovell, L. & Rennie, M.J. (1984). Protein synthesis measured in vivo in muscle and liver of chachetic tumor-bearing mice. *Cancer Res*, 44,2779-2784.

[68] McPherron, A.C., Lawler, A.M., & Lee S.J. (1997). Regulation of skeletal muscle mass in mice by a new TGF-beta superfamily member. *Nature*, 387,83-90.

[69] Costelli, P., Muscaritoli, M., Bonetto, A., Penna, F., Reffo, P., Bossola, M., Bonelli, G., Doglietto, G.B., Baccino, F.M., & Rossi Fanelli, F. (2008). Muscle myostatin signalling is enhanced in experimental cancer cachexia. *Eur J Clin Invest*, 38, 531-538.

[70] Langley, B., Thomas, M., Bishop, A., Sharma, M., Gilmour, S., & Kambadur, R. (2002). Myostatin inhibits myoblast differentiation by down-regulating MyoD expression. J Biol Chem, 277,49831-49840.

[71] Amirouche, A., Durieux, A.C., Banzer, S., Koulmann, N., Bonnefoy, R., Mouret, C., Bigard, X., Peinnequin, A., & Freyssenet, D. (2009). Down-regulation of Akt/mammalian target of rapamycin signaling pathway in response to myostatin overexpression in skeletal muscle. *Endocrinoloy*, 150,286-294.

[72] McFarlance, C., Plummer, E., Thomas, M., Hennebry, A., Ashby, M., Ling, N., Smith, H., Sharma, M., & Kambadur, R. (2006). Myostatin induces cachexia by activating the ubiquitin proteolytic system through an NF-κB-independent, FoxO1-dependent mechanism. *J Cell Physiol*, 209,501-514.

[73] Marks, D.L., Ling, N., & Cone, R.D. (2001). Role of the central melanocortin system in cachexia. Cancer Res, 61,1432-1438.

[74] Nicholson, J.R., Kohler, G, Schaerer, F,Sebb, C., Wevermann, P., & Hofbauer, K.G. (2006). Peripheral administration of amelanocortin 4-receptor inverse agonist prevents loss of lean body mass in tumor-bearing mice. *J Pharmacol Exp Ther*, 317,771-777.

[75] Dass, N.B., Munonyara, M., Bassil, A.K., Hervieu, G.J., Osbourne, S., Corcoran, S., Morgan, M., & Sanger, G.J. (2003). Growth hormone secretagogue receptors in rat and human gastrointestinal tract and the effects of ghrelin. *Neuroscience*, 120,443-453.

[76] Wiedenmann, B., Malfertheiner, P., Friess, H., Ritch, P., Arseneau, J., Mantovani, G., Caprioni, F., Van Cursem, E., Richel, D., DeWitte, M., Qi, M., Robinson, D, Jr., Zhong, B., DeBoer, C., Lu, J.D., Prabhaker, U., Corringham, R., Von Hoff, D. (2008). A multicenter, phase II study of infliximab plus gemcitabine in pancreatic cancer cachexia. *J Support Oncol*, 6,18-25.

[77] Clarke, S.J., Smith, J.T., Gebbie, C., Sweeney, C., & Olszewski, N. (2009). A phase I, pharmacokinetic (PK), and preliminary efficacy assessment of ALD518, a humanized anti-IL-6 antibody, in patients with advanced cancer. *J Clin Oncol*, 27,3025.

[78] Smith, H.J., Lorite, M.J., & Tisdale, M.J. (1999). Effect of cancer cachectic factor on protein synthesis/degradation in murine C2C12 myoblasts: modulation by eicosapentaenoic acid. *Cancer Res*, 59,5507-5513.

[79] Barber, M.D., Ross, J.A., Voss, A.C., Tisdale, M.J., & Fearon, K.C. (1999). The effect of an oral nutritional supplement enriched with fish oil on weight-loss in patients with pancreatic cancer. *Br J Cancer*, 81,80-86.

[80] Wigmore, S.J., Barber, M.D., Ross, J.A., Tisdale, M.J., & Fearon, K.C. (2000). Effect of oral eicosapentaenoic acid on weight loss in patients with pancreatic cancer. *Nutr Cancer*, 36,177-184.

[81] Bruera, E., Strasser, F., Palmer, J.L., Willey, J., Calder, K., Amyotte, G., & Baracos, V. (2003). Effect of fish oil on appetite and other symptoms in patients with advanced cancer and anorexia/cachexia: a double-blind, placebo-controlled study. *J Clin Oncol*, 21,129-134.

[82] Jatoi, A., Rowland, K., Loprinzi, C., Sloan, J.A., Dakhil, S.R., MacDonald, N., Gagnon, B., Novotny, P.J., Mailliard, J.A., Bushey, T.I., Nair, S., Christensen, B.; & North Central Cancer Treatment Group. (2004). An eicosapentaenoic acid supplement versus megestrol acetate versus both for patients with cancer-associated wasting: A North Central Cancer Treatment Group and National Cancer Institute of Canada collaborative effort. *J Clin Oncol*, 22,2469-2476.

[83] Reyes-Teran, G., Sierra-Madero, J., Martinez del Cerro, V., Arroyo-Figueroa, H., Pasquetti, A., Calva, J.J., & Ruiz-Palacios, G.M. (1996). Effects of thalidomide on HIV associated wasting syndrome: a randomized double blind placebo controlled clinical trial. AIDS, 10,1501-1507.

[84] Haslett, P., Hempstead, M., Seidman, C., Diakun, J., Vasquez, D., Freedman, V.H., & Kaplan, G. (1997). The metabolic and immunologic effects of short term thalidomide treatment of patients infected with the human immunodeficiency virus. *AIDS Res Hum Retroviruses*, 13,1047-1054.

[85] McMillan, D.C., Leen, E., Smith, J., Sturgeon, C., Preston, T., Cooke, T.G., & McArdle, C.S. (1995). Effect of extended ibuprofen administration on the acute phase protein response in colorectal cancer patients. *Eur J Surg Oncol*, 21,531-534.

[86] Preston, T., Fearon, K.C., McMillan, D.C., Winstanley, F.P., Slater, C., Shenkin, A., & Carter, D.C. (1995). Effect of ibuprofen on the acute-phase response and protein metabolism in patients with cancer and weight loss. *Br J Surg*, 82,229-234.

[87] Wigmore, S.J., Falconer, J.S., Plester, C.E., Ross, J.A., Maingay, J.P., Carter, D.C., & Fearon, K.C. (1995). Ibuprofen reduces energy expenditure and acute-phase protein production compared with placebo in pancreatic cancer patients. *Br J Cancer*, 72,185-188.

[88] McMillan, D.C., Wigmore, S.J., Fearon, K.C., & O'Gorman, P., Wright, C.E. & McArdle, C.S. (1999). A prospective randomized study of megestrol acetate and ibuprofen in gastrointestinal cancer patients with weight loss. *Br J Cancer*, 79,495-500.

[89] Mantovani, G., Macciò, A., Madeddu, C., Serpe, R., Antoni, G., Massa, E., Dessì, M., & Panzone, F. (2010). Phase II nonrandomized study of the efficacy and safety of COX-2 inhibitor celecoxib on patients with cancer cachexia. *J Mol Med*, 88,85-92.

[90] Huang, J.S., Wilke, S.J., Dolan, S., Gallafent, J.H., Aliabadi, N., Sullivan, M.P., & Grinspoon, S. (2003). Reduced testosterone levels in human immunodeficiency virus-infected women with weight loss and low weight. *Clin Infec Dis*, 36,499-506.

[91] Fearon, K.C.H., Hansell, D.T., Preston, T., Plumb, J.A., Davies, J., Shapiro, D., Shenkin, A., Calman, K.C., & Burns, H.J. (1988). Influence of whole protein turnover rate on resting energy expenditure in patients with cancer. Cancer Res, 48,2590-2595.

[92] Rabkin, J.G., Rabkin, R., & Wagner, G. (1995). Testosterone replacement therapy in HIV illness. *Gen Hosp Psych*, 17, 37-42.

[93] Kong, A., & Edmonds, P. (2002. Testosterone therapy in HIV wasting syndrome: systemic review and meta-analysis. *Lancet*, 2,692-699.

[94] Strawford, A., Barbieri, T., Neese, R., Van Loan, M., Christiansen, M., Hoh, R., Sathyan, G., Skowronski, R., King, J., & Hellerstein, M. (1999). Effects of nandrolone decanoate therapy in borderline hypogonadal men with HIV-associated weight loss. *J Acquir Immune Defic Syndr Hum Retrovirol*, 20,137-146.

[95] Sattler, F.R., Jaque, S.V., Schroeder, E.T., Olson, C., Dube, M.P., Martinez, C., Briggs, W., Horton, R., & Azen, S. (1999). Effects of pharmacological doses of nandrolone decanoate and progressive resistance training in immunodeficient patients infected with human immunodeficiency virus. J Clin Endocrinol Metab, 84,1268-1276.

[96] Chlebowski, R.T., Herrold, J., Ali, I., Oktay, E., Chlebowski, J.S., Ponce, A.T., Heber, D., & Block, J.B. (1986). Influence of nandrolone decanoate on weight loss in advanced non-small cell lung cancer. *Cancer*, 58,183-186.

[97] Hengge, U.R., Stocks, K., Wiehler, H., Faulkner, S., Esser, S., Lorenz, C., Jentzen, W., Hengge, D., Goos, M., Dudley, R.E., & Ringham, G. (2003). Double-blind, randomized, placebo-controlled phase III trial of oxymetholone for the treatment of HIV wasting. *AIDS*, 17,699-710.

[98] Von Roenn, J., Tchekmedyian, S., & Ottery, F.D. Oxandrolone increases weight, lean tissue, performance status and quality of life scores in cancer related weight loss. *Support Care Cancer*, 2002 Abstract.

[99] Edwards, J.P., West, S.P., Pooley, C.L., Marschke, K.B., Farmer, L.J., & Jones, T.K. (1998). New nonsteroidal androgen receptor modulators based on 4-(trifluorometyl)-2(1H)-pyrrolidino[3.2-g] quinolinone. *Bioorg Med Chem Lett*, 8,745-750.

[100] Miner, J.N., Chang, W., Chapman, M.S., Finn, P.D., Hong, M.H., López, F.J., Marschke, K.B., Rosen, J., Schrader, W., Turner, R., van Oeveren, A., Viveros, H., Zhi, L., & Negro-Vilar, A. (2006). An orally-active selective androgen receptor modulator is efficacious on bone, muscle and sex function with reduced impact on prostate. *Endocrinology*, 148.363-373.

[101] Yin, D., Gao, W., Kearby, J.D., Xu, H., & Dalton, J.T. (2003). Pharmacodynamics of slective androgen receptor modulators. *J Pharmacol Exp Ther*, 304,1334-1340.

[102] Gao, W., Reiser, P.J., Coss, C.C., Phelps, M.A., Kearbey, J.D., Miller, D.D. & Dalton, J.T. (2005). Selective androgen receptor modulator (SARM) treatment improves muscle strength and body composition, and prevent bone loss in orchidectomized rats. *Endocrinology*, 146,4887-4896.

[103] Hanada, K., Furuya, K., Yamamoto, N., Nejishima, H, Ichikawa, K., Nakamura, T., Miyakawa, M., Amano, S., Sumita, Y., & Oguro, N. (2003). Bone anabolic effects of S-40503, a novel nonsteroidal selective androgen receptor modulator (SARM), in rat models of osteoporosis. *Biol Pharm Bull*, 26,1563-1569.

[104] Mantovani, G., Macciò, A., Madeddu, C., Serpe, R., Massa, E., Dessì, M., Panzone, F., & Contu, P. (2010). Randomized phase III clinical trial of five different arms of treatment in 332 patients with cancer cachexia. *Oncologist.*, 15,200-211.

[105] Seruga, B., Zhang, H., Bernstein, L.J., & Tannock, I.F. (2008) Cytokines and their relationship to the symptoms and outcome of cancer. *Nat Rev Cancer*, 8,887-899.

[106] Galvaoo, D.A.,& Newton, R.U. (2005). Review of exercise intervention studies in cancer patients. *J Clin Oncol*, 23,899-909.

[107] Roubenoff, R., & Wilson, I.B. (2001). Effect of resistance training on self-reported physical functioning in HIV infection. *Med Sci Sport Exerc*, 33,1811-1817.

[108] Strawford, A., Barbieri, T., Van Loan, M., Parks, E., Catlin, D., Barton, N., Neese, R., Christiansen, M., King, J., & Hellerstein, M.K. (1999). Resistance exercise and supraphysiologic androgen therapy in eugonadal men in HIV-related weight loss: a randomized controlled trial. *JAMA*, 281,1282-1290.

[109] Gerber, L.H. (2001). Cancer rehabilitation into the future. *Cancer*, 92,975-979.

[110] Van Weert, E., Hoekstra-Weebers, J.E.H.M., Grol, B.M.F., Otter, R., Arendzen, J.H., Postema, K., & van der Schans, C.P. (2004). Physical functioning and quality of life after cancer rehabilitation. *Inter J Rehabil Res*, 27,27-35.

[111] Deuster, P.A., Morrison, S.D., & Ahrens, R.A. (1985). Endurance exercise modifies cachexia of tumor growth in rats. *Med Sci Sports Exer*, 17,385-392.

[112] Singh, N.A., Clements, K.M., & Fiatarone, M.A. (1997). A randomized controlled trial of progressive resistance training in depressed elders. *J Gerontol A Biol Sci Med Sci*, 52,M27-M35.

[113] Mock, V., Dow, K.H., Meares, C.J., Grimm, P.M., Dienermann, J.A., Haisfield-Wolfe, M.E., Quitasol, W., Mitchell, S., Chakravarthy, S., & Gage, I. (1997). Effects of exercise on fatigue, physical functioning, and emotional distress during radiation therapy for breast cancer. *Oncol Nurs Forum*, 24,991-1000.

[114] Mock, V., Pickett, M., Ropka, M.E., Muscari Lin, E., Stewart, K.J., Rhodes, V.A., McDaniel, R., Grimm, P.M., Krumm, S., & McCorkle, R. (2001). Fatigue and quality of life outcomes of exercise during cancer treatment. *Cancer Practice*, 9,119-127.

[115] Schwartz, A.L. (1999). Fatigue mediates the effects of exercise on quality of life. *Qual Life Res*, 8,529-538.

In: Handbook of Fatigue in Health and Disease
Editor: Howard S. Smith
ISBN 978-1-61761-920-5

Chapter 6

FATIGUE, SLEEPINESS AND SLEEP DISORDERS

***Aaron E. Sher*[1] *and Howard S. Weiss*[2]**

[1] Associate Medical Director
Associate Clinical Professor, Albany Medical Center
St. Peter's Sleep Center, Pine West Plaza #1
Washington Avenue Extension
Albany , NY 1220, USA
[2] St. Peter's Sleep Center, Pine West Plaza #1
Washington Avenue Extension
Albany , NY 12205, USA

ABSTRACT

Sleep appears to be crucial to optimal functioning of higher level mammals. Disturbed sleep may be vitally important in contributing to fatigue. Although, both sleep and fatigue may be extremely similar and overlapping perceptions they are two distinct concepts. Multiple instruments may be utilized in efforts to assess sleep disorders as well as fatigue or the interaction of the two. Various sleep disorders especially those associated with nonrestorative sleep may contribute to fatigue. Behavioral medicine therapy, improving sleep hygiene, as well as specific treatment sdirected towards any particular sleep disorders (e.g. stimulants, continuous positive airway pressure (CPAP)) and/or circadian therapy may be beneficial for certain patients with sleep-related fatigue.

[1] Phone: (518) 464-9999
Email: docsher2002@yahoo.com
[2] Phone: (518) 464-9999
Email: hweiss@stpetershealthcare.org

Introduction

Sleep medicine, a newly recognized medical specialty, is made up of researchers and clinicians who initially specialize in primary disciplines (including, but not limited to internal medicine, pulmonary medicine, neurology, psychiatry, otolaryngology-head and neck surgery, and pediatrics), then sub-specialize in sleep medicine. Their work focuses on differences between the states of sleep and wake: characteristics that define and distinguish these states, mechanisms that regulate them, and their impact on other bodily systems. Sleep specialists diagnose and treat disorders that primarily affect the integrity of the states of sleep and wakefulness, disorders of other body systems that affect the integrity of sleep and wakefulness, and disorders of other body systems resulting from dysfunction of the sleep/wake axis.

In disorders in which there is disruption of sleep physiology (sleep architecture is fragmented), sleepiness and/or fatigue may be prominent features. In other disorders, sleepiness and/or fatigue may occur despite relatively intact sleep (at least as defined by contemporary measures of sleep physiology), and the problem may be viewed as a disorder of wakefulness. In some cases, morbidity may result only from intrinsic factors (resulting from bodily causes), while in other cases, extrinsic factors (resulting primarily from outside, or environmental, causes) may be important. For example, circadian rhythm disorders result from a mismatch between the body's internal clock and the geophysical environment. A circadian rhythm disorder may result from primary malfunction of the biological clock (e.g., advanced or delayed sleep phase). On the other hand, it may also be secondary to external forces that result in a shift in the environment causing a normally functioning body clock to be out of phase with the environment, (e.g. circadian rhythm malfunctions resulting from jet-lag or shift work).

While sleepiness is a prominent feature of many sleep disorders, so also is fatigue. Though not synonymous, fatigue and sleepiness are related. This chapter will discuss the relationship between sleepiness and fatigue, and present, in encapsulated form, some illustrative sleep disorders in which sleepiness and fatigue occur: obstructive sleep apnea syndrome (in which respiratory dysfunction degrades sleep/wake integrity), narcolepsy (in which neurological dysfunction degrades sleep/wake integrity), and delayed sleep phase (a circadian rhythm disorder in which primary malfunction of the biological clock causes it to be out of phase with normal environmental cues, resulting in degradation of sleep/wake integrity). Though, clearly, sleepiness and fatigue occur in many other sleep/wake disorders, consideration of these three will suggest the range of types of these disorders in which sleepiness and fatigue may be symptoms.

Sleepiness and Fatigue

Sleepiness can be defined in different ways. It can be defined as the tendency to fall asleep, or sleep propensity (SP). The measure of SP can be "objective" or "subjective". SP (and hence sleepiness) can also be defined in terms of "state" SP (reflecting specific conditions at a specific given time) or "trait" SP (reflecting a variety of conditions over a prolonged time). In lieu of measures of SP, sleepiness can, alternatively, be defined in terms of other symptoms believed to reflect sleepiness. These often overlap with symptoms believed to reflect fatigue. The varied nature of definitions of sleepiness has resulted in the evolution of varied assessment instruments for sleepiness [1].

The distinction between subjective and objective SP is demonstrated by a comparison of two instruments: Multiple Sleep Latency Test (MSLT) and Epworth Sleepiness Scale (ESS). The fact that onset of sleep can be objectively and precisely measured electroencephalographically (EEG) has resulted in defining "objective" SP in terms of *the rapidity and frequency of sleep onset as determined by EEG under designated test conditions*. This is the basis of the MSLT, the validated objective test of "excessive sleepiness" regarded as a "gold standard". Following a night of physiologically monitored sleep, the patient is given five *nap opportunities* at 2 hour intervals across the day, beginning 2 hours after the EEG-documented morning awakening. Each nap opportunity consists of 20 to 30 minutes of physiological monitoring (including EEG) while the individual lies in a quiet, darkened room. *Sleep latency* for each of the naps is the elapsed time from lights out to the first 30 second EEG epoch scored as sleep. MSLT provides 5 sleep latencies across the day, and the average sleep latency over the 5 nap opportunities is taken to be an *objective* measure of average SP. In contrast, the ESS represents a *subjective* measure of SP. The ESS is a self completed questionnaire that asks the subject to rate the likelihood (under conditions of "usual way of life in recent times") of falling asleep or dozing, on a likelihood scale of 0 to 3 (ranging from never to high likelihood) in 8 relatively specific circumstances (sitting and reading, watching TV, sitting---inactive in a public place, as a passenger in a car for an hour without a break, lying down to rest in the afternoon when circumstances permit, sitting and talking to someone, sitting quietly after lunch without alcohol, in a car while stopped for a few minutes in traffic) [3]. After summation of the scores of all 8 items, values over 10-11 (based on validation studies) are taken to indicate abnormal *subjective* sleepiness characterized by elevated SP (the maximum score achievable is 24) [1- 3].

The distinction between characterizing sleepiness as a "state" vs. a "trait" is illustrated by comparison of ESS with the Stanford Sleepiness Scale (SSS), a 7-point self-evaluation scale (Table 1) [4]. Sleepiness, as measured by ESS, is considered to be a measure of "trait" sleepiness (characterizing the individual's level of sleepiness over an extended time period and under many different circumstances). SSS questions the individual about his perceptions at the moment of execution of the task (the moment of completing the SSS), and the response to the instrument is taken to measure sleepiness *at that moment and under the specific circumstances at that moment* (This reflects state sleepiness, and is likely influenced by factors such as the quality and quantity of sleep the preceding night, the hour of day at which the questionnaire is being completed, and the level of external stimulation at the time of completing the questionnaire). Trait sleepiness would appear to be more relevant from a clinical perspective than state sleepiness, which defines the quality only within a very narrow time frame and in specific circumstances surrounding that time frame. Trait sleepiness is more likely to determine the presence of sleep/wake pathology and (if defined by SP) predict whether sleep onset is likely to occur at inappropriate times [1, 3, 4].

Table 1. Stanford Sleepiness Scale (SSS) [4]

For the following scale please check the one statement that best describes you at present.	
1	Feel active and vital; alert, wide awake
2	Functioning at a high level, but not at peak, able to concentrate
3	Relaxed; awake; not at full alertness, responsive
4	A little foggy, not at peak; let down
5	Fogginess; beginning to lose interest in remaining awake; slowed down
6	Sleepiness; prefer to be lying down; fighting sleep; woozy
7	Almost in reverie; sleep onset soon; lost struggle to remain awake

Both sleep deprivation and sleep fragmentation increase SP, and negatively impact cognitive performance, motor performance, and mood, resulting in increased negative mood states, feelings of fatigue, loss of vigor, sleepiness, and confusion. Feelings of irritability, anxiety, and depression are believed to result from inadequate or fragmented sleep. Sleep fragmentation differs from sleep restriction in that adequate overall hours of sleep are obtained, but the sleep is characterized by frequent "arousals" (not awakenings to a conscious level, but 3- second periods of increased cortical EEG frequency indicative of subclinical alerting or lightening of sleep). Such arousals have been associated with increased SP, cognitive performance deficits, and mood alterations. Studies show that sleep fragmentation has the same effect as sleep deprivation on waking behavior. Involuntary microsleeps occur. Attentiveness is unstable. Cognitive slowing occurs, and time pressure increases cognitive errors. Response time, short-term recall, and working memory decline. Response perseveration on ineffective solutions increases. Increased compensatory effort is required to remain behaviorally effective. Tasks may be begun well, but performance deteriorates as task duration increases. There is growing neglect of activities inappropriately judged to be nonessential [1, 5].

The contrast between instruments defining sleepiness only in terms of SP and those which define it in terms of other qualities reflective of sleepiness is illustrated by comparison of ESS and SSS. ESS is a subjective measure of sleepiness defined by SP. SSS is a subjective measure of sleepiness defined not only in terms of SP ("wide awake; fighting sleep; sleep onset soon; last struggle to remain awake"), but also in terms of other subjective sensations and feelings relating to the transitional state between wakefulness and sleep: ("functioning; not at peak; not at full alertness; foggy; let down; losing interest in remaining awake; slowed down; prefer to be lying down; woozy") [1, 3, 4].

Terms regarding fatigue and sleepiness are frequently used interchangeably or in the context of 'tired', or 'drowsy'. Once the definition of sleepiness is broadened beyond SP, it incorporates many symptoms associated also with fatigue: including those reflective of decrements in cognitive performance, motor function, and mood changes. In the absence of generally accepted *objective* measures of fatigue, fatigue is frequently characterized by using a number of *subjective* scales, such as the Fatigue Severity Scale (Table 2) and the Fatigue Scale (Table 3). Like sleepiness, fatigue can be considered as a state (acute) phenomenon or a trait (chronic) phenomenon. It can be defined in psychological and/or physical terms, reflecting its heterogeneous nature. Therefore, attempts to clarify the interaction of sleepiness and fatigue would likely utilize subjective scales of sleepiness and of fatigue [1, 5-7].

The distinction between fatigue and sleepiness is not well delineated. Each phenomenon is complex and multi-dimensional. Each can result from sleep restriction, sleep fragmentation or other compromise in the mechanisms regulating sleep and wakefulness. However, while related and probably overlapping, they are not one entity. Despite the development of a number of objective and subjective tools for measuring sleepiness, and numerous scales defining and measuring fatigue, there is no universally agreed upon definition of either phenomenon. In the case of fatigue, the lack of a "gold standard" and, indeed, the lack of an objective measure, reflects and has contributed to the lack of consensus. The importance of future work to develop a clear conceptualization of sleepiness and fatigue, independent of each other, and then to strive to clarify points of overlap and points of distinction has been suggested [1].

A recent attempt to assess fatigue and sleepiness simultaneously as two separate but interacting processes, is referred to as FACES [8]. FACES represents a 50-item self-report questionnaire. The FACES consists of five subscales: Fatigue, Anergy, Consciousness, Energized and Sleepiness. The Fatigue subscale includes 15 items (fatigued, worn-out, exhausted, wacked-out, drained, pooped, overtired, weary, tired, spent, bushed, out of steam, frazzled, limited endurance, achy muscles), and the sleepiness subscale includes 10 items (snoozy, sleepy, drowsy, slumber, heavy-eyed, half-awake, yawning, dozy, somnambulant, sluggish). Convergent and discriminate validity were evaluated by calculating correlations between FACES subscales and a number of independent indices. The results suggest that FACES offers a promising self-report instrument for the measurement of fatigue, sleepiness and related subjective experiences [1, 8].

Neu and colleagues used Rasch analysis-based methods to study the interrelations of fatigue, sleepiness and nonrestorative sleep (NRS) in 150 subjects (mean age = 39.3 years, range = 18-65) from a community sample [9]. They found that NRS complaints can simultaneously present with higher daytime fatigue and sleepiness levels but the associative relationships between fatigue and sleepiness remain relatively unaffected by NRS [9]. Although participants might not present adequate differentiation, fatigue and sleepiness seem to relate to different underlying concepts [9].

Examples of Sleep Disorders Characterized by Sleepiness/Fatigue

To demonstrate the broad range of sleep disorders which can result in sleepiness and fatigue, three examples will be briefly highlighted: obstructive sleep apnea syndrome (in which respiratory dysfunction degrades sleep/wake integrity), narcolepsy (in which neurological dysfunction degrades sleep/wake integrity), and delayed sleep phase (a primary circadian rhythm disorder in which malfunction of the biological clock causes it to be out of phase with environmental cues, resulting in degradation of sleep/wake integrity).

Table 2. Fatigue Severity Scale (FSS) *

Using the following scale, circle the most appropriate number in the chart (1-7):
1=Completely disagree; 4=Neither agree nor disagree; 7=Completely agree

	Completely Disagree		Neither Agree or Disagree			Completely Agree	
	1	2	3	4	5	6	7
During the past week, I have found:							
1. My motivation is lower when I am fatigued	0	0	0	0	0	0	0
2. Exercise brings on my fatigue	0	0	0	0	0	0	0
3. I am easily fatigued	0	0	0	0	0	0	0
4. Fatigue interferes with my physical functioning	0	0	0	0	0	0	0
5. Fatigue causes frequent problems for me	0	0	0	0	0	0	0
6. My fatigue prevents sustained physical functioning	0	0	0	0	0	0	0
7. Fatigue interferes with carrying out certain duties and responsibilities	0	0	0	0	0	0	0
8. Fatigue is among my three most disabling symptoms	0	0	0	0	0	0	0
9. Fatigue interferes with my work, family, or social life	0	0	0	0	0	0	0
10. 100 mm VAS rating of fatigue intensity **No Fatigue--Worst Fatigue**							

* Based on ref 6 (Krupp 1989).

Table 3. Fatigue Scale (FS) *

Using the following scale, circle the most appropriate number in the chart (0-3):
0=No; 1=Mildly; 2=Moderately; 3=Markedly

	0	1	2	3
During the past week, I have found:				
1. Do you have problems with tiredness?	0	0	0	0
2. Do you need to rest more?	0	0	0	0
3. Do you feel sleepy or drowsy?	0	0	0	0
4. Do you have problems starting things?	0	0	0	0
5. Are you lacking in energy?	0	0	0	0
6. Do you have less strength in your muscles?	0	0	0	0
7. Do you feel weak?	0	0	0	0
8. Do you have difficulty concentrating?	0	0	0	0
9. Do you have problems thinking clearly?	0	0	0	0
6. Do you have less strength in your muscles?	0	0	0	0
6. Do you have less strength in your muscles?	0	0	0	0

* Based on ref 7 (Chalder 1993).

This review is intended to point up the diversity of sleep pathology that can produce these common endpoints.

Obstructive Sleep Apnea Syndrome

Obstructive sleep apnea syndrome (OSAS) is found in 2-4% of the population [10]. As increased body weight is a risk factor, its incidence and prevalence is likely increasing with ongoing increase of obesity in the population. The pathophysiological event characterizing OSAS is pharyngeal collapse occurring only while the individual sleeps [11]. Airway collapse occurring at the termination of expiration is reinforced by negative pressure introduced at the start of the next inspiratory effort. In essence, the airway is sucked shut. The fundamental defect in OSAS is excessive pharyngeal collapsibility, most commonly the consequence of pharyngeal anatomical restriction, increased body weight, or both. Anatomical restriction may result from specific space occupying pathological lesions of the pharyngeal airway (benign or malignant), but more commonly results from soft tissue variations (e.g. hypertrophic tonsils, elongated soft palate, prominent tongue) or skeletal variations (e.g. mandibular or maxillary deficiency compromising the pharyngeal space by impacting spatial relationships of attached soft tissues) [12]. These anatomical factors collectively determine the threshold of body weight at which airway collapse (ranging from snoring to severe obstructive apnea) occurs. If the patient exceeds the weight threshold at which snoring commences, snoring progresses to OSAS, which, in turn, progresses in severity with further weight gain. Patient specific variation in respiratory control is likely to play a secondary etiological role.

Notably, OSAS patients do *not* experience airway obstruction when *awake*. At such time, inspiratory negative pressure triggers reflex contraction of muscles whose vector of action prevents pharyngeal collapse. Sleep, on the other hand, is characterized by loss of skeletal muscle tone, including tone in muscles which reflexively dilate the pharyngeal airway.

Each obstructed inspiratory effort may result in hypoxemia and hypercarbia, elevation of systemic and pulmonary blood pressure, robust sympathetic and parasympathetic activation, and, ultimately, arousal. Arousal, a direct result of increased respiratory effort, is likely to be brief (cortically or subcortically detected), but generally not to the level of a conscious awakening. Therefore, the patient remains subjectively "asleep", even in the presence of hundreds of partial "arousals". Only occasionally will there be a full awakening to the point of awareness. It is the (generally unconscious) arousal that triggers a brief increment in pharyngeal muscle tone sufficient to reopen the airway and allow for recovery of ventilation.

Associated with OSAS is cardiovascular risk, believed to result from associated blood gas abnormality, including hypoxemia, and stress related to recurrent airway obstruction and recurrent arousal. These include systemic and pulmonary hypertension, cardiac arrhythmia (most notably, atrial fibrillation unresponsive to therapy), congestive heart failure, myocardial infarction and stroke. Insulin resistance and diabetes mellitus is associated.

Behavioral, consequences likely relate more directly to sleep instability and frequent arousal (although ventilatory insufficiency and blood gas abnormality may also play a role). Over the course of a night, the patient may experience hundreds of obstructed breaths, triggering an equal number of arousals [13]. The primary complaints of patients with OSAS are frequently sleepiness and fatigue. Severely affected patients may experience uncontrolled sleep attacks under bizarre circumstances, such as standing at a podium delivering a lecture (not unlike a patient with narcolepsy). Other patients have much more subtle daytime complaints, including various manifestations of fatigue. Complaints include tiredness, "fatigue", inattentiveness, lack of ambition, and dysphoria. In children and some adults, the clinical picture may be similar to that associated with attention deficit disorder, and inattentiveness may be more prominent that frank sleepiness or fatigue [12]. A worrisome outcome of the inattentiveness and sleepiness/fatigue associated with OSAS is increased risk of automobile crashes secondary to inattentiveness, poor coordination, or episodes of frank dozing at the wheel.

OSAS is diagnosed by means of continuous physiological monitoring during a night of sleep (PSG) (Table 4).

Table 4. Polysomnography (PSG)

1.	EEG (electroencephalography)
2.	EMG (electromyography)
3.	EOG (electrooculography)
4.	EKG (electrocardiography)
5.	Airflow
6.	Respiratory effort
7.	Oximetry
8.	Body position

Treatments for OSAS are varied. Weight loss (achieved through behavioral means or bariatric surgery) is therapeutic when OSAS is associated with excess body weight. Mechanical measures can "brace" the airway in sleeping patients, thereby eliminating the obstructive phenomenon. These include application of mandibular advancement devices (which anchor the mandible in an advanced "pseudoprognathic" position) by articulating with the mandibular and maxillary teeth while the patient sleeps [13]. More widely applicable are positive pressure devices that stent the pharyngeal airway with an air column of supra-atmospheric air pressure (delivered to the nose or nose and mouth via a soft, pliable interface) while the patient sleeps [13]. The pressure applied is the minimal pressure capable of maintaining a patent airway during all stages of sleep and in all body positions, and is determined by titrating pressure against airway obstruction while the patient is monitored by PSG during a night of sleep [13]. More recently, autotitrating devices have been introduced. Surgical measures can diminish pharyngeal collapsibility through extirpation or alteration of the soft tissues which abut the pharynx or through modification (osteotomy and/or transposition) of the maxilla, mandible, and hyoid. As a last resort, in cases not amenable to the above measures, tracheotomy can successfully bypass the obstructing pharynx.

NARCOLEPSY

Narcolepsy is a syndrome characterized by excessive daytime sleepiness associated with manifestations related to rapid eye movement (REM) sleep, including cataplexy, sleep paralysis and hypnogogic or hypnopompic hallucinations [14]. The prevalence is estimated at 1/2000 in North American and Western European countries [15]. While genetic factors play a significant role, reflected by a 40-fold increased risk in first degree relatives, other influences are likely present [16]. This is supported by studies in monozygotic twins, demonstrating that when one twin has narcolepsy, the second twin is affected only 25% of the time [15].

The underlying mechanism of narcolepsy is one of instability between wakefulness, non-REM, and REM sleep, whereby an inappropriately low threshold exists to transition between these states [17]. Innervation of wakefulness and sleep (REM vs. non-REM) appear to be distinct. Areas in the brain involved in promoting wakefulness include cholinergic neurons in the laterodorsal and pedunculopontine tegmental nuclei, noradrenergic neurons in the locus ceruleus, serotonergic neurons in the dorsal raphe nuclei, histaminergic neurons in the tuberomamillary nucleus, and perhaps dopaminergic neurons in the periaqueductal gray matter [17]. With one exception, all of these neurons have their highest firing rates during wakefulness, are slower during non-REM sleep, and are silent during REM sleep (the exception being a distinct population of cholinergic neurons which have a high firing rate during REM sleep and are responsible for the generalized muscle atonia associated with this state) [17]. In addition to the high firing rates seen during wakefulness, noradrenergic and serotonergic neurons also inhibit REM sleep-producing neurons during this state [17]. Conversely, gabaergic neurons in the ventrolateral preoptic area are responsible for generating sleep and are specifically most active during non-REM sleep [17]. In addition to actively promoting sleep, these neurons serve to inhibit firing of wake-promoting neurons during this stage [17].

While this mutually inhibitory circuit does aid in consolidating states of sleep and wakefulness, an additional important stabilizing influence is needed. This role is played by orexin, also known as hypocretin, and its recent discovery has dramatically enhanced our understanding of the neurobiology underlying narcolepsy [18]. Orexin is a neuropeptide produced in the posterior and lateral hypothalamus and serves to promote wakefulness and inhibit REM sleep.

It is now believed that narcolepsy develops on the basis of an acquired loss of orexin neurons. Narcoleptic patients with cataplexy have impaired orexin signaling. 90% have low or no detectable orexin-A in their cerebrospinal fluid (CSF), and, with rare exceptions, this is a finding not seen in other neurologic diseases [19]. The explanation for the loss of orexin neurons has not been elucidated. While autoimmune destruction has been proposed as the causative mechanism, there is little evidence to support this theory.

Narcolepsy is characterized primarily by excessive daytime sleepiness and cataplexy. While sleepiness, sleep paralysis, hypnogogic and hypnopomic hallucinations may be seen in patients with various other sleep disorders and in normal individuals, cataplexy is unique to narcolepsy. It represents an abrupt and reversible decrease in or loss of skeletal muscle tone, most frequently elicited by emotional responses such as laughter, anger, or surprise. Most typically, the jaw sags, the head falls forward, the arms drop to the side, and the knees unlock or buckle. Cataplexy reflects the intrusion of REM sleep related muscle atonia into wakefulness [20].

While unequivocal cataplexy may be sufficient to establish a diagnosis of narcolepsy in a pathologically sleepy patient, it is frequently unclear whether the subtle symptoms described by many patients actually represent cataplexy [20]. Accordingly, the diagnosis of narcolepsy should, whenever possible, be confirmed by nocturnal PSG followed immediately by MSLT on the subsequent day [20]. The PSG excludes other etiologies of sleepiness (e.g. sleep disordered breathing, periodic limb movement disorder) and confirms that sufficient sleep (>6 hours) has been obtained on the night before the MSLT. The MSLT permits measurement of mean sleep latency, and documents the presence or absence of sleep onset REM periods (SOREMPs). The presence of 2 or more SOREMPs, in association with a mean sleep latency of <8 minutes is considered diagnostic of narcolepsy [20]. During the week preceeding PSG/MSLT testing, the patient's sleep pattern and adequacy are established through the use of sleep logs or actigraphy (continuously clocked and recorded measurement of body motion by a device generally worn on the wrist, establishing sleep-wake periodicity through detection of sleep-related immobility and wakefulness-related motion). All pharmacological agents that may affect REM sleep or sleepiness are discontinued for an appropriate time period preceeding PSG/MSLT testing so as not to obscure the test results.

Other diagnostic modalities available include human leukocyte antigen (HLA) testing and CSF examination for orexin levels. Almost all patients with narcolepsy with cataplexy show the presence of HLA DQB1*0602, but the finding is of limited diagnostic value given the widespread presence of this marker in individuals without narcolepsy. A negative result is more meaningful clinically (to rule out narcolepsy in equivocal cases) than is a positive result. CSF orexin levels may prove helpful in the future as 90% of patients with narcolepsy with cataplexy have levels below 110 pg/ml.

Behavioral treatment of narcolepsy includes assuring adequate sleep and applying strategically planned naps, but is rarely sufficient to manage the sleepiness [21]. The mainstay of therapy consists of stimulant medications including modafanil, methylphenidate, and methamphetamine [21]. Given the relative lack of side effects of modafanil compared with other stimulants, including minimal, if any, effect on blood pressure and a low potential for addiction and abuse, modafanil is generally considered first line. Medications used in the treatment of cataplexy primarily include antidepressants including fluoxetine, venlafaxine, and clomipramine (among other tricyclic antidepressants), applied primarily for their ability to inhibit the reuptake of norepinephrine and, to a lesser extent, serotonin [21]. While methylphenidate and methamphetamine may possess some mild anti-cataplectic properties, modafanil does not. A new drug, sodium oxybate (which may function through activation of the GABA-B receptor), has been approved by the Food and Drug Administration as treatment for both the EDS and cataplexy associated with narcolepsy. While the compound has shown efficacy, its use is limited by the requirement of a repeat dose 2 to 4 hours after bedtime, the potential for abuse (with a notorious history as the "date rape" drug), and the large salt load that accompanies the medication (requiring caution in the face of renal insufficiency and/or congestive heart failure) [22]. The development of orexin agonists will likely represent a primary goal of future research aimed at improving our armamentarium.

Circadian Rhythm Disturbance: Delayed Sleep Phase

Circadian rhythms are biological cycles that have a length of approximately 24 hours and are generated by an endogenous clock. Examples of physiological variables which fluctuate with this rhythmicity include body temperature, cortisol level, and the sleep-wake cycle. In humans, the "master" internal clock responsible for their timing lies in the suprachiasmatic nucleus (SCN) of the anterior hypothalamus. It has recently additionally been discovered that many tissues and organs generate circadian rhythms independent of the SCN. While circadian rhythms persist regardless of whether external stimuli are present or not, they are generally synchronized, or entrained, with the external environment, primarily through exposure to light. When the sleep-wake cycle is out of synchrony with the external environment, manifestations including fatigue, sleepiness, and insomnia may develop and have a significant negative impact on education, work, mood and social life.

A mismatch between the body's endogenous clock and external environment can lead to inappropriately late sleep and wake times, as in the delayed sleep phase syndrome (DSPS), or inappropriately early sleep and wake times, as in the advanced sleep phase syndrome (ASPS) [23]. With both of these conditions individuals experience a normal quality and duration of sleep with a schedule that is consistent from day to day if circumstances permit. However, if the "natural" bedtime of an individual with DSPS is 3 AM, and the "natural" wake up time is 11 AM, it is easy to understand how sleepiness and fatigue may develop when a school or work schedule requires the individual to awaken at 6 AM. The patient will be deprived of the last 5 hours of his "natural" sleep period. Furthermore, if an attempt is made to force a 10 PM bedtime, in an effort to obtain 8 hours of sleep, insomnia is likely to result as the patient's intrinsic rhythm would favor bedtime at 3AM.

Similar problems with misalignment between the body's internal clock and external environment may occur when the environment itself is drastically changed. One common example is jet lag syndrome, which develops as a result of eastward or westward air travel across multiple time zones. Another example is shift work sleep disorder seen in people working night shifts. Their plight may become further complicated if they attempt to routinely reverse their sleep/wake schedules from daytime sleep on workdays to nighttime sleep on days off.

While a thorough history is imperative in establishing a diagnosis of circadian rhythm disturbance, it is recommended that the diagnosis be supported by sleep logs to accurately document an individual's sleep/wake schedule. Alternatively, this may be more objectively accomplished through the use of actigraphy [24]. Note, however, that actigraphy may not adequately differentiate rest from sleep, nor is it able to differentiate among various stages of sleep [24].

Treatment options for the various circadian rhythm disturbances include chronothereapy, properly timed bright light exposure, and melatonin administration. Chronotherapy refers to a strategy whereby a patient's bedtime is successively delayed (moved clockwise) by 3 hours per night, in the case of DSPS, or advanced by 3 hours per night (moved counter-clockwise) in the cases of ASPS, until the desired bedtime is achieved. The treatment course takes approximately 6-7 days. Bedtime is moved in the directions described because patients with DSPS find it easier to go to bed at a later hour, and those with ASPS prefer an earlier hour.

Light exposure can produce a shift in the endogenous circadian phase by activating the SCN through a direct connection involving the retinohypothalamic tract [25]. Depending on the timing of light exposure, dramatic phase delays or advances may occur. Melatonin, while somewhat less potent than light in its ability to shift the circadian phase, may also be useful, particularly in producing phase advances [25]. Melatonin may also facilitate entrainment to new environments, as in jetlag syndrome and shift work sleep disorder [26]. As with light exposure, it is crucial that melatonin administration be properly timed in each individual to achieve the desired effect [26].

Conclusion

Sleepiness and fatigue are related, but probably distinct, phenomena occurring in diverse sleep and wake disorders. Sleep restriction (inadequate sleep for any reason) may be the problem. On the other hand, sleep may be adequate in quantity, but of poor quality. In some cases, sleep may appear adequate in quantity and quality. In such cases, the problem may lie primarily in mechanisms maintaining *wakefulness* rather than sleep. Morbidity may be intrinsic to the body, lodging within structures housing the mechanisms which maintain sleep and wakefulness (e.g. narcolepsy). On the other hand, it may be intrinsic to the body, but lodging within structures remote from mechanisms which maintain sleep and wakefulness, thereby *indirectly* disrupting those mechanisms (e.g. obstructive sleep apnea syndrome). Finally, interaction between bodily mechanisms and the environment may result in sleepiness and fatigue (e.g. circadian rhythm disturbances). Where does fatigue end and sleepiness begin? Only future work will give us the answer.

References

[1] Shen, J., Barbera, J., & Shapiro, C.M. (2006). Distinguishing sleepiness and fatigue: Focus on definition and measurement. *Sleep Medicine Reviews*, 10,63-76.

[2] Carscadon, M.A., Dement, W.C., Mitler, M.M., Roth, T., Westbrook, P.R., & Keenan, S. (1986). Guidelines for the multiple sleep latency test (MSLT): A standard measure of sleepiness. *Sleep*, 9,519-524.

[3] Johns, M.W. (1991). A new method for measuring daytime sleepiness: the Epworth Sleepiness Scale. *Sleep*, 14,540-545.

[4] Hoddes, E., Zarcone, V., Smythe, H., Phillips, R., & Dement, W.C. (1973). Quantification of sleepiness: A new approach. *Psychophysiology*, 10,431-436.

[5] Durmer, J.S., & Dinges, D.F. (2005). Neurocognitive consequences of sleep deprivation. *Seminars in Neurology*, 1,117-129.

[6] Krupp, L.B., LaRocca, N.G., Muir-Nash, J., & Steinberg, A.D. (1989). The fatigue severity scale: application to patients with multiple sclerosis and systemic lupus erythematosus. *Ach Neurol*, 46,1121-1123.

[7] Chalder, T., Berelowitz, G., Pawlikowska, T., Watts, L., Wessely, S., Wright, D., & Wallace, E.P. (1993). Development of a fatigue scale. *J Psychosom Res*, 37,147-153.

[8] Shapiro, C.M., Flanigan, M., Fleming, J.A.E., Morehouse, R., Moscovitch, A., Plamondon, J., Reinish, L., & Devins, G.M. (2002). Development of an adjective checklist to measure five FACES of fatigue and sleepiness: Data from a national survey of insomniacs. *J Psychosom Res*, 52,467-473.

[9] Neu, D., Mairesse, O., Hoffman, G., Valsamis, J.B., Verbanck, P., Linkowski, P, & Le Bon, O. (2010). Do 'Sleepy' and 'Tired' Go Together? Rasch Analysis of the Relationships between Sleepiness, Fatigue and Nonrestorative Sleep Comlpaints in a Nonclinical Population Sample. *Neuroepidemiology*, 35,1-11.

[10] Young, T., Palta, M., Dempsey, J., Skatrud, J., Weber, S., & Badr, S.(1993). The occurrence of sleep-disordered breathing among middle aged adults. *New Eng J Med*, 328,1230-1235.

[11] International classification of sleep disorders. Second Edition. Westchester, IL: American Academy of Sleep Medicine; 2005; 51-59.

[12] Marcus, C.L. (2000). Pathophysiology of childhood obstructive sleep apnea: Current concepts. *Respir Physiol*, 119,143-154.

[13] Sanders, M.H., & Givelber, R.J. Overview of obstructive sleep apnea in adults. In: Lee-Chiong, T.L., Editor. Sleep: A comprehensive handbook. Hoboken, NJ: Wiley-Liss; 2006; 231-240.

[14] Guilleminault, C., & Fromherz, S. Narcolepsy: diagnosis and treatment. In: Kryger, M.H., Dement, W., & Roth, T., Editors. Principles and Practice of Sleep Medicine. 4th ed. Philadelphia, Pa: Elsevier Saunders; 2005; 780-790.

[15] Hublin, C., Kaprio, J., Partinen, M., Koskenvuo, M., Heikkila, K., Koskimies, S., & Guilleminault, C. (1994). The prevalence of narcolepsy: An epidemiological study of the Finnish twin cohort. *Ann Neurol*, 35,709-716.

[16] Mignot, E. (1998). Genetic and familial aspects of narcolepsy. *Neurology*, 50,S-116-122.

[17] Scammel, T. (2003). The neurobiology, diagnosis and treatment of narcolepsy. *Ann Neurol*, 53,154-166.

[18] Nishino, S., Ripley, B., Overeem, S., Lammers, G.J., & Mignot, E. (2000). Hypocretin (orexin) deficiency in human narcolepsy. *Lancet*, 355,39-40.

[19] Ripley, B., Overeem, S., Fujiki, N., Nevsimalova, S., Uchino, M., Yesavage, J., Di Monte, D., Dohi, K., Melberg, A., Lammers, G.J., Nishida, Y., Roelandse, F.W., Hungs, M., Mignot, E., & Nishino, S. (2001). CSF hypocretin/orexin levels in narcolepsy and other neurologic conditions. *Neurology*, 57,2253-2258.

[20] Aldrich, M.S., Chervin, R.D., & Malow, B.A. (1997). Value of the multiple sleep latency test (MSLT) for the diagnosis of narcolepsy. *Sleep*, 20,620-629.

[21] Mignot, E., & Nishino, S. (2005). Emerging therapies in narcolepsy-cataplexy. *Sleep*, 28,754-763.

[22] Littner, M., Johnson, S.F., McCall, W.V., Anderson, W.M., Davila, D., Hartse, S.K., Kushida, C.A., Wise, M.S., Hirshkowitz, M., Woodson, B.T.; & Standards of Practice Committee. (2001). AASM Standards of Practice Committee. Practice parameters for the treatment of narcolepsy: An update for 2000. Sleep, 24,451-466.

[23] Regestein, Q.R., & Monk, T.H. (1995). Delayed sleep phase syndrome: A review of its clinical aspects. *Am J Psychiatry*, 152,602-608.

[24] Sadeh A, Hauri, P., Kripke, D.F., & Lavie, P. (1995). The role of actigraphy in the evaluation of sleep disorders. Sleep, 18,288-302.

[25] Chesson, A.L. Jr., Wise, M., Davila, D., Johnson, S., Littner, M., Anderson, W.M., Hartse, K., & Rafecas, J. (1999). Practice parameters for the use of light therapy in the treatment of sleep disorders. *Sleep*, 22,641-648.

[26] Mundey, K., Benloucif, S., Harsanyi, K., Dubocovich, M.L., & Zee, P.C. (2005). Phase-dependent treatment of delayed sleep phase syndrome with melatonin. *Sleep*, 28,1271-127.

In: Handbook of Fatigue in Health and Disease
Editor: Howard S. Smith
ISBN 978-1-61761-920-5

Chapter 7

FATIGUE IN HEART DISEASE

Andrew L. Clark[*]

Honorary Consultant Cardiologist, Academic Cardiology
Castle Hill Hospital
Castle Road
Cottingham, Hull HU16 5JQ, UK

ABSTRACT

Heart disease, and particularly chronic heart failure, is intimately linked to the sensation of fatigue. Many factors contribute to fatigue, including the underlying disease processes, associated co-morbid conditions, the central responses to the presence of disease, and drugs used to treat heart disease. Beta blockers, statins and diuretics are particularly likely to be associated with fatigue. Treatment aimed at improving cardiac function may help relieve fatigue, as with positive inotropic drugs (which worsen prognosis) and resynchronisation pacemakers (which improve prognosis). However, aerobic exercise training is far easier to apply widely to cardiac patients and is associated with marked improvement in symptoms in clinical trials. Training might even improve cardiac function, and there are very few patients for whom exercise is not appropriate.

INTRODUCTION

Fatigue is an almost universal symptom in cardiology clinics. Indeed, the presence of fatigue does not seem to be related to the severity of any underlying heart disease, and is often overwhelmingly present in patients in whom there is no detectable pathology. Overwhelmingly present, yet under-researched. It is important to draw a distinction between the general fatigue suffered by many patients as a condition of their daily life ("I'm tired all the time, doctor"), sometimes described as "vital exhaustion", and the symptoms of fatigue

[*] Email: a.l.clark@hull.ac.uk
Phone:+44 1482 624012

that limit exercise. Smith et al defined distinct trajectories of fatigue for exertion fatigue and for general fatigue. Both severe exertion fatigue and severe general fatigue trajectories predicted an increased mortality rate and conversely, the low exertion fatigue trajectory was associated with better survival [1].

There are several possible causes for fatigue in heart disease: 1. the underlying disease processes themselves; 2. associated conditions, such as peripheral vascular disease; 3. a central response to the presence of disease; and 4. drugs used to treat heart disease.

EXERTIONAL FATIGUE

Chronic Heart Failure

Chronic heart failure (CHF) is the cardiac condition *par excellence* associated with exertional fatigue. Unlike for many other diseases, indeed, a defining part of the chronic heart failure syndrome is the presence of symptoms: unless the patient has complained of some symptom, he or she does not have heart failure. I shall focus on chronic heart failure as the exemplar of the relation between cardiac disease and exertional fatigue, as most research has been done in this area. Some of the underlying pathophysiological features apply to other cardiac conditions.

The commonest symptoms in CHF are breathlessness and fatigue. Early notions of the pathophysiology of CHF were that the failing left ventricular myocardium required an ever higher filling pressure to maintain cardiac output. During exercise, the filling pressure rises progressively, ultimately leading to the development of pulmonary oedema as the cost of keeping up cardiac output. At the least, the resulting stiff lungs would cause breathlessness, as would frank fluid in the alveolar spaces. In this understanding of heart failure, fatigue arises from the damaged left ventricle failing to perfuse exercising skeletal muscle. The combination of stiff lungs and reduced muscle perfusion was presumed to result in hypoxia, acidosis and lactate accumulation, causing the sensation of fatigue.

We have shown that there is little physiological difference between those patients with fatigue as their dominant symptom and those with breathlessness [2]. This finding leads to the suggestion that there is a common process underlying both symptoms.

Assessing Symptoms in Chronic Heart Failure

As most symptoms are related to exertion, objective assessment usually takes the form of an exercise test. Corridor walk tests, particularly the six minute walk test, are commonly used and are cheap and simple to administer [3, 4]. A more profound physiological insight can be gained from maximal incremental testing with metabolic gas exchange measurements. The patient exercises with a close fitting mask allowing all expired air to be collected. Ventilation (VE), carbon dioxide production (VCO_2) and oxygen consumption (VO_2) can then be measured. In a typical test in a heart failure patient, the maximal, or peak, VO_2 is reduced and the slope of the relation between ventilation and carbon dioxide production (VE/VCO_2 slope) is increased. Thus, for any given level of carbon dioxide production, the ventilatory response is greater for a heart failure patient (See Figure 1).

A variety of different protocols, both treadmill and cycle, has been used in heart failure research. To help to try and analyse symptoms, some modification of the Borg score is often used with patients asked to score their symptoms at the end of each stage.

Maximal incremental testing is a highly abnormal test in the sense that most patients simply don't perform this type of exercise in daily life. Nevertheless, it is interesting to note that the exercise responses are abnormal from the onset of exercise – thus, for instance, the increased VE/VCO_2 slope is apparent from the beginning. Peak VO_2 is a useful measurement in clinical practice, for example, in helping to define the patient population with most to gain from cardiac transplantation and for stratifying prognosis [5-7].

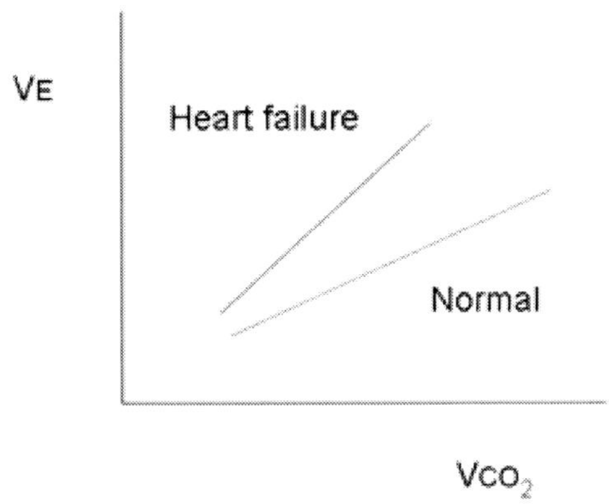

Figure 1. Ventilatory response to exercise. VE is ventilation and VCO_2 is carbon dioxide production. Note that in the heart failure patient, the slope of the line is steeper, so that for any given level of carbon dioxide production, the ventilatory response is greater.

A first observation that can be made is that different exercise testing regimes result in different symptoms. Lipkin et al. [8] showed that more rapidly incremental tests were likely to be terminated by breathlessness, whereas a slower test, although patients reached the same peak VO_2, was more likely to be terminated by fatigue. This is despite the fact that pulmonary capillary wedge pressure was the same in both exercise tests. However, in the rapid tests, patients had a greater fall in arterial pH and a higher lactate level at peak exercise, suggesting that the sensation of breathlessness might be mediated by stimulation of peripheral chemoreceptors.

Cycle exercise is more often stopped by fatigue than breathlessness [9] and we have shown that cycle exercise in heart failure patients is associated with a lower VE/VCO_2 slope than treadmill exercise, despite similar peak oxygen consumption [10]. Thus the sensation of breathlessness appears to be related to the ventilatory response to exercise rather than to the level of exercise *per se*. Fatigue is the sensation left when breathlessness is not prominent.

Origin of Symptoms in CHF

Why are patients with heart failure limited? At first sight, this seems a simple question: impaired cardiac output causes impaired exercise capacity. However, many studies have shown that there is no correlation between indices of cardiac function at rest and exercise performance [11, 12]. More tellingly, acute changes in haemodynamics, either pharmacological [9] or by cardiac transplantation [13], do not affect exercise performance.

The central nervous system can be abnormal in chronic heart failure with accelerated cognitive decline [14]. This appears to be related to a decline in cerebral vasoreactivity [15], and the degree of impairment is related to both the severity of left ventricular dysfunction and the level of symptoms. Thus more severely fatigued patients have worse cerebral perfusion [15], and the impairment in cerebral perfusion and fatigue can be corrected by heart transplantation [16]. Part of the fatigue problem might therefore be related to impaired cerebral perfusion.

There are pulmonary changes in chronic heart failure, and there has been much debate as to the relevance of the changes to exercise performance. There appears to be some increase in dead space ventilation, with consequent "inefficient" ventilation, although the significance of this has been questioned [17]. One difficulty with accepting that abnormal pulmonary function and metabolic gas exchange is responsible for symptoms is the observation that during exercise, patients with chronic heart failure have partial pressures of carbon dioxide lower, and oxygen higher, than normal subjects [18]: in other words, what signal could the body be sensing that caused breathlessness or fatigue if gas exchange is the problem?

More recently, attention has focussed on the periphery as the source of heart failure symptoms. A key observation is that patients without peripheral changes have near normal exercise capacity, despite severely impaired left ventricular function [19]. In particular, skeletal muscle has been investigated intensively as the factor limiting exercise performance [20].

Skeletal Muscle in CHF

Skeletal muscle in CHF is abnormal. Early in the progression of the disease, there is loss of muscle bulk [21], and exercise capacity is related to both muscle strength and bulk [22]. Muscle strength is reduced [23], as is endurance [24]. From a the patient's point of view, the ability to perform repeated submaximal exercise is more important than peak force generation, and early quadriceps fatiguability has been reported [24, 25]. The reduction in endurance correlates with exercise performance [25].

Fatigue appears to be independent of acute changes in blood flow [24, 27] and of central factors [26]. Fatiguability has been shown in a very small muscle group [22] in which blood flow is unlikely to be limited by cardiac reserve, suggesting that intrinsic muscle factors mediate fatiguability of muscle.

Skeletal muscle becomes histologically abnormal with a shift towards type II muscle fibres [25, 28]. Mitochondrial structure is abnormal [29], with a reduction in volume of the cristae, and there are reductions in enzyme content, particularly of the enzymes of the Kreb's cycle and in the oxidative chain [30, 31]. The changes in muscle structure and ultrastructure are reflected in changes in muscle metabolism. Magnetic resonance spectroscopy can be used to examine intracellular phosphate metabolism, which has been shown to be abnormal in chronic heart failure with more rapid depletion of phosphocreatine and early acidosis compared with normal [32, 33].

These changes could be related to the sensation of fatigue. Ultimately, that sensation is generated centrally, and it is possible that there is some biochemical released by fatigued muscle that causes the perception. In chronic heart failure, for example, early lactic acidosis and a lower than normal anaerobic threshold have been described [34, 35]. However, Wilson et al showed that reduction in lactate by dichloroacetate infusion had no effect on exercise performance [36].

We found evidence for neural signalling from skeletal muscle that at least in part is responsible for driving the ventilatory response to exercise. In normal subjects, leg exercise with a cuff inflated to suprasystolic blood pressure around the thighs caused an increase in V_E/V_{CO_2} slope [37]. Arm exercise at the same workload causes an increase in V_E/V_{CO_2} slope [36]. It is difficult to explain this other than by invoking a neural pathway. Exercising muscle in some way detects activity and sends a neural signal to the central nervous system that in turn modifies ventilatory responses to exercise.

The Ergoreflex

Ergoreceptors in skeletal muscle respond to work performed and transmit a signal [38], transmitted to the lateral spinothalamic tracts via small unmyelinated or poorly myelinated fibres [39]. Their stimulation is responsible in part for mediating adrenergic activation during exercise [40-42].

Piepoli and co-workers used arm exercise to assess the ergoreflex contribution to the ventilatory response to exercise [42]. Subjects exercised to exhaustion using a hand-grip dynamometer. At peak exercise, a cuff was inflated to suprasystolic pressure around the exercising arm, thereby entrapping the metabolic products of exercise in the forearm. Metabolic gas exchange and other variables can then be measured during the recovery period, and compared with recovery from a separate bout of exercise without cuff inflation (See Figure 2).

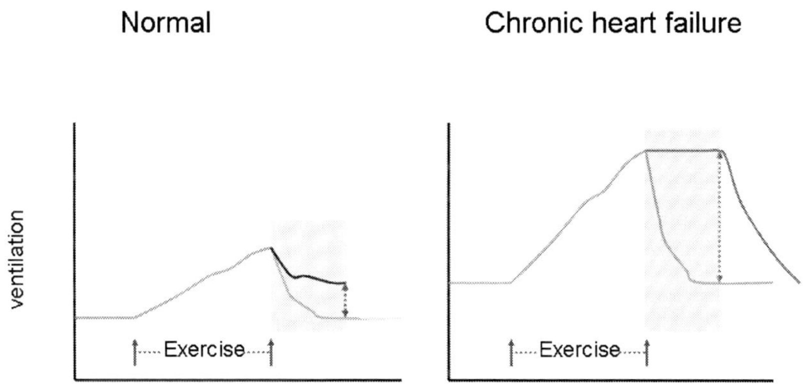

Figure 2. The ergoreflex. Ventilation is measured continuously and increases during exertion. At peak exercise a cuff is inflated for the initial recovery period (dark blue line) or not (green line). The difference in ventilation after 3 minutes can be used to quantify the ergoreflex response. Note that in heart failure the initial ventilatory response is greater, and the ergoreflex contribution to ventilation more marked.

In patients with chronic heart failure, there appears to be a much enhanced ergoreflex response to exercise [43, 44], and the degree of ergoreflex activation correlates strongly with the degree of functional limitation [45]. Piepoli was further able to show that the signal was related to the degree of metabolic stimulation of receptors rather than simply being a mechanoreceptor response [46]. It thus seems the case that the skeletal muscle in heart failure patients sends an abnormal signal to the central nervous system. It is not an overly sensitive response to limb movement, but rather an increased response to metabolic stimulation. This could be due to increased sensitivity to a given stimulus, or an increase in the stimulus *per se*.

Possible stimuli are likely to be products of metabolism, such as hydrogen ion. In a series of experiments involving infusions of different test chemicals, Scott *et al* showed that reducing hydrogen ion concentration with bicarbonate reduced the ergoreflex response to arm exercise [47]. Direct measurement of blood draining the exercising limb suggested that prostaglandins may also have a role in ergoreflex activation [48].

Respiratory Muscle

The muscles of respiration are also abnormal in chronic heart failure. There is increased diaphragmatic work and accessory muscle deoxygenation [49, 50], and reduced respiratory muscle strength [51, 52]. These findings may, in part, explain the similarity of the sensation of fatigue and that of shortness of breath.

Origins of Muscle Changes

How does skeletal muscle come to be abnormal in heart failure? The changes must ultimately be related to the heart failure syndrome itself, and the obvious candidate is decreased peripheral perfusion. The oxygen saturation in veins draining exercising muscle of heart failure patients can be very low indeed [53, 54], suggesting that the system is limited by the failure of the circulation to deliver oxygen to the tissues.

The peripheral resistance is greatly increased in heart failure patients [55], but the relation between blood flow and exercise capacity is complex. Acute changes in blood flow induce no change in lactate production at matched workload, highlighting the possible distinction between "nutritive flow" and mere blood flow [56]. Some patients have normal blood flow, but abnormal metabolism [57].

Some of the pathophysiology of chronic heart failure is similar to the effects of de-training in normal subjects. Common to both are skeletal muscle wasting and depletion of oxidative enzymes [58, 59] and activation of the sympathetic [60] and renin-angiotensin [61] systems. However, disuse is unlikely to be the only contributor to muscle changes. In normals undergoing de-training, there is little evidence of the fibre-type shift seen in heart failure, and as the heart failure muscle changes are seen in small muscles unlikely to be affected by disuse, there is likely to be a systemic cause for the heart failure myopathy.

Anabolic-Catabolic Imbalance in Chronic Heart Failure

Far from being a "haemodynamic" disease, heart failure is increasingly recognised to be a multisystem disease with changes in most body systems studied. Cardiac cachexia has been recognised since the time of Hippocrates [62], and has latterly been shown to be associated with a particularly poor outcome [63]. As previously noted, loss of muscle bulk happens early in the course of heart failure [21] and, indeed, excess weight is associated with improved survival [64]. The weight loss appears to affect all body compartments [65].

Although the cause is not known, there is a general change in the balance between catabolic and anabolic factors in the chronic heart failure syndrome. Thus, for example, mass sympathetic stimulation (as seen in heart failure) is catabolic, causes an increase in the basal metabolic rate [66, 67], causes glycogenolysis, both through a direct effect and via inhibition of insulin secretion and promotion of glucagon secretion [68], and lipolysis [69].

Insulin is a vital anabolic hormone, and insulin resistance is common in heart failure patients [70, 71]. The insulin resistance is characterised by high circulating levels of insulin, and normal fasting glucose. Insulin levels appear to be higher in heart failure patients with cachexia than in those without [72], and body mass index is related to the degree of insulin resistance [73]. Similarly, the catabolic steroid cortisol can be grossly elevated in untreated patients with chronic heart failure, and the anabolic steroid precursor, DHEA is low [72]. There is thus a rise in the *ratio* of cortisol to DHEA in chronic heart failure patients [74, 75], which correlates negatively with body mass index (the higher the BMI, the lower the ratio of catabolic to anabolic steroid). Growth hormone resistance is also common [76].

Fatigue in Chronic Heart Failure

We can now formulate a general path by which chronic heart failure might lead to fatigue (and breathlessness) (See Figure 3). The catabolic responses caused by many insults to the internal milieu, which have evolved to mobilise resources to deal with damage, are persistently activated as the original stimulus, heart failure, persists. The alteration in catabolic:anabolic balance leads to skeletal muscle changes, in some patients amounting to a myopathy.

The abnormal skeletal muscle in turn is limited in its capacity to perform work. It signals its distress to the central nervous system via the ergoreflex, a reflex system responsive to the metabolic products of exercise. Under some circumstances, the signal is interpreted as breathlessness and in others as fatigue.

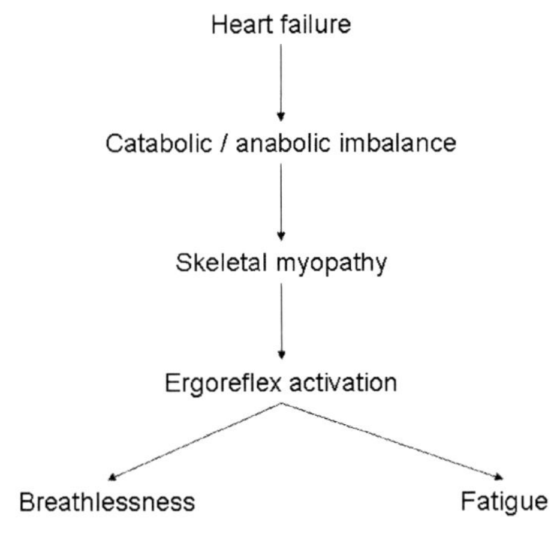

Figure 3. Schematic representation of the origin of fatigue and breathlessness in chronic heart failure.

Ischaemic Heart Disease

Vital Exhaustion

"Vital exhaustion" is a psychological state characterized by unusual fatigue, irritability, and feelings of demoralization. Women report more fatigue than men as a manifestation of acute coronary syndromes [77, 78]. This may be related to personality type, with a type D ("distressed") personality more prone to "vital exhaustion", and women more likely to be classified as type D personalities [79]. Interestingly, in this study of patients with chronic stable angina, improving the angina had no effect on symptoms of exhaustion [79]. The effects of psychological well-being on fatigue are difficult to disentangle: depression correlates with fatigue in patients with stable ischaemic heart disease, but correlation cannot tell which (if either) causes the other [80].

The presence of fatigue as a prominent symptom is predictive of a worse symptomatic outcome following treatment for coronary disease, both with coronary artery bypass surgery [81] and coronary artery angioplasty [82]. Fatigue is very weakly associated with the burden of atherosclerotic disease, but is much more closely related to adverse outcomes following intervention [82]. The absence of fatigue is related to the ability to return to employment following bypass surgery [83]. Fatigue is also related to the risk of development of coronary disease [84]. In a population of patients with risk factors for coronary disease, raised levels of TNFα and interleukin -10 were associated with fatigue. [85] For an interesting discussion of the relation between coronary disease and vital exhaustion, see reference [86].

The limiting symptom doesn't appear to alter the exercise performance of patients with coronary disease, whether it is angina, fatigue or breathlessness [87].

Other Heart Disease

Other heart diseases are associated with exhaustion. Arrhythmia, particularly sustained atrial fibrillation, can reduce exercise tolerance; the underlying pathophysiology is presumably similar to that underlying fatigue in heart failure. Valvular heart disease and pericardial disease, such as constrictive pericarditis, cause fatigue, again presumably by the same mechanism. Occasional patients with complete heart block present with fatigue, presumably due to low cardiac output.

Some patients with a permanent pacemaker develop a symptom cluster collectively known as "pacemaker syndrome". Some authorities believe that the syndrome can arise when a patient has normal atrial electrical activity but asynchronous right ventricular pacing. The mechanism is believed to be loss of the normal contribution of atrial transport to cardiac output, and thus some of the mechanisms invoked to explain fatigue in heart failure come into play. In addition, symptoms can be caused by atrial contraction against a closed atrio-ventricular valve. Fatigue can be a prominent part of the syndrome [88, 89], but its true frequency (given the vagueness and lack of specificity of its symptoms) is unclear [90].

Patients with infective endocarditis often have profound fatigue as part of their presentation, but the diagnosis is usually suggested by other features such as fever, peripheral stigmata of endocarditis and the presence of heart murmurs. An exception can be endocarditis due to *Coxiella burnetti* which can cause profound fatigue with little else initially to suggesting the underlying diagnosis [91]. There has been some suggestion that atherosclerotic disease might be related to chronic infection, particularly by *Chlamydia* [92], which might be related to the vital exhaustion suffered by some patients. However, support for the hypothesis is waning [93], particularly given the disappointing results of intervention trials [94].

MEDICAL THERAPY

Many of the drugs used for treating heart disease are said to cause fatigue. The most widely known are the beta adrenoceptor antagonists (β blockers).

β Bblockers

β blockers are a heterogenous group of drugs with different pharmacological properties. The earliest agents were non-selective, blocking both the predominantly cardiac β_1 receptors and the peripheral β_2 receptors. β_1-selective blockade may reduce cardiac output, and consequently both cerebral and peripheral perfusion; β_2-selective blockade causes vasoconstriction, and may thereby reduce peripheral perfusion.

Fatigue is said to be very common with β blockade. This is of major importance when considering β blockers for conditions such as hypertension which of themselves don't cause symptoms. Thus, for example, calculations from the MRC hypertension trial results [95] suggest that for every heart attack or stroke prevented, seven patients withdrew from the trial because of fatigue [96]. However, despite the widespread perception of β blockers as being a major factor in causing fatigue, meta-analysis of randomized trials suggest that although fatigue is present, the incidence is low and is equivalent to 1 additional report of fatigue for every 57 patients treated per year with β-blockers [97]. It's important to note here that the frequency of fatigue was very high in both β blocker and placebo groups (33.4% and 30.4% respectively) [97].

In patients being treated for angina, higher doses of β-blocker are more likely to cause fatigue without necessarily improving symptoms [98]. The β blocker, celiprolol, which has β_1-selective antagonist, but β_2-selective agonist properties, is a peripheral vasodilator. It causes less fatigue than conventional β blockers [99]. Verapamil produces less fatigue than propranolol in patients with chronic stable angina on treadmill testing [100]. These findings suggest that the mechanism of fatigue is, at least in part, related to the effects on the peripheral circulation rather than to a reduction in cardiac output.

The relation between medication and fatigue may be of less importance when the β blockers are being prescribed for more serious illness: in chronic heart failure, fatigue might be the commonest cause for withdrawal of β blocker therapy, but that only affects fewer than 10% of patients [101]. Clinical trials of carvedilol in patients with very severe heart failure have shown that the withdrawal rate from the treated group was lower than for the placebo group [102, 103]. The overall effect of β blockers in heart failure is to improve symptoms [104-106].

Statins

The cholesterol-reducing drugs, HMGCoA reductase inhibitors, or statins, are becoming very widely prescribed. There is a general belief that these are "miracle drugs" that will prevent most heart disease, but there are some sceptical voices. Very few patients continue to take statins long term [107], and even in clinical trials, many patients drop out due to side-effects. In the Heart Protection Study, one third of patients dropped out in the run-in phase [108]. Common side-effects are muscle pains, but also a more generalised fatigue.

Statins reduce the body content of coenzyme Q10 [109]. Use of coenzyme Q10 dramatically reduces the incidence of fatigue following myocardial infarction [110].

There is also some evidence that statins can affect cognitive function, also perhaps via their effect on coenzyme Q10. There is some evidence at least that the adverse effects of statins can be mitigated by coenzyme Q10 supplements [111].

Other Drugs

Almost all cardiovascular drugs can be associated with fatigue in some patients. Diuretics can cause fatigue, possibly in association with biochemical alterations (particularly hyponatraemia and hypokalaemia. Acetazolamide, used to treat altitude sickness, increases fatigue, perhaps by slowing carbon dioxide production and acidosis [112]. Torasemide is less associated with fatigue than furosmide in heart failure patients [113].

Treatment of Fatigue in Chronic Heart Failure

Drug treatment in the modern era of heart failure management has primarily been aimed at addressing mortality as a clinical end-point, rather than symptom relief, and few trials have looked specifically at fatigue.

Much of the reason for this comes from disappointing experience with positive inotropic agents. These drugs improve the contractile function of the heart, and appear thereby to relieve fatigue, but have uniformly demonstrated an adverse effect on outcome [114-116]. There has been much subsequent debate about whether in an individual patient's case, it might be justifiable to give an agent to improve symptoms even though it might shorten life [117].

The drugs most commonly prescribed for chronic heart failure are angiotensin converting enzyme inhibitors (ACEi) and β blockers (discussed above). ACEi have a vasodilating effect, but the effect need not necessarily underlie their mortality benefit. Indeed, other vasodilators, such as hydralazine-nitrate combination, may have a greater *symptomatic* benefit than ACEi, but are less effective in reducing mortality [118]. This leads to the suggestion that whilst vasodilation may improve symptoms, it is the neurohormonal effects of ACEi that improve outcome. ACEi inhibitors do improve symptoms, but require some months before their full effect is apparent [119].

The muscle hypothesis for the generation of symptoms in chronic heart failure offers some possible therapeutic options. Exercise training regimes, aimed at improving skeletal muscle function rather than central haemodynamic function, can improve exercise capacity [120, 121] which persists for up to a year if the training continues [122]. Importantly, training improves patient well-being scores and reduces symptoms [121-123]. Training induces no great change in haemodynamics, but improves skeletal muscle functioning [124] and causes the ergoreflex activation to return towards normal [43]. Although a meta-analysis of early small-scale studies suggested that training might improve prognosis, [125] the HF-ACTION study in 2331 patients with chronic heart failure randomized to training or usual care did not show any convincing effect of training on the outcome of all-cause mortality or hospitalization [126]. However, there was a striking improvement in quality of life seen from early in the course of the study and persisting for the three years of follow up, [127] lending powerful support to the idea that exercise training programmes have much to offer patients with chronic heart failure.

More recently, there has been a return to a more haemodynamics-focused strategy. The technique of biventricular pacing offers potential benefits to patients with chronic heart failure and very broad QRS complexes on the surface electrocardiogram. In addition to conventional pacing leads implanted in the right ventricular apex and the right atrial appendage, a third lead is manipulated via the coronary sinus into a vein draining the left ventricle (See Figure 4). This lead can then be used to deliver a pacing stimulus synchronous with the right ventricular apex, thus "resynchronising" the heart. Resynchronisation improves exercise tolerance and quality of life in ambulatory patients with severe symptoms [128]. In some patients, there can be a dramatic symptomatic benefit, even in those who are dependent upon continuous infusion of positive inotropic drugs [129]. Recent evidence demonstrates a profound mortality benefit from resynchronization therapy, too [130].

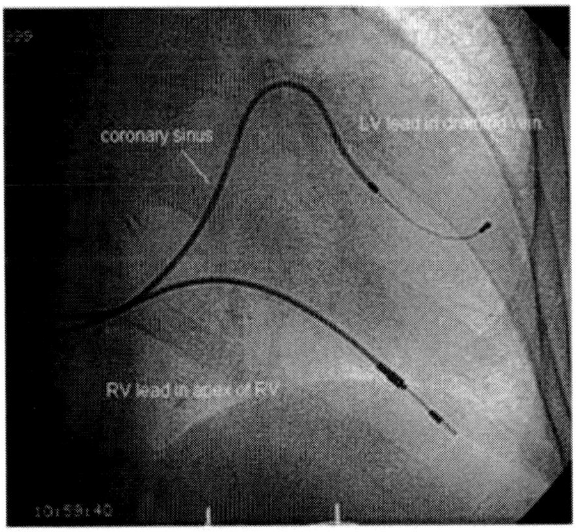

Figure 4. A biventricular pacing system in situ. The course of the two ventricular leads is labelled.

A more dramatic possibility for very symptomatic patients is the left ventricular assist device (LVAD). There is some evidence that in patients with end-stage heart failure LVADs provide a mortality benefit [131]. In selected cases, there is no doubt that an LVAD can result in dramatic resolution of heart failure symptoms, including fatigue [132]. The most intractable problem with LVADs has been that of drive line infection, but that now seems to have been addressed, and LVADs as "destination therapy" [133] are likely to be developed further and become more widespread.

Conclusion

Fatigue is an almost universal symptom of heart disease. It is most prevalent in patients with chronic heart failure. The pathophysiological processes underlying fatigue are not clearly delineated, but involve an initial haemodynamic insult resulting in complex peripheral changes, particularly to skeletal muscle. In turn, abnormal skeletal muscle causes abnormal signalling to the central nervous system during exercise, resulting in the perception of fatigue.

Successful treatment of cardiac fatigue has usually been based around training skeletal muscle; pharmacological treatment aimed at improving cardiac function has been unsuccessful. More recently, haemodynamic improvement with device therapy has enjoyed much success, and is likely to be much more widely used.

References

[1] Smith O.R., Kupper, N, de Jonge, P. & Denollet, J. (2010). Distinct trajectories of fatigue in chronic heart failure and their association with prognosis. *Eur J Heart Fail*, In Press.

[2] Clark, A.L., Sparrow, J.L., & Coats, A.J.S. (1995). Muscle fatigue and dyspnoea in chronic heart failure: two sides of the same coin? *Eur Heart J*, 16,49-52.

[3] Olsson, L.G., Swedberg, K., Clark, A.L., Witte, K.K., & Cleland JG. (2005). Six minute corridor walk test as an outcome measure for the assessment of treatment in randomized, blinded intervention trials of chronic heart failure: a systematic review. *Eur Heart J*, 26,778-793.

[4] Ingl, L., Shelton, R.J., Rigby, A.S., Nabb, S., Clark, A.L., & Cleland, J.G. (2005). The reproducibility and sensitivity of the 6-min walk test in elderly patients with chronic heart failure. *Eur Heart J*, 26,1742-1751.

[5] Szlachcic, J., Massie, B.M., Kramer, B.L., Topic, N., & Tubau J. (1985). Correlates and prognostic implication of exercise capacity in chronic congestive heart failure. *Am J Cardiol*, 55,1037-1042.

[6] Cohn, J.N., Johnson, G.R., Shabetai, R., Loeb, H., Tristani, F., Rector, T., Smith, R., & Fletcher, R. (1993). Ejection fraction, peak exercise oxygen consumption, cardiothoracic ratio, ventricular arrhythmias, and plasma norepinephrine as determinants of prognosis in heart failure. The V-HeFT VA Cooperative Studies Group. *Circulation.*, 87,VI5-16.

[7] Parameshwar, J., Keegan, J., Sparrow, J., Sutton, G.C., & Poole-Wilson, P.A. (1992). Predictors of prognosis in severe chronic heart failure. *Am Heart J*, 123,421-426.

[8] Lipkin, D.P., Canepa-Anson, R., Stephens, M.R., & Poole-Wilson, P.A. (1986). Factors determining symptoms in heart failure: comparison of fast and slow exercise tests. Br Heart J, 55,439-445.

[9] Fink, L.I., Wilson, J.R., & Ferraro, N. (1986). Exercise ventilation and pulmonary artery wedge pressure in chronic stable congestive heart failure. *Am J Cardiol*, 57,249-253.

[10] Witte, K.K.A., & Clark, A.L. (2005). Cycle exercise causes a lower ventilatory response to exercise in chronic heart failure. *Heart*, 91,225-226.

[11] Franciosa, J.A., Park, M., & Levine, T.B. (1981). Lack of correlation between exercise capacity and indexes of resting left ventricular performance in heart failure. Am J Cardiol, 47,33-39.

[12] Clark, A.L., Swan, J.W., Laney, R., Connelly, M., Somerville, J., & Coats, A.J. (1994). The Role of right and left ventricular function in the ventilatory response to exercise in chronic heart failure. *Circulation*, 89,2062-2069.

[13] Marzo, K.P., Wilson, J.R., & Mancini, D.M. (1992). Effects of cardiac transplantation on ventilatory response to exercise. *Am J Cardiol*, 69,547-553.

[14] Zuccala, G., Cattel, C., Manes-Gravina, E., Di Niro, M.G., Cocchi, A., & Bernabei, R. (1997). Left ventricular dysfunction : a clue to cognitive impairment in older patients with heart failure. *J Neurol Neurosurg Psychiatry*, 63,509–512.

[15] Georgiadis, D., Sievert, M., Cencetti, S., Uhlmann, F., Krivokuca, M., Zierz, S., & Werdan, K.. (2000). Cerebrovascular reactivity is impaired in patients with cardiac failure. *Eur Heart J*, 21,407–413.

[16] Gruhn, N., Larsen, F.S., Boesgaard, S., Knudsenm G.M., Mortensen, S.A., Thomas, G., & Aldershvile, J. (2001). Cerebral blood flow in patients with chronic heart failure before and after heart transplantation. *Stroke*, 32,2530-2533.

[17] Clark, A.L., Chua, T.P., & Coats, A.J.S. (1995). Anatomical dead space, ventilatory pattern and exercise capacity in chronic heart failure. *Br Heart J*, 74,377-380.

[18] Clark, A.L., & Coats, A.J.S. (1994). Usefulness of arterial blood gas estimations during exercise in patients with chronic heart failure. *Br Heart J*, 71,528-530.

[19] Harrington, D., Anker, S.D., & Coats, A.J. (2001). Preservation of exercise capacity and lack of peripheral changes in asymptomatic patients with severely impaired left ventricular function. *Eur Heart J*, 22,392-399.

[20] Clark, A.L., Poole-Wilson, P.A., & Coats, A.J.S. (1996). Exercise limitation in chronic heart failure: The central role of the periphery. *J Am Coll Cardiol*, 28,1092-1102.

[21] Mancini, D.M., Walter, G., Reichnek, N., Lenkinski, R., McCully, K.K., Mullen, J.L., Wilson, J.R. (1992). Contribution of skeletal muscle atrophy to exercise intolerance and altered muscle metabolism in heart failure. *Circulation*, 85,1364-1373.

[22] Volterrani, M., Clark, A.L., Ludman, P.F., Swan, J.W., Adamopoulos, S., Piepoli, M., & Coats, A.J. (1994). Predictors of exercise capacity in chronic heart failure. *Eur Heart J*, 15,801-809.

[23] Buller, N.P., Jones, D., & Poole-Wilson, P.A. (1991). Direct measurements of skeletal muscle fatigue in patients with chronic heart failure. *Br Heart J*, 65,20-24.

[24] Minotti, J.R., Pillay, P., Chang, L., Wells, L., & Massie, B.M. (1992). Neurophysiological assessment of skeletal muscle fatigue in patients with congestive heart failure. Circulation, 86,903-908.

[25] Lipkin, D., Jones, D., Round, J., & Poole-Wilson, P. (1988). Abnormalities of skeletal muscle in patients with chronic heart failure. *Int J Cardiol*, 18,187-195.

[26] Wilson, J.R., Mancini, D.M., & Simson, M. (1992). Detection of skeletal muscle fatigue in patients with heart failure using electromyography. *Am J Cardiol*, 70,488-493.

[27] Minotti, J.R., Christoph, I., Oka, R., Weiner, M.W., Wells, L., & Massie, B.M. (1991). Impaired skeletal muscle function in patients with congestive heart failure. Relationship to systemic exercise performance. *J Clin Invest*, 88,2077-2082.

[28] Mancini, D.M., Coyle, E., Coggan, A., Beltz, J., Ferraro, N., Montain, S., & Wilson, J.R. (1989). Contribution of intrinsic skeletal muscle changes to 31P NMR skeletal muscle abnormalities in patients with chronic heart failure. *Circulation*, 80,1338-1346.

[29] Drexler, H., Riede, U., Munzel, T., König, H., Funke, E., & Just, H. (1992). Alterations of skeletal muscle in chronic heart failure. *Circulation*, 85,1751-1759.

[30] Wilson, J.R., Martin, J.L., & Ferraro, N. (1984). Impaired skeletal muscle nutritive flow during exercise in patients with congestive heart failure: role of cardiac pump dysfunction as determined by the effect of dobutamine. *Am J Cardiol*, 53,1308-1315.

[31] Sullivan, M.J., Green, H.J., & Cobb, F.R. (1990). Skeletal muscle biochemistry and histology in ambulatory patients with long-term heart failure. *Circulation*, 81,518-527.

[32] Massie, B.M., Conway, M., Yonge, R., Frostick, S., Ledingham, J., Sleight, P., Radda, G., & Rajagopalan, B. (1987). Skeletal muscle metabolism in patients with congestive heart failure: relation to clinical severity and blood flow. *Circulation*, 76,1009-1019.

[33] Massie, B.M., Conway, M., Yonge, R., Frostick, S., Sleight, P., Ledingham, J., Radda, G., & Rajagopalan, B. (1987). 31P nuclear magnetic resonance evidence of abnormal skeletal muscle metabolism in patients with congestive heart failure. *Am J Cardiol*, 60,309-315.

[34] Reddy, H.K., Weber, K.T., Janicki, J.S., & McElroy, P.A. (1988). Hemodynamic, ventilatory and metabolic effects of light isometric exercise in patients with chronic heart failure. *J Am Coll Cardiol*, 12,353-358.

[35] Weber, K.T., Wilson, J.R., Janicki, J.S., & Likoff, M.J. (1984). Exercise testing in the evaluation of the patient with chronic cardiac failure. *Am Rev Respir Dis*, 129,S60-S62.

[36] Wilson, J.R., Mancini, D.M., Ferraro, N., & Egler, J. (1988). Effect of dichloroacetate on the exercise performance of patients with heart failure. *J Am Coll Cardiol*, 12,1464-1469.

[37] Clark, A.L., Piepoli, M., & Coats, A.J.S.(1995). Skeletal muscle and the control of ventilation on exercise; evidence for metabolic receptors. *Eur J Clin Invest*, 25,299-305.

[38] Rowell, L.B., & O'Learly, D.S. (1990). Reflex control of the circulation during exercise: chemoreflexes and mechanoreflexes. *J Appl Physiol*, 69,407-418.

[39] McCloskey, D.I., & Mitchell, J.H. (1972). Reflex cardiovascular and respiratory responses originating in exercising muscle. *J Physiol*, 224,173-187.

[40] Hultman, E., & Sjoholm, H. (1982). Blood pressure and heart rate response to voluntary and nonvoluntary static exercise in man. *Acta Physiol Scand*, 115,499-501.

[41] Gandevia, S.C., & Hobbs, S.F. (1990). Cardiovascular responses to static exercise in man: central and reflex contributions. *J Physiol*, 430,105-117.

[42] Piepoli, M., Clark, A.L., & Coats, A.J.S. (1995). Muscle metaboreceptors in the hemodynamic, autonomic and ventilatory responses to exercise in man. *Am J Physiol*, 269,H1428-436.
[43] Piepoli, M., Clark, A.L., Volterrani, M., Adamopoulos, S., Sleight, P., & Coats, A.J. (1996). Contribution of muscle afferents to the hemodynamic, autonomic, and ventilatory responses to exercise in patients with chronic heart failure: effects of physical training. *Circulation*, 93,940-952.
[44] Grieve, D.A.A., Clark, A.L., McCann, G.P., & Hillis, W.S. (1999). The Ergoreflex in patients with chronic stable heart failure. *Int J Cardiol*, 68,157-164.
[45] Piepoli, M., Ponikowski, P., Clark, A.L., Banasiak, W., Capucci, A., & Coats, A.J. (1999). A neural link to explain the "muscle hypothesis" of exercise intolerance in chronic heart failure. *Am Heart J*,137,1050-1056.
[46] Scott, A.C.., Francis, D.P., Davies, L.C., Ponikowski, P., Coats, A.J., & Piepoli, M.F. (2000). Contribution of skeletal muscle 'ergoreceptors' in the human leg to respiratory control in chronic heart failure. *J Physiol*, 529,863-870.
[47] Scott, A.C., Wensel, R., Davos, C.H., Georgiadou, P., Kemp, M., Hooper, J., Coats, A.J., & Piepoli, M.F. (2003). Skeletal muscle reflex in heart failure patients: role of hydrogen. *Circulation*, 107,300-306.
[48] Scott, A.C., Wensel, R., Davos, C.H., Kemp, M., Kaczmarek, A., Hooper, J., Coats, A.J., & Piepoli, M.F. (2002). Chemical mediators of the muscle ergoreflex in chronic heart failure: a putative role for prostaglandins in reflex ventilatory control. *Circulation*, 106,214-220.
[49] Mancini, D.M., Ferraro, N., Nazzaro, D., Chance. B., & Wilson, J.R. (1991). Respiratory muscle deoxygenation during exercise in patients with heart failure demonstrated with near-infrared spectroscopy. *J Am Coll Cardiol*, 18,492-498.
[50] Mancini, D.M., Henson, D., LaManca, J., & Levine, S. (1992). Respiratory muscle function and dyspnea in patients with chronic congestive heart failure. *Circulation*, 86,909-919.
[51] Hammond, M.D., Bauer, K.A., Sharp, J.T., & Rocha, R.D. (1990). Respiratory muscle strength in congestive heart failure. *Chest*, 98,1091-1094.
[52] McParland, C., Krishnan, B., Wang, Y., & Gallagher, C.G. (1992). Inspiratory muscle weakness and dyspnea in chronic heart failure. *Am Rev Respir Dis*, 146,467-472.
[53] Herrlin, B., & Sylven, C. (1991). Increased arterial oxygen content - an important compensatory mechanism in chronic moderate heart failure. *Cardiovasc Res*, 25,384-390.
[54] Clark, A.L., Volterrani, M., Swan, J.W., Hue, D., Hooper, J., & Coats, A.J.(1996). Leg blood flow, metabolism and exercise capacity in chronic stable heart failure. Int J Cardiol, 55,127-135.
[55] LeJemtel, T.H., Maskin, C.S., Lucido, D., & Chadwick, B.J. (1986). Failure to augment maximal limb blood flow in response to one-leg versus two-leg exercise in patients with severe heart failure. *Circulation*, 74,245-251.
[56] Wilson, J.R., Martin, J.L., & Ferraro, N. (1984). Impaired skeletal muscle nutritive flow during exercise in patients with congestive heart failure: role of cardiac pump dysfunction as determined by the effect of dobutamine. *Am J Cardiol*, 53,1308-1315.
[57] Wilson, J.R., Mancini, D.M., & Dunkman, W.B. (1993). Exertional fatigue due to skeletal muscle dysfunction in patients with heart failure. *Circulation*, 87,470-475.

[58] Holloszy, J.O. (1976). Adaptations of muscular tissue to training. *Prog Cardiovasc Dis*, 18,445-458.

[59] Refenberick, D.H., Gamble, J.G., & Max, S.R. (1973). Response of mitochondrial enzymes to decreased muscular activity. *Am J Physiol*, 225,1295-1259.

[60] Cooksey, J.D., Reilly, P., Brown, S., Bomze, H., & Cryer, P.E. (1978). Exercise training and plasma catecholamines in patients with ischemic heart disease. *Am J Cardiol*, 42,372-376.

[61] Hespel, P., Lijnen, P., Van Hoof, R., Fagard, R., Goossens, W., Lissens, W., Moerman, E., & Amery, A.. (1988). Effects of physical endurance training on the plasma renin-angiotensin-aldosterone system in normal man. *J Endocr*,116, 443-449.

[62] Katz, A.M., & Katz, P.B. (1962). Disease of the heart in works of Hippocrates. *Br Heart J*, 24,256-264.

[63] Anker, S., Ponikowski, P., Varney, S., Chua, T.P., Clark, A.L., Webb-Peploe, K.M., Harrington, D., Kox, W.J., Poole-Wilson, P.A., & Coats, A.J. (1997). Wasting as an independent risk factor for mortality in chronic heart failure. *Lancet*, 349,1050-1053.

[64] Davos, C.H., Doehner, W., Rauchhaus, M., Cicoira, M., Francis, D.P., Coats, A.J., Clark, A.L., & Anker, S.D. (2003). Body mass and survival in patients with chronic heart failure without cachexia: the importance of obesity. *J Cardiac Failure*, 9,29-35.

[65] Anker, S.D., Clark, A.L., Teixeira, M.M., Hellewell, P.G., & Coats, A.J. (1999). Loss of bone mineral in patients with cachexia due to chronic heart failure. *Am J Cardiol*, 83,612-615.

[66] Staten, M.A., Matthews, D.E., Cryer, P.E., & Bier, D.M. (1987). Physiological increments in epinephrine stimulate metabolic rate in humans. *Am J Physiol*, 253,E322-E330.

[67] Simonsen, L., Bulow, J., Madsen, J., & Christensen, N.J. (1992). Thermogenic response to epinephrine in the forearm and abdominal subcutaneous adipose tissue. *Am J Physiol*, 263,E850-855.

[68] Webber, J., & Macdonald, I.A. (1993). Metabolic actions of catecholamines in man. Baillieres Clin Endocrinol Metab, 7, 93-413.

[69] Lafontan, M., & Berlan, M. (1993). Fat cell adrenergic receptors and the control of white and brown fat cell function. *J Lipid Res*, 34,1057–1091.

[70] Swan, J.W., Walton, C., Godsland, I.F., Clark, A.L., Coats, A.J., & Oliver, M.F. (1994). Insulin resistance in chronic heart failure. *Eur Heart J*, 15,1528-1532.

[71] Swan, J.W., Anker, S.D., Walton, C., Godsland, I.F., Clark, A.L., Leyva, F., Stevenson, J.C., & Coats, A.J. (1997). Insulin resistance in chronic heart failure: relation to severity and aetiology of heart failure. *J Am Coll Cardiol*, 30,527-532.

[72] Anker, S.D., Chua, T.P., Ponikowski, P., Harrington, D., Swan, J.W., Kox, W.J., Poole-Wilson, P.A., & Coats, A.J. (1997). Hormonal changes and catabolic/anabolic imbalance in chronic heart failure and their importance for cardiac cachexia. Circulation, 96,526-534.

[73] Sabelis, L.W., Senden, P.J., Zonderland, M.L., van de Wiel, A., Wielders, J.P., Huisveld, I.A., van Haeften, T.W., & Mosterd, W.L. (2003). Determinants of insulin sensitivity in chronic heart failure. *Eur J Heart Fail*, 5,759-765.

[74] Anker, S.D., Clark, A.L., Kemp, M., Salsbury, C., Teixeira, M.M., Hellewell, P.G., & Coats, A.J. (1997). Tumour necrosis factor and steroid metabolism in chronic heart failure: possible relation to muscle wasting. *J Am Coll Cardiol*, 30,997-1001.

[75] Anker, S.D., Ponikowski, P.P., Clark, A.L., Leyva, F., Rauchhaus, M., Kemp, M., Teixeira, M.M., Hellewell, P.G., Hooper, J., Poole-Wilson, P.A., & Coats, A.J. (1999). Cytokines and neurohormones relating to body composition alterations in the wasting syndrome of chronic heart failure. *Eur Heart J*, 20,683-693.

[76] Niebauer, J., Pflaum, C-D., Clark, A.L., Strasbruger, C.J., Hooper, J., Poole-Wilson, P.A., Coats, A.J., & Anker, S.D. (1998). Deficient insulin-like growth factor-I in chronic heart failure predicts altered body composition, anabolic deficiency, cytokine and neurohormonal activation. *J Am Coll Cardiol*, 32,393-397.

[77] Devon, H.A., & Zerwic, J.J. (2002). Symptoms of acute coronary syndromes: are there gender differences? A review of the literature. *Heart Lung*, 31,235-245.

[78] Patel, H., Rosengren, A., & Ekman, I. (2004). Symptoms in acute coronary syndromes: does sex make a difference? *Am Heart J*, 148,27-33.

[79] Pedersen, S.S., & Middel, B. (2001). Increased vital exhaustion among type-D patients with ischemic heart disease. *J Psychosom Res*, 51,443-449.

[80] Sullivan, M.D., LaCroix, A.Z., Russo, J.E., & Walker, E.A. (2001). Depression and self-reported physical health in patients with coronary disease: mediating and moderating factors. *Psychosom Med*, 63,248-256.

[81] Jenkins, C.D., Jono, R.T., & Stanton, B.A. (1996). Predicting completeness of symptom relief after major heart surgery. *Behav Med*, 22,45-57.

[82] Appels, A., Kop, W., Bar, F., de Swart, H., & Mendes de Leon, C.(1995). Vital exhaustion, extent of atherosclerosis, and the clinical course after successful percutaneous transluminal coronary angioplasty. *Eur Heart J*, 16,1880-1885.

[83] Stanton, B.A., Jenkins, C.D., Denlinger, P., Savageau, J.A., Weintraub, R.M, & Goldstein, R.L. (1983). Predictors of employment status after cardiac surgery. *JAMA*, 1983, 249,907-911.

[84] Appels, A., & Mulder, P. (1989). Fatigue and heart disease. The association between 'vital exhaustion' and past, present and future coronary heart disease. *J Psychosom Res*, 33,727-738.

[85] Meyer, T., Stanske, B., Kochen, M.M., Cordes, A., Yüksel, I., Wachter, R., Lüers, C., Scherer, M., Binder, L., Pieske, B., & Herrmann-Lingen, C. (2010). Elevated serum levels of interleukin-10 and tumor necrosis factor are both associated with vital exhaustion in patients with cardiovascular risk factors, *Psychosomatics*, 51,248-256.

[86] Appels, A. (2004). Exhaustion and coronary heart disease: the history of a scientific quest. *Patient Educ Couns*, 55, 223-229.

[87] Eldridge, J.E., Ramsey-Green, C.L., & Hossack, K.F. (1986). Effects of the limiting symptom on the achievement of maximal oxygen consumption in patients with coronary artery disease. *Am J Cardiol*, 57,513-517.

[88] Heldman, D., Mulvihill, D., Nguyen, H., Messenger, J.C., Rylaarsdam, A., Evans, K., & Castellanet, M.J. True incidence of pacemaker syndrome. (1990). *Pacing Clin Electrophysiol*, 13,1742-1750.

[89] Oldroyd, K.G., Rae, A.P., Carter, R., Wingate, C., & Cobbe, S.M. (1991). Double blind crossover comparison of the effects of dual chamber pacing (DDD) and ventricular rate adaptive (VVIR) pacing on neuroendocrine variables, exercise performance, and symptoms in complete heart block. *Br Heart J*, 65,188-193.

[90] Sulke, N., Dritsas, A., Bostock, J., Wells, A., Morris, R., & Sowton, E. (1992). "Subclinical" pacemaker syndrome: a randomised study of symptom free patients with

ventricular demand (VVI) pacemakers upgraded to dual chamber devices. *Br Heart J*, 67,57-64.

[91] Madariaga, M.G., Rezai, K., Trenholme, G.M., & Weinstein, R.A. (2003). Q fever: a biological weapon in your backyard. *Lancet Infect Dis*, 3,709-721.

[92] Libby, P., Egan, D., & Skarlatos, S. (1997). Roles of infectious agents in atherosclerosis and restenosis: an assessment of the evidence and need for future research. *Circulation*, 96,4095-4103.

[93] Ieven, M.M., & Hoymans, V.Y. (1997). Involvement of Chlamydia pneumoniae in atherosclerosis: more evidence for lack of evidence. *J Clin Microbiol*. 2005, 43,19-24.

[94] O'Connor, C.M., Dunne, M.W., Pfeffer, M.A., Muhlestein, J.B., Yao, L., Gupta, S., Benner, R.J., Fisher, M.R., Cook, T.D., & Investigators in the WIZARD Study. (2003). Azithromycin for the secondary prevention of coronary heart disease events: the WIZARD study: a randomized controlled trial. *JAMA*, 290,1459-1466.

[95] Medical Research Council Working Party. (1985). MRC trial of treatment of mild hypertension: principal results. *Br Med J*, 291,97–104.

[96] Messerli, F.H., & Grossman, E. (2002). Beta-blocker therapy and depression. *JAMA*, 288,1845–1846.

[97] Ko, D.T., Hebert, P.R., Coffey, C.S., Sedrakyan, A., Curtis, J.P., & Krumholz, H.M. (2002). **β**-Blocker therapy and symptoms of depression, fatigue, and sexual dysfunction. *JAMA* , 288,351-357.

[98] Rod, J.L., Admon, D., Kimchi, A., Gotsman, M.S., & Lewis, B.S. (1979). Evaluation of the beta-blocking drug acebutolol in angina pectoris. *Am Heart J*; 98,604-612.

[99] Dargie, H.J., Grant, S., & McLenachan, J. (1991). Angina, ischemia, and effort tolerance with vasodilating beta-blockers. *Am Heart J*, 121,1017-1020.

[100] Roubin, G.S., Sadick, N.A., Anderson, Devenish-Meares, S., Harris, P.J., & Kelly, D.T. (1987). Effect of propranolol and verapamil on oxygen utilization, acidosis and fatigue during exercise in stable angina pectoris. *Am J Cardiol*, 60,249-255.

[101] Butler, J., Khadim, G., Belue, R., Chomsky, D., Dittus, R.S., Griffin, M., & Wilson, J.R. (2003). Tolerability to beta-blocker therapy among heart failure patients in clinical practice. *J Card Fail*, 9,203-209.

[102] Packer, M., Coats, A.J., Fowler, M.B., Katus, H.A., Krum, H., Mohacsi, P., Rouleau, J.L., Tendera, M., Castaigne, A., Roecker, E.B., Schultz, M.K., DeMets, D.L.; & Carvedilol Prospective Randomized Cumulative Survival Study Group. (2001). Effect of carvedilol on survival in severe chronic heart failure. *N Engl J Med*, 344,1651–1658.

[103] Krum, H., Roecker, E.B., Mohacsi, P., Rouleau, J.L., Tendera, M., Coats, A.J., Katus, H.A., Fowler, M.B., Packer, M.; & Carvedilol Prospective Randomized Cumulative Survival (COPERNICUS) Study Group. (2003). Effects of initiating carvedilol in patients with severe chronic heart failure: results from the COPERNICUS Study. *JAMA*, 289,712–718.

[104] Bristow, M.R., Gilbert, E.M., Abraham, W.T., Adams, K.F., Fowler, M.B., Hershberger, R.E., Kubo, S.H., Narahara, K.A., Ingersoll, H., Krueger, S., Young, S., & Shusterman, N. (1996). Carvedilol produces dose-related improvements in left ventricular function and survival in subjects with chronic heart failure. MOCHA Investigators. *Circulation*, 94,2807-2816.

[105] Packer, M., Colucci, W.S., Sackner-Bernstein, J.D., Liang, C.S., Goldscher, D.A., Freeman, I., Kukin, M.L., Kinhal, V., Udelson, J.E., Klapholz, M., Gottlieb, S.S.,

Pearle, D., Cody, R.J., Gregory, J.J., Kantrowitz, N.E., LeJemtel, T.H., Young, S.T., Lukas, M.A., & Shusterman, N.H.. (1996). Double-blind, placebo-controlled study of the effects of carvedilol in patients with moderate to severe heart failure. The PRECISE Trial. Prospective Randomized Evaluation of Carvedilol on Symptoms and Exercise. *Circulation*, 94,2793-2799.

[106] Waagstein, F., Bristow, M.R., Swedberg, K., Camerini, F., Fowler, M.B., Silver, M.A., Gilbert, E.M., Johnson, M.R., Goss, F.G., & Hjalmarson, A. (1993). Beneficial effects of metoprolol in idiopathic dilated cardiomyopathy. Metoprolol in Dilated Cardiomyopathy (MDC) Trial Study Group. *Lancet*, 342,1441-1446.

[107] Benner, J.S., Glynn, R.J., Mogun, H., Neumann, P.J., Weinstein, M.C., & Avorn, J. (2002). Long-term persistence in use of statin therapy in elderly patients. *JAMA*, 288,455-461.

[108] Heart Protection Study Collaborative Group. (2004). Effects of cholesterol-lowering with simvastatin on stroke and other major vascular events in 20536 people with cerebrovascular disease or other high-risk conditions. *Lancet*, 363,757-767.

[109] Jula, A., Marniemi, J., Huupponen, R., Virtanen, A., Rastas, M., & Rönnemaa, T. (2002). Effects of Diet and Simvastatin on Serum Lipids, Insulin, and Antioxidants in Hypercholesterolemic Men. *JAMA*, 287,598-605.

[110] Singh, R.B., Neki, N.S., Kartikey, K., Pella, D., Kumar, A., Niaz, M.A., & Thakur, A.S. (2003). Effect of coenzyme Q10 on risk of atherosclerosis in patients with recent myocardial infarction. *Mol Cell Biochem*, 246,75-82.

[111] Langsjoen, P.H., & Langsjoen, A.M. (2003). The clinical use of HMG CoA-reductase inhibitors and the associated depletion of coenzyme Q10. A review of animal and human publications. *Biofactors*, 18,101-111.

[112] Garske, L.A., Brown, M.G., & Morrison, S.C. (2003). Acetazolamide reduces exercise capacity and increases leg fatigue under hypoxic conditions. *J Appl Physiol*, 94,991-996.

[113] Murray, M.D., Deer, M.M., Ferguson, J.A., Dexter, P.R., Bennett, S.J., Perkins, S.M., Smith, F.E., Lane, K.A., Adams, L.D., Tierney, W.M., & Brater, D.C. (2001). Open-label randomized trial of torsemide compared with furosemide therapy for patients with heart failure. *Am J Med*, 111,513-520.

[114] Packer, M., Carver, J.R., Rodeheffer, R.J., Ivanhoe, R.J., DiBianco, R., Zeldis, S.M., Hendrix, G.H,, Bommer, W.J., Elkayam, U., Kukin, M,L. & et al. (1991). Effect of oral milrinone on mortality in severe chronic heart failure. The PROMISE Study Research Group. *N Engl J Med*, 325,1468-1414.

[115] (1993). Flosequinan for chronic heart failure. *Drugs Ther Bull*, 31, 47-48.

[116] The Xamoterol in Severe Heart Failure Study Group. (1990). Xamoterol in severe heart failure. *Lancet*, 336,1-6.

[117] Cowley, A.J., & Skene, A.M., on behalf of the Enoximone Investigators. (1994). Treatment of severe heart failure: quantity or quality of life? A trial of enoximone. *Br Heart J*, 72,226-230.

[118] Cohn, J.N., Johnson, G., Ziesche, S., Cobb, F., Francis, G., Tristani, F., Smith, R., Dunkman, W.B., Loeb, H., Wong, M., & et al. (1991). A comparison of enalapril with hydralazine-isosorbide dinitrate in the treatment of chronic congestive heart failure. *N Engl J Med*, 325,303-310.

[119] Drexler, H., Banhardt, U., Meinertz, T., Wollschläger, H., Lehmann, M., & Just, H. (1989). Contrasting peripheral short-term and long-term effects of converting enzyme inhibition in patients with congestive heart failure. A double-blind, placebo-controlled trial. *Circulation*, 79,491-502.

[120] Coats, A.J., Adamopoulos, S., Meyer, T., Conway, J., & Sleight, P. (1990).Effects of physical training in chronic heart failure. *Lancet*, 335,63-66.

[121] Meyer, K., Schwaibold, M., Westbrook, S., Beneke, R., Hajric, R., Görnandt, L., Lehmann, M., & Roskamm, H. (1996). Effect of short-term exercise training and activity restriction on functional capacity in patients with severe chronic congestive heart failure. *Am J Cardiol*, 78,1017-1022.

[122] Kavanagh, T., Myers, M.G., Baigrie, R.S., Mertens, D.J., Sawyer, P., & Shephard, R.J. (1996). Quality of life and cardiorespiratory function in chronic heart failure: effects of 12 months' aerobic training. *Heart*, 76,42-49.

[123] Coats, A.J., Adamopoulos, S., Radaelli, A., McCance, A., Meyer, T.E., Bernardi, L., Solda, P.L., Davey, P., Ormerod, O., Forfar, C., & et al. (1992). Controlled trial of physical training in chronic heart failure: exercise performance, hemodynamics, ventilation, and autonomic function. *Circulation*, 85,2119-2131.

[124] Hambrecht, R., Niebauer, J., Fiehn, E., Kälberer, B., Offner, B., Hauer, K., Riede, U., Schlierf, G., Kübler, W., & Schuler G. (1995). Physical training in patients with stable chronic heart failure: Effects on cardiorespiratory fitness and ultrastructural abnormalities of leg muscles. *J Am Coll Cardiol*, 25,1239-1249.

[125] Piepoli, M.F., Davos, C., Francis, D.P., Coats, A.J.; & ExTraMATCH Collaborative. (2004). Exercise training meta-analysis of trials in patients with chronic heart failure (ExTraMATCH). *Br Med J*, 328,189.

[126] O'Connor, C.M., Whellan, D.J., Lee, K.L., Keteyian, S.J., Cooper, L.S., Ellis, S.J., Leifer, E.S., Kraus, W.E., Kitzman, D.W., Blumenthal, J.A., Rendall, D.S., Miller, N.H., Fleg, J.L., Schulman, K.A., McKelvie, R.S., Zannad, F., Piña. I,L,; & HF-ACTION (2009). Investigators. Efficacy and safety of exercise training in patients with chronic heart failure: HF-ACTION randomized controlled trial. *JAMA*, 301,1439-1450.

[127] Flynn, K.E., Piña, I.L., Whellan, D.J., Lin, L., Blumenthal, J.A., Ellis, S.J., Fine, L.J., Howlett, J.G., Keteyian, S.J., Kitzman, D.W., Kraus, W.E., Miller, N.H., Schulman, K.A., Spertus, J.A., O'Connor, C.M., Weinfurt, K.P.; & HF-ACTION Investigators. (2009). Effects of exercise training on health status in patients with chronic heart failure: HF-ACTION randomized controlled trial. *JAMA*, 301,1451-1459.

[128] Cazeau, S., Leclercq, C., Lavergne, T., Walker, S., Varma, C., Linde, C., Garrigue, S., Kappenberger, L., Haywood, G.A., Santini, M., Bailleul, C., Daubert, J.C.; & Multisite Stimulation in Cardiomyopathies (MUSTIC) Study Investigators. (2001). Effects of multisite biventricular pacing in patients with heart failure and intraventricular conduction delay. *N Engl J Med*, 344,873-880.

[129] Cowburn, P.J., Patel, H., Jolliffe, R.E., Wald, R.W., & Parker, J.D. (2005). Cardiac resynchronization therapy: an option for inotrope-supported patients with end-stage heart failure? *Eur J Heart Fail*, 7,215-217.

[130] Cleland, J.G., Daubert, J.C., Erdmann, E., Freemantle, N., Gras, D., Kappenberger, L., Tavazzi, L,; & Cardiac Resynchronization-Heart Failure (CARE-HF) Study Investigators. (2005). The effect of cardiac resynchronization on morbidity and mortality in heart failure. *N Engl J Med*, 352,1539-1549.

[131] Rose, E.A., Gelijns, A.C., Moskowitz, A.J., Heitjan, D.F., Stevenson, L.W., Dembitsky, W., Long, J.W., Ascheim, D.D., Tierney, A.R., Levitan, R.G., Watson, J.T., Meier, P., Ronan, N.S., Shapiro, P.A., Lazar, R.M., Miller, L.W., Gupta, L., Frazier, O.H., Desvigne-Nickens, P., Oz, M.C., Poirier, V.L.; & Randomized Evaluation of Mechanical Assistance for the Treatment of Congestive Heart Failure (REMATCH) Study Group. (2001). Long-term mechanical left ventricular assistance for end-stage heart failure. *N Engl J Med*, 345,1435-1443.

[132] Westaby, S., Banning, A.P., Jarvik, R., Frazier, O.H., Pigott, D.W., Jin, X.Y., Catarino, P.A., Saito, S., Robson, D., Freeland, A., Myers, T.J., & Poole-Wilson, P.A. (2000). First permanent implant of the Jarvik 2000 Heart. *Lancet*, 356,900-903.

[133] Park, S.J., Tector, A., Piccioni, W., Raines, E., Gelijns, A., Moskowitz, A., Rose, E., Holman, W., Furukawa, S., Frazier, O.H., & Dembitsky. W. (2005). Left ventricular assist devices as destination therapy: a new look at survival. *J Thorac Cardiovasc Surg*, 129,9-17.

In: Handbook of Fatigue in Health and Disease
Editor: Howard S. Smith
ISBN 978-1-61761-920-5

Chapter 8

FATIGUE AND CHRONIC RENAL FAILURE

George H. Eisele*

Professor of Medicine; Division Head of Nephrology
Albany Medical College
47 New Scotland Avenue, MC 69
Albany, NY, 12208, USA

ABSTRACT

Chronic kidney disease (CKD) is a spectrum associated with various degrees of abnormal pathophysiology. CKD is not uncommon and in a significant proportion of patients with CKD, the cause is uncertain. Fatigue is present in many patients with CKD, both initiation of dialysis and afterwards. Furthermore, the presence of severity of fatigue appears unrelated to the type of dialysis (e.g. hemodialysis, continuous ambulatory peritoneal dialysis) as well as whether the patient is pre- or post-dialysis. Increasing hemoglobin values by transfusion or by the administration of erythropoiesis-stimulating agents (ESAs) may improve symptoms of profound fatigue in certain patients. Optimal values for hemoglobin, electrolytes, or values/parameters of other substances remain uncertain.

INTRODUCTION

The kidneys are organs central to the maintenance of the internal milieu of the body. Homeostasis requires renal operations that are both conservative and execratory in nature.

* Phone: (518) 262-5176
Fax: (518) 262-5573
Email: eiseleg@mail.amc.edu

The excretion of urea best exemplifies the excretory functions of the kidney. After growth is completed the adult body does not store the daily intake of protein. Daily protein metabolism entails repair and turnover of enzymes, structural and other proteins that generate nitrogen-bearing wastes. These wastes, if not excreted, accumulate in blood and tissues and cause cellular and organ dysfunction. The body converts most nitrogen bearing waste compounds to urea. In the early nineteenth century, Richard Bright working in London examined young adults dying with kidneys found to be shriveled at autopsy. He identified urea as a substance found in great abundance in the blood of these patients. Thus began the paradigm of renal failure as a state of autointoxication from retained nitrogenous wastes (i.e. uremia). So fundamental, a metabolic derangement would be expected to cause protean clinical pathology. At very high blood levels of urea, coma, respiratory depression and death occur. It is not hard to imagine that at somewhat lower urea levels many clinical manifestations, including fatigue would be present.

The kidneys also have important conservative functions. All cells of the body with access to the circulation are bathed in a solution of many chemicals, which support their proper function. Crucial among these are ions such as potassium, sodium, magnesium, calcium and bicarbonate. The kidney is the central organ charged with maintaining blood levels of these and many other necessary substances within tight physiologic bounds. Alteration of blood potassium levels, for example, has a marked and immediate effect upon muscle function, including the cardiac muscle. As kidneys fail, the level of potassium rises. At high enough blood levels skeletal muscle becomes flaccid and patients become unable to stand, walk, lift or even breathe. While some patients inevitably will experience these symptoms as fatigue, this may not be a good model for the fatigue of chronic renal failure. Cardiac muscle is equally sensitive to potassium levels and when skeletal muscle is so affected that it no longer contracts, then cardiac flaccidity (and death) is usually not far behind. Still, less extreme derangements of the many ions crucial for normal cell functioning could contribute to dysfunction and dysphoria, including the subjective sensation of fatigue.

The third major area of normal renal function, which bears upon the issue of fatigue, is renal endocrinology. Broadly speaking, a hormone is a chemical substance produced by one body organ, which is exported (usually by the circulation) to affect the operation of a target organ physically distant from the endocrine organ. Thyroid hormone, excreted by the small organ in the neck, has profound influence upon most organs of the body including the brain and the bowel. The kidney acts as an endocrine organ at several levels. In response to poor circulation to the kidney (low perfusion pressure), the kidney manufactures renin and excretes it into the central circulation via the renal veins and the inferior vena cava. Through a series of enzymatic steps the release of renin results in the production of angiotensin II. This hormone reaches the blood bathing the adrenal glands and induces the formation of aldosterone, which in turn circulates to the kidney causing it to retain sodium and intravascular volume, raising renal perfusion pressure. This decreases renal renin production and closes a classic endocrine feedback loop.

Another example of renal endocrinology involves erythropoiten. In response to a drop in the red blood cell count-anemia- the kidney secretes erythropoietin into the circulation. When this hormone reaches the bone marrow, it stimulates the manufacture of new red blood cells. Once the hematocrit is high enough, the kidney ceases production of erythropoietin and new red blood cells. Even at relatively preserved levels of glomerular filtration, damaged kidneys frequently decrease the production of

Erythropoietin. For most, although not for all renal failure patients, anemia is an early and persistent component of the disease. At ESRD (end stage renal disease, or a dialysis requirement) most patients suffer from profound anemia, with hematocrit values of 20 or less (normal is above 40). Typically these patients are not iron deficient and have no other cause for their profound anemia. Absent erythropoietin, no therapeutic approach can adequately correct the anemia. Human recombinant erythropoietin was released for use in American dialysis patients in 1989, and the result was revolutionary.

End Stage Renal Disease and Fatigue

Patients at or near ESRD frequently experience a constellation of dysphoric symptoms, which have traditionally been attributed to uremia. These symptoms include anorexia, weight loss, profound fatigue and lassitude, coldness even in warm environments, distortions of taste and smell, sleep disturbance, shortness of breath (fluid overload), and a decrease of mental acuity ("fuzziness"). Bossola and colleagues found that depression, anxiety, number and severity of comorbidities and IL-6 levels are significantly correlated with fatigue in end-stage renal disease patients receiving chronic hemodialysis [1]. Correction of anemia by the transfusion of red blood cells alleviates symptoms very effectively in the short term. Symptoms of cold and fatigue rapidly improve and the sense of well being returns. Beyond the issue of cost, the strategy of frequent transfusion is quite problematic. More transfusions create a greater the risk of transfusion reactions. The typical lifespan of red blood cells in normals is about 120 days. In uremic patients this lifespan is reduced significantly [1]. This means that the clinical improvement afforded by a red cell transfusion has a significant time limit. Each transfusion of red cells, however thoroughly washed and separated, invariably leads to introduction of at least a few donor white cells. White cells are immunogenic; they contain surface proteins, which stimulate an immune response in the recipient. Once a patient's immune system reacts to these foreign proteins and cells, the patient may develop antibodies to the same immunogenic proteins which appear on a donor kidney. Transplant surgeons are reluctant to transplant a kidney into a recipient whose blood contains antibodies preformed to reject it. While different individuals have differing propensities to form antibodies, the greater the number of transfusions, the greater is the difficulty in finding a donor kidney whose immunologic structure is compatible with the recipient.

As transfused red blood cells age and breakdown, the iron, which they contain, remains in the body. Dialysis does not eliminate it. Multiple transfusions, even if spaced over years, have a cumulative effect in this regard. Secondary hemachromatosis may cause serious damage to liver and heart. "Bronze diabetes" can occur. This reflects both iron discoloration of the skin and the damage which iron can cause to the insulin producing cells of the pancreas. The strategy of frequent transfusion, while effective in alleviating symptoms, has significant clinical limitations and dangers.

ERYTHROPOIESIS-STIMULATING AGENTS (ESAs)

The widespread use of EPO occurred very quickly after its approval by the Food and Drug Administration. The sustained improvement in hematocrit soon revealed that many of the symptoms so closely tied to uremia are actually manifestations of anemia alone. Symptoms such as coldness, mental sluggishness, exercise intolerance and fatigue show dramatic and sustained improvement [3]. Of course some symptoms, such as metallic taste, nausea and vomiting do not respond to EPO. Still by 1991-1992 articles documenting the remarkable symptomatic improvements afforded by EPO began to fill the medical literature [4-6]. At present more than 90% of chronic dialysis patients in the US receive EPO [7].

Nearly 90% of patients with glomerular filtration rates of less than 25-30 ml/min have hemoglobin levels of less than 10 g/dl [8]. The World Health Organization defines anemia as hemoglobin less than 13.0 g/dl in adult males and postmenopausal women. The limit is less than 12.0 g/dl in adult premenopausal women. Although one source estimates that only 35% of anemic chronic renal failure patients receive therapy [9], EPO is now frequently given to patients with chronic renal failure long before they reach a dialysis requirement. Occasionally this results in an irony wherein the physician, notes the profound decline in renal function documented by blood tests and recommends staring dialysis. The patient rejects the advice because he or she simply feels too well (personal observation)!

There has long been discussion in the literature about the optimal goal hematocrit for EPO therapy. This controversy continues to the present. While there is some data and some theoretical concern about completely normalizing hematocrit in hemodialysis patients, it is fair to say that third party payers strongly influence this decision. Lead by CMS, the agency which pays for Medicaid, third party payers will not pay for enough EPO to completely normalize hematocrit, but set hematocrit goals below this. US Government estimates put the annual cost of EPO therapy for hemodialysis patients at $1.5 billion [10]. The current goal set by CMS is hemoglobin of 11-12 with potential financial penalties if the hemoglobin exceeds 12.5 over a 90-day rolling average. There is consensus about the lower limit of the current hemoglobin target but disagreement about the optimal upper limit. A Spanish study published in 2000 treated dialysis patients without diabetes mellitus or known cardiovascular disease to a goal of 12.5 hemoglobin [11]. Those that achieved the goal showed improved quality of life and functional status. Over a six-month period there were no deaths and hospitalizations were fewer than the previous six-month experience. A Scandinavian study randomized patients to a goal hemoglobin of either 9-12 or 13.5-15 g/dl in women or 14.5-15 in men [12]. Fatigue occurred less in the higher hemoglobin group. Higher hemoglobin levels did not incur greater risk of adverse events. Other studies have raised concern about attempting to normalize hemoglobin in hemodialysis patients. The US Normal Hematocrit Study took hemodialysis patients with known cardiovascular disease and compared outcomes of groups treated to a goal of either hemoglobin of 14 or 10 [13]. The study was terminated early when a trend to an increased incidence of either death or nonfatal myocardial infarction was noted. Cardiovascular disease is common in dialysis populations and studies suggesting worse cardiovascular outcomes at normal hemoglobin have left the issue of optimal hemoglobin open for further study. What data there is does support the idea that less anemic patients feel better and report less fatigue.

Very recent reports and editorials have only served to sharpen the debate over the optimal use of erythropoietin stimulating agents. Essentially the arguments come down to a risk/benefit analysis. Publishing in the American Journal of Kidney Disease (2006) [14], the study group organized by the National Kidney Foundation advocated for treatment of anemia in chronic renal failure patients not yet in need of dialysis. This comprehensive set of guidelines addressed many issues besides anemia and is known as KDOQI, the Kidney Disease Outcomes Quality Initiative. These recommendations incorporate data published in the nephrology literature, but are influenced heavily by best practices advocated by invited panels of experts. These guidelines, along with earlier similar guidelines focused on chronic dialysis patients (DOQI--Dialysis Outcomes Quality Initiative) have quickly become de facto standards of care for American nephrologists and very influential with the international community. KDOQI recommends a goal hemoglobin level of at least 11.0 but less than 13.

Writing in the January 21, 2010 edition of the New England Journal of Medicine, Unger lays out in forceful detail the contemporary arguments against the use of ESAs to address the anemia of chronic renal failure [15]. This argument is founded upon the observations reported in several recent well conducted randomized clinical trials which compare matched cohorts treated to "normal" hematocrits, usually between 40-42, vs. a cohort treated to a hematocrit in the 30-33 range. As a first order summary, most of these trials show an increased cardiovascular morbidity and mortality burden in those treated to the higher hematocrit goals. In the Correction of Hemoglobins and Outcomes in Renal Insufficiency (CHOIR) trial [16], 1432 patients with chronic kidney disease not yet requiring dialysis were randomized to a goal hemoglobin of either 13.5 or 11.3. All participants had not previously received any ESA. The study composite end point was death/myocardial infarction/hospitalization for congestive heart failure/ or stroke. With a median follow-up of 16 months, the composite end point was reached in 17.5% of the high hemoglobin group and 13.5 % of the low hemoglobin (hgb) group. The statistically significant risk ratio was 1.34%.

The TREAT study [17] enrolled 4038 patients with type 2 diabetes and chronic kidney disease. 2012 received darbopoeitin alpha and 2026 received placebo. At 29 months the mean hemoglobin achieved in the treated group was 12.5. Death or a non-fatal cardiovascular event occurred in 31.4% of the treated group and 29.7 % of the placebo group. These differences were not statistically significant unlike the clear outcome differences in the earlier CHOIR trial and the much earlier NORMAL trial [18] the editorial writers Unger et. Al.. emphasizes not only the potential risks of ESAs, but also the modest reported benefits in these trials. Medical Outcomes Study 36-item Short Form General Health Survey (SF-36) and other quality of life indexes did not show impressive improvements with anemia correction.

A cursory interpretation of all this might quickly lead to the conclusion that the accumulated wisdom gleaned from 15 to 20 years of clinical experience with ESAs was refuted within the last 5 to 10 years by a few well structured clinical trials. This clearly is the editorial position of Ungerer et. al. Reality however may not be so monochromatic. In the same edition of the New England Journal which reported the CHOIR trial, there appeared the formal publication of the CREATE trial [19]. This European study enrolled anemic patients with chronic kidney disease stage 3 or 4—pre dialysis. The target hemoglobin range was 13 to 15, significantly higher than goal hemoglobin for other contemporaneous studies. Unlike the results of other studies, the high hemoglobin group did not suffer excess morbidity/ mortality. Furthermore some quality of life metrics were improved by normalization of RBC counts. There is no consensus regarding an explanation for these differences in outcome. But there were some interesting differences in methodology. The European study, CREATE used smaller, more frequent dosing regimens which may have corrected anemia more gradually—or even more "gently". Whether these minute differences in methodology really are of significance, they do serve to highlight how much clinical uncertainty has crept into an area of clinical medicine which seemed to be a settled arena just a few years previously. In the future the use of orally active prolyl-hydroxylase inhibitors (e.g. FG-2216) to stabilize hypoxia-inducible transcription factor (HIF) with resultant stimulation of endogenous EPO production may be utilized.

The very positive experience with improvement of anemia over the past fifteen years has not abolished fatigue from treated populations. Many other factors have received attention. Current dialysis therapy does not fully compensate the loss of renal function. As previously discussed, the kidneys are charged with excretion of nitrogen bearing wastes which accumulate daily as part of normal bodily function. Standard hemodialysis involves three treatments a week spaced two or three days apart. Typically the patient dialyzes for three to four hours on Monday, Wednesday and Friday, or Tuesday, Thursday and Saturday. A unitless parameter has been developed to assess the adequacy of each dialysis treatment. This parameter, kT/V, should exceed 1.2 to satisfy current theory and government regulation. T is the time on dialysis in minutes. V is the volume of distribution of urea in the patient's body and k is a urea permeability factor characteristic of the particular dialysis cartridge being used for the treatment. This value of 1.2 correlates approximately with a urea reduction ratio of 65%. Suppose that the urea level in the patient's blood at the start of a dialysis treatment is exactly 100 mg/dl. The treatment is considered adequate if blood level of urea at the end of dialysis is below 35 mg/dl. During the time between treatments, the level of urea continuously increases, so that the average blood level is between the two treatment extremes. A normal value of urea in the blood is around 10 mg/dl. Thus a patient considered well dialyzed by conventional standards always retains urea and other nitrogenous wastes well above the levels achieved by normal renal function. Data published over two decades ago show that patients whose dialysis prescription results is a kT/V of 1.2 or greater suffer less mortality and fewer hospitalizations than patients whose kT/V is less than 1.2 [20]. Patients receiving more intensive dialysis (kT/V > 1.2) had no improvement in these outcomes.

Recently more intensive dialysis prescriptions have been offered to selected patients. One schedule calls for patients to dialyze at home while they sleep for as much as 7-9 hours per night. There are 5 or 6 nightly treatments a week. This translates to kT/V values above 3 and average urea values close to normal. While proponents of this approach to hemodialysis are quick to note these metabolic improvements, there is no good comparative data to show that mortality and morbidity are improved. Patients often report feeling better and more alert, but anecdotal experience in selected patient groups does not constitute hard evidence that subjective symptoms such as fatigue are reliably improved.

Sleep disturbance is a significant factor in the chronic fatigue of renal failure, both before and during the time of dialysis. A recent Canadian study of chronic kidney patients not yet on dialysis employed the Pittsburgh Sleep Quality Index to investigate the prevalence of "poor sleep" in 120 patients. Sixty-three patients had a global PQSI score above 5 [21]. Only a history of depression was an independent predictor of "poor sleep". Blood urea nitrogen levels and serum creatinine levels, which are traditional markers of severity of kidney disease, did not correlate significantly with "poor sleep". A sleep questionnaire administered to chronic hemodialysis patients in a Hong Kong dialysis center revealed a prevalence of daytime sleepiness of 74% [22]. Other studies [23] have placed the prevalence of sleep disorders [24] in dialysis patients at 50-80% [25].

Before turning to several specific causes of sleep disturbance well documented in the literature, consider a factor little mentioned in this context but obvious to any clinician familiar with hemodialysis patients.

A major charge of the kidneys is to maintain fluid balance. In normals the amount of fluid consumed daily is excreted daily, once losses through the skin, lungs and bowel are accounted for. Dialysis patients early in the course of their disease sometimes retain the ability to produce some urine.

Only rarely can the kidneys of dialysis patients excrete volumes in excess of 2 liters a day, though some will respond to very large doses of diuretics. Almost all dialysis patients will gradually lose responsiveness to diuretics over time and eventually fail to excrete any urine at all. Patients eventually become fully dependent upon their dialysis treatments to remove fluid taken in during the interdialytic interval. Hemodialysis machines remove fluid from the body by ultrafiltering the blood. In brief, the blood that passes out of the body and through the dialysis cartridge is maintained at a higher hydraulic pressure than the dialysis fluid on the other side of the dialysis membrane (usually at atmospheric pressure). Depending upon the surface area and the hydraulic permeability characteristic of the dialysis membrane material, a fixed amount of fluid leaves the blood each hour and is discarded along with the spent dialysate. The membrane is designed to hold back critical blood proteins such as albumin and immunoglobulins, as well as red cells, white cell and platelets. The time on dialysis and the adjustable transmembrane pressure dictate how much fluid will be removed during the dialysis treatment. The fluid goal so determined is one of the components of the physician's dialysis prescription. The dialysis machine can remove far more fluid during a treatment than the patient can comfortably tolerate. Too rapid a rate of fluid removal can result in severe and sudden hypotension. This would occur when the rate of ultrafiltration from the intravascular volume exceeds the rate of refilling of the blood compartment by the capillary uptake from the tissues (interstitial space). The nursing personnel quickly respond to sudden drops in blood pressure by turning off ultrafiltration and infusing saline very rapidly into the circulation, reversing the hypotension and also reducing the net fluid removal. Dialysis nurses and technicians will respond the same way when the manifestation of overly rapid and aggressive fluid removal results in severe, very painful cramps. While individual tolerance of fluid removal is quite variable, for a specific patient there is a practical limit to the amount of fluid removal which a given dialysis treatment can achieve. As a rough guideline this limit is in the range of 3-4 liters per treatment. If the patient chooses to ingest more than 2 liters per day, then he will exceed the realistic capacity of the treatment to maintain him at an optimal fluid weight. This will lead to a state of chronic excess hydration.

The retained fluid has three major consequences. First the patient may manifest significant peripheral swelling of the extremities or trunk (edema). Secondly, blood pressure elevation can be quite elevated and resistant to conventional antihypertensive medications. Finally, if the patient does not have normal cardiac function, the fluid will build up in the lungs, which in the severest circumstance is known as pulmonary edema. Wet heavy lungs are difficult to inflate and this increased work of breathing is subjectively sensed as dyspnea or shortness of breath. The work of breathing is less in the upright than the supine position, so patients with congestive heart failure cannot tolerate lying flat and at night will try to sleep sitting up (orthopnea). If the situation is severe enough and sufficiently longstanding, the patient will be unable to sleep. Chronic sleep deprivation will lead to daytime somnolence and chronic fatigue. In principle this entire pathologic sequence is fully avoidable: the patient limits interdialytic fluid intake to technically manageable volumes and the situation does not arise. Experience in the dialysis unit quickly teaches the profound difficulty which many dialysis patients have with fluid limitation and the clinical consequences thereof. Hemodialysis regimens that feature more frequent treatments, such as nightly dialysis therapy allow much more time for fluid removal. Over hydration is much less common in these circumstances, even with the lifting of recommended fluid restrictions. Peritoneal dialysis, which gently removes fluid over much longer treatment times, also markedly reduces the prevalence of over hydration and its consequences.

Obstructive sleep apnea (OSA) is common in the dialysis population. The Hong Kong study mentioned above estimates the prevalence of OSA in its dialysis unit at 49% on the basis of a variety of symptoms such as witnessed apnea and disruptive snoring [26]. Other studies have estimated prevalence at 50-70% [27]. There is no clear explanation for such high rates of prevalence. One report in 2001 showed improvement in a population of patients undergoing nocturnal hemodialysis compared to reported rates in conventional dialysis [28].

Restless leg syndrome (RLS) is a movement disorder, which features a subjective drive to keep the legs moving. The patient expresses a compulsive need to get up and walk around. This typically occurs at night though it is not difficult to find restless legs during daytime dialysis treatments. The International RLS Study Group devised a questionnaire to diagnose the syndrome on clinical grounds [29]. Each of the four criteria should be present:

1) A sensation of an urge to move the limbs (usually legs)
2) Motor restlessness to reduce sensations.
3) Onset of worsening of symptoms when at rest
4) Marked circadian variation in occurrence or severity of symptoms.

Sabbatini et al. noted the prevalence of insomnia in 311 of 694 Italian hemodialysis patients [30]. Using a less strict case definition of RLS, these workers diagnosed RLS in 52% of the insomniacs. RLS can be difficult to treat, though dialysis patients sometimes respond to therapies such as Sinemet and codeine, which work in nondialysis patients.

Sabbitini et al. pointed out other interesting features of their multicenter study. The overall incidence of insomnia was more frequent in the elderly, those with longer dialysis times and those with high parathyroid hormone levels. There was no correlation with anemia, EPO use, and calcitriol or hypertensive drugs. Cigarette smoking, caffeine and alcohol intake were not different between insomniac and unaffected dialysis patients. Creatinine and urea levels were lower in the insomnia group. The authors cited pruritis as another factor in insomnia. This is a common and very difficult to manage problem in dialysis patients. It is sometimes but not always associated with hyperparathyroidism.

L-carnitine deficiency has been proposed as a cause of chronic fatigue in dialysis patients. L-carnitine (molecular weight 162 D) is important in the beta-oxidation of fatty acids. Carnitine helps in the transport of fatty acids into mitochondria and thus participates significantly in cellular energy production. It is estimated that a typical dialysis treatment can reduce blood levels of carnitine by 40%. Skeletal muscle is a storage depot for carnitine and chronic dialysis patients have depleted stores [31]. Studies conducted over the years suggest that carnitine deficiency could play a role in numerous problems in dialysis patients including lethargy, muscle weakness, muscle cramps, erythropoietin resistant anemia, cardiac arrthymias, and intradialytic hypotension. L-carnitine is available as an intravenous preparation, which can be administered at the conclusion of a hemodialysis treatment. Brass, Adler et.al noted in 2001 that exercise capacity in ESRD patients remains impaired despite correction of anemia [32]. They assessed fatigue by the Kidney Disease Questionnaire. Maximal O2 consumption was used to measure exercise capacity. In one portion of the study 28 patients received carnitine intravenously thrice weekly at a dose of 20 mg/kg. 28 other patients received placebo. In a second portion of the study 32 patients received carnitine at a dose of 20 mg/kg, 32 patients received a dose of 40 mg/kg and another 32 received placebo. The study duration was again 24 weeks. Carnitine appeared to offer a small benefit in preserving the maximal O2 uptake but did show a statistically significant improvement in the fatigue domain of the KDQ. As of January 1, 2003 CMS began to reimburse intravenous carnitine administration in chronic hemodialysis patients for the indications erythropoietin resistant anemia or symptomatic intradialytic hypotension. Evidence of low serum carnitine deficiency must also be documented for reimbursement to occur. Several authors have subsequently questioned this entire approach. Writing in April 2003, Steinman, Nissenson, Glassock, et.al state "Careful review of all available clinical trials of L-carnitine leads to the conclusion that there is insufficient evidence to support the routine use of L-carnitine for any indication in dialysis patients. The literature suffers from a lack of adequately designed studies, and many of the studies, which supposedly justify payment for L-carnitine supplementation, are more than ten years old. While some studies support a subjective improvement in symptoms after a few months of L-carnitine treatment, there is little confirming objective data? ... A major criticism is that many if the reported symptoms could be attributed to anemia, which at the time the L-carnitine studies were taking place, was generally being corrected with EPO" [33].

An alternate perspective on carnitine therapy comes from the Carnitine Consensus Conference of the National Kidney Foundation. Among other recommendations for carnitine therapy in dialysis patients, this committee supports the use of carnitine for alleviation of fatigue:

"The administration of L-carnitine is recommended for selected patients with symptoms such as muscle weakness and fatigability that affect their quality of life. L-carnitine should be reserved for those patients in whom other causes have been excluded and who have been unresponsive to standard therapies. Response to L-carnitine should be evaluated at 3-month intervals with an appropriate objective instrument. The same instrument should be used before and during therapy. L-carnitine therapy should be discontinues if no clinical improvement has occurred within 9-12 months.

The available evidence is weakest for the response of muscle weakness and functional well being to L-carnitine therapy. However, the central role of L-carnitine in muscle function and the limited number of reports showing improvement in muscle strength and functional well being following L-carnitine justify consideration of treatment of selected patients' [34].

Post dialytic fatigue is a symptom limited to dialysis patients treated with chronic intermittent dialysis therapy. Its appearance is unpredictable and its treatment uncertain. Some patients at the conclusion of a dialysis session experience extreme fatigue and lethargy. Post dialysis hypotension is an explanation for some patients. There remains a small cohort of patients who manifest these symptoms and complaints without anemia or hypotension. Fatigue is sometimes so extreme that patients sleep as soon as they return to their homes and many patients are so weak as to be incapacitated until sometime the next day. In 1996 Sklar, et.al. studied 85 patients on conventional maintenance hemodialysis [35]. They used a validated questionnaire as a survey tool and found that 43 patients reported significant fatigue related to their dialysis treatment. Twenty-eight of these fatigued patients reported that their symptoms occurred with about 80% of their treatments. 28 patients reported that the fatigue started with the first dialysis treatment. They needed an average of 4.8 hours of sleep to overcome the post dialysis fatigue, though some required 24 hours to recover. Sklar et.al noted that the Beck depression score yielded more positive results in the fatigue patients than the 42 unaffected patients (p=0.02). The two groups did not differ with respect to many other parameters, including age, sex, cause of ESRD, the presence of ischemic or congestive heart failure, lung disease, anemia, albumin, urea or creatinine blood levels, or parathyroid hormone levels.

In a later study Sklar et.al examined the potential effect of dialyzer membrane type upon post dialysis fatigue [36]. For many years conventional hemodialysis employed membranes constructed of cellulose or a processed form of cellulose known as cuprophane. While these materials are still in use, synthetic membranes such as polymethylmethacrylate, polysulfone or polyacrylonitrile find increasing use. These materials are generally held to be more "biocompatible". This concept stems from a number of observations about interactions between cellulosic membranes and blood components. Cellulosic membranes often activate the complement cascade during dialysis and can cause temporary redistribution of white blood cells from the peripheral circulation to the lungs during the first hour of conventional dialysis [37]. Such events do not occur with the synthetic membranes. Noting that tumor necrosis factor can cause somnolence and is found in the circulation of dialysis patients treated with cuprophane membranes, Sklar et.al. conducted a crossover trial with a week of dialysis treatments using either cuprophane or polymethymethacrylate [36]. These investigators found no difference in fatigue symptoms, but studied only sixteen patients in total.

In a still later study Sklar et.al examined sodium profiling and ultrafiltration effects upon fatigue symptoms [38]. Traditionally the concentration of sodium in the dialysate delivered to the membrane has been somewhat less than the normal blood sodium concentration. These differences are not large, but are enough to establish an osmotic gradient between the patient's blood and the fluid on the other side of the dialysis membrane. Sodium profiling is a scheme wherein the initial concentration of sodium in the dialysate is slightly hypertonic to the body during the early dialysis run but drops during the treatment according to a variety of algorithms. The drop in sodium concentration is sometimes done in stepwise fashion or may model an exponential decay curve. The proponents of these approaches assert that they reduce the frequency of abrupt severe drops in blood pressure and severe cramps, which bedevil so many patients treated with conventional hemodialysis. Sklar et.al. found in this small study of 12 hemodialysis paitents that those patients who experienced sodium profiling reported less post dialysis fatigue than those not so treated. In 1993 Sadowski et.al reported that sodium profiling reduced the incidence of intradialytic cramps, headaches, nausea and vomiting as well as post dialysis fatigue [39]. The study involved sixteen patients between the ages of 16 and 32. These observations have never been validated in large-scale clinical trials: sodium profiling is commonly but not universally applied today. These findings do suggest benefit from longer duration treatments such as peritoneal dialysis or nocturnal daily dialysis. In these modalities the osmotic and hemodynamic shifts are minimized.

The path from onset of kidney disease to a dialysis requirement may be short or very long. Some patients require dialysis within days of trauma, nephrotoxic exposure, or surgical complication. Diabetic nephropathy, the most common cause for ESRD in the U.S., typically has a slow course measured in years or even decades. For many, the slow deterioration of renal function goes on unnoticed and undetected. Whether it comes as an abrupt shock or the final culmination of a multi-year dread, the institution of chronic dialysis represents a major alteration of lifestyle and self-perception. In a sense the initiation of dialysis represents the substitution of a less lethal but often highly morbid chronic disease for the much more lethal disease of uremia. Depression often accompanies the advent of hemodialysis or peritoneal dialysis. Depression can present in many ways, including lassitude, altered sleep patterns and fatigue. Complaints of fatigue in someone at or near a dialysis requirement should always prompt a consideration of a diagnosis of depression. Clinicians often employ anti-depressant medication with significant benefit. Cho and Tsay recently reported that a month long course of acupressure massage reduced the common problems of fatigue and depression in 62 Taiwanese hemodialysis patients [40]. Many studies employing physical therapy and various exercise regimens have documented improvement in physical activity. Some, such as the 1993 study by Brunier and Graydon correlate low levels of physical activity with fatigue [41].

CONCLUSION

Renal failure and chronic dialysis are states, which expose patients to profound metabolic, hemodynamic and psychosocial challenges. Along with many other symptoms, fatigue is predictably common. Less predictable are which of the many potential factors causing or promoting fatigue is present in an individual patient. Many of these factors are not well understood and some cannot be avoided easily given current therapeutic options. The diligent search for root causes of fatigue in chronic renal failure can bring rewards to both patients and clinicians.

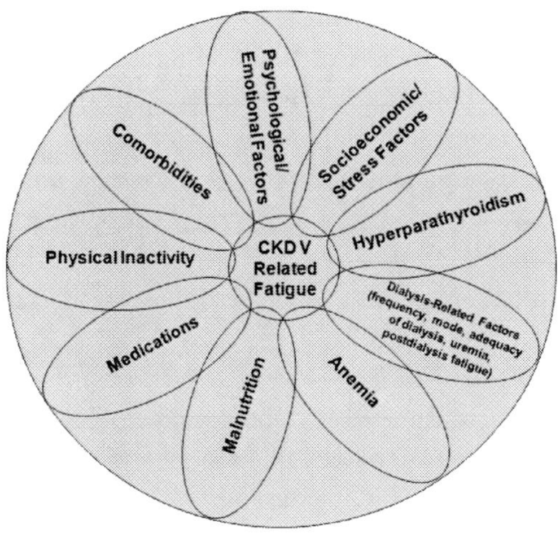

Figure 1. Factors contributing to Fatigue in CKD V.

References

[1] Bossola, M., Luciani, G., & Tazza, L. (2009). Fatigue and its correlates in chronic hemodialysis patients. *Blood Purif*, 28,245-252.

[2] Eshbach, J.W., Haley, N.R., & Adamson, J.W. (1990). The anemia of chronic renal failure: pathophysiology and effects of recombinant erythropoietin. *Contrib Nephrol*, 78,24-37.

[3] Ross, S.D., Fahrbach, K., Frame, D., Scheye, R., Connelly, J.E., & Glaspy, J. (2003). The effect of anemia treatment on selected health related quality of life domains: a systematic review. *Clin Ther*, 25,1786-1803.

[4] Evans, R.W., Rader, B., Mannimen, D.L., & the Cooperative Multicenter EPO Clinical Trial Group. (1990). The quality of life of hemodialysis recipients treated with recombinant human erythropoietin. *J Am Med Assoc*, 263,825-830.

[5] Barany, P., Pettersson, E., & Konarski-Svensson, J.K. (1993). Long term effects on quality of life in hemodialysis patients of correction of anemia with erythropoietin. *Nepohrol Dial Transplant*, 8,426-432.

[6] Canadian Erythropoietin Study Group. (1990). Association between recombinant human erythropoietin and quality of life and exercise capacity of patients receiving haemodialysis. *BMJ*, 300,573-578.

[7] Berns, J.S. (2005). Should the Target Hemoglobin for Patients with Chronic Kidney Disease Treated with Erythropoietin Replacement Therapy be changed? *Sem Dial*, 18,22.

[8] Kazmi, W.H., Kausz, A.T., Khan, S., Abichandani, R., Ruthazer, R., Obrador, G.T., & Pereira, B.J. (2001). Anemia: an early complication of chronic renal insufficiency. *Am J Kidney Dis*, 38,803-812.

[9] (2003). USRDS: the United States Renal Data System. *Am J Kidney Dis*, 42,1-230.

[10] ibid.

[11] Moreno, F., Sany-Guajardo, D., Lopez-Gomez, J.M., Jofre, R., & Valdernabano, F. (2000). Increasing the hematocrit has a beneficial effect on quality of life and is safe in selected hemodialysis patients. Spanish Cooperative Renal Patients Quality of Life. Study Group of the Spanish Society of Nepohrology. *J Am Soc Nepohrol*, 11,335-342.

[12] Furland, H., Linde, T., Ahlmen, J., Christensson, A., Strombom, U., & Danielson, B.G. (2003). A randomized controlled trial of haemoglobin normalization with epoietin alpha in pre dialysis and dialysis patients. *Nephrol Dial Transplant*, 18,353-361.

[13] Besarab, A., Bolton, W.K., Browne, J.K., Egrie, J.C., Nissenson, A.R., Okamoto, D.M., Schwab, S.T., & Goodkin, D.A. (1998). The effects of normal as compared with low hematocrit values in patients with cardiac disease who are receiving hemodialysis and epoietin. *N Eng J Med*, 339,584-590.

[14] (2006). *American Journal of Kidney Disease*, 47, S11-S145.

[15] E. F. Unger, A. M. Thompson, M. J. Blank, and R. Temple. (2010). Erythropoiesis-Stimulating Agents — Time for a Reevaluation. *New Engl J Med*, 362,189-192.

[16] Singh, A.K., Szczech, L. Tang, K.L., Barnhart, H., Sapp, S. Wolfson, M., Reddan, D., & CHOIR Investigators. (2006). Correction of anemia with epoetin alfa in chronic kidney disease. N Engl J Med, 355,2085-2098.

[17] Pfeffer, M.A., Burdmann, E.A., Chen, C.Y., Cooper, M.E., de Zeeuw, D., Eckardt, K.U., Feyzi, J.M., Ivanovich, P., Kewalramani, R., Levey, A.S., Lewis, E.F., McGill, J.B., McMurray, J.J., Parfey, P., Parving, H.H., Remuzzi, G., Singh, A.K. Solomon, S. D., Toto, R. & TREAT Investigators. (2009). A trial of darbepoetin alfa in type 2 diabetes and chronic kidney disease. *N Engl J Med*, 361,2091-2032.

[18] Besarab, A., Bolton, W.K., Browne, J.K., Egrie, J.C., Nissenson, A.R., Okamoto, D.M., Schwab, S.J.., & Goodkin, D.A. (1998). *N Engl J Med*. 339,584-590.

[19] Drüeke, T.B., Locatelli, F., Clyne, N., Eckardt, K.U., Macdougall, I.C., Tsakiris, D., Burger, H.U., Scherhag, A., & CREATE Investigators. (2006). Normalization of hemoglobin level in patients with chronic kidney disease and anemia. *N Engl J Med*, 355,2071-2084.

[20] Gotch, F.A., & Sargent, J.A. (1985).A mechanistic analysis of the National cooperative Dialysis Study (NCDS). Kidney Int, 28,526-534.

[21] Iliescu, E.A., Yeates, K.E., & Holland, D.C. (2004). Quality of sleep in patients with chronic kidney disease. *Nephrol Dial Transplant*, 19,95-99.

[22] Hul, D.S.C., Wong, T.Y.H., Li, T.S.T., Ko, F.W.S., Choy, D.K.L., Szeto, C.C., & Li, P.K.T. (2002). Prevalence of Sleep disturbances in Chinese patient with End Stage Renal Failure on maintenance hemodialysis. *Med Sic Monit*, 8,CR331-336.

[23] Hanly, P. (2004). Sleep Apnea and Daytime Sleepiness in End Stage Renal Disease. *Semen Dial*, 17,109-114.

[24] Parker, K.P., Bliwise, D.L., Bialy, J.L & Rye, D.B. (2003). Daytime sleepiness in stable hemodialysis patients. *Amer J Kid Dis*, 41,394-402.

[25] Sabbatini, M., Minale, B., Crispo, A., Pisani, A., Rigosta, A., Esposito, R., Cesaro, A., Cianciaruso, B., & Andreucci, V.F. (2002). Insomnia in Maintenance hemodialysis patients. *Nephrol Dial Transplant*, 17,852-856.

[26] Hui, D.S.C., Wong, T.Y.H., Li, T.S.T., Ko, F.W.S., Choy, D.K.L., Szeto, C.C., Lui, S.F., & Li, P.K.T. (2002). Prevalence on sleep disturbances in Chinese patients with End Stage Renal Failure on maintenance hemodialysis. *Med Sci Monit*, 8,CR331-336.

[27] Fletcher, E.C. (1993). Obstructive sleep apnea and the kidney. *J Am Soc Nephrol*, 4,1111-1121.

[28] Hanly, P.J., Gabor, J.Y., Chan, C., & Pierratos, A. (2003). Daytime sleepiness in patients with CRF: impact on nocturnal hemodialysis. *Am J Kidney Dis*, 41,403-410.

[29] Walters, A.S., & the International Restless Leg Study Group. (1995). Toward a better definition of the [restless] leg syndrome. *Mov Disord*, 10,634-642.

[30] Sabbatini, M., Minale, B., Crispo, A., Pisani, A., Ragosta, A., Esposito, R., Cesaro, A., Cianciaruso, B., & Andreucci, V.E. (2002). Insomnia in Maintenance hemodialysis patients. *Nephrol Dial Transplant*, 17,852-856.

[31] Huroi, J.M., Cuchert, M., Haugh, M., & Fouque D. (2002). Effects of L-carnitine Supplementation in Maintenance Hemodialysis Patients: A systematic Review. *J Am Soc Nephrology*, 13,708-714.

[32] Brass, E.P., Adler, S., Sietsema, K.E., Hiatt, W.R., Orland, A.M., & Amato, A. (2001). Intravenous L-carnitine increases plasma carnitine, reduces fatigue, and may preserve exercise capacity in hemodialysis patients. *Am J Kidney Dis*, 37,1018-1028.

[33] Steinman, T.I., Nissenson, A.R., Glassick, R.J., Dickmeyer, J., Mattern, W.D., Parker, T.F., & Hull, A.R. (2003). L-carnitine use in dialysis patients: is national coverage for supplementation justified? *Nephrol News and Issues*, 17,10-11.

[34] Eknoyan, G., Latos, D.L., & Lindberg, J. (2003). Practice recommendations for the use of L-carnitine in Dialysis Related Carnitine Disorder. National Kidney Foundation Carnitine Consensus Conference. *Am J Kidney Dis*, 41,868-875.

[35] Sklar, A.H., Riesenberg, L.A., Silber, A.K., Ahmed, W., & Ali, A. (1996). Postdialysis fatigue. *Am J Kidney Dis*, 28,732-736.

[36] Sklar, A.H., Beezhold, D.H., Newmon, N., Hendrickson, T.,& Driesbach, A.W. (1998). Postdialysis Fatigue: lack of effect of a biocompatible membrane, *Am J Kidney Dis*, 31,1007-1010.

[37] Koller, H., Hochegger, K., Zlabinger, G.J., Lhotta, K., Mayer, G., & Rosenkranz, A.R. (2004). Apoptosis of human polymorphonuclear neutrophils accelerated by dialysis membranes via the activation of complement. *Nephrol Dial Transplant*, 19,3104-3111.

[38] Sklar, A., Newman, N., Semenyuk, L., Schultz, J., & Fiacco, V. (1999). Identification of factors responsible for postdialysis fatigue. *Am J Kidney Dis*, 34,464-470.

[39] Sadowski, R.N., Allred, E.N., & Jabs, K. (1993). Sodium modeling ameliorates intradialytic and interdialytic and interdialytic symptoms in young hemodialysis patients. *J Am Soc Nephrol*, 4,1192-1198.

[40] Cho, Y.C., & Tsay, Y.L. (2004). The effect of acupressure with massage on fatigue and depression in patients with end-stage renal disease. *J Nurs Res*, 12,51-59.

[41] Brunier, G.M., & Graydon, J. (1993). The influence of physical activity on fatigue in patients with ESRD on hemodialysis. *ANNA J*, 20, 457-461.

In: Handbook of Fatigue in Health and Disease
Editor: Howard S. Smith

ISBN 978-1-61761-920-5

Chapter 9

FATIGUE AND DEPRESSION

L. J. Norelli[a,b*] ***and S. K. Harju***[c+]

[a] Capital District Psychiatric Center, 75 New Scotland, Albany, NY 12208, USA
[b] Department of Psychiatry, Albany Medical Center, Albany, NY, USA
[c] Department of Psychology, University of Joensuu, Joensuu, Finland

ABSTRACT

Major depressive disorder (MDD) is a common and potentially debilitating illness for millions of subjects throughout the world. MDD is typically episodic but 60% of patients have a recurrence within 5 years of their index episode and it may become a chronic condition in up to a third of patients. Fatigue is a core symptom of depression and can accompany any phase of the disorder - prodromal, acute, and during recovery. The neurobiology of fatigue associated with depression is poorly understood. Despite improved treatment strategies, partial response and persistence of residual symptoms remains common. Thus, with treatment, mood and aspects of MDD may improve without concomitant improvement in fatigue. In fact, residual fatigue may be predictive of relapse, or chronicity with subsequent severe psychosocial dysfunction. No specific robust evidence exists with respect to treating the fatigue associated with MDD.

* Corresponding author:
Lisa Norelli, MD, MPH, MRCPsych
Chief of Psychiatry, Capital District Psychiatric Center, Albany, New York
Assistant Professor, Department of Psychiatry, Albany Medical College, Albany, New York
Capital District Psychiatric Center
75 New Scotland Avenue, Albany NY 12208
tel 518 447 9611
fax 518 447 9630
Email: cdfmljn@omh.ny.gov
+ Post Office Box 771
Clifton Park, New York 12065
Email: sharju@earthlink.net

INTRODUCTION

There is growing recognition of depression as a significant global public health problem. According to the World Health Organization (WHO) depression is estimated to affect 121 million people worldwide and is one of the most disabling conditions in both developed and developing nations [1-3]. Depression typically manifests as an episodic disorder; and for a significant portion of patients it develops into a chronic condition. About sixty percent of patients experience a recurrence within five years of the index episode, and up to one third develops chronic depression following a single episode [4-7].

The current editions of the American Psychiatric Association Diagnostic and Statistical Manual of Mental Disorders (DSM-IV-TR) and the WHO International Classification of Disease (ICD-10) are two internationally accepted psychiatric diagnostic nosologies [8, 9]. Both employ similar symptom criteria for the diagnosis of a unipolar depressive episode in the context of persistently depressed mood, or loss of interest or pleasure. Table 1 compares the DSM-IV-TR and ICD-10 symptom criteria for a depressive episode. In both systems, fatigue is one of the core symptoms of depression. In DSM-IV-TR, major depressive disorder is characterized by depressive episodes of at least 2 weeks duration with at least five out of nine criterion symptoms. In ICD-10, the diagnosis of a depressive episode and recurrent depressive disorder is more descriptive and less criterion-specific. Depressive disorder excludes depression caused by the direct physiological effects of a substance (e.g. drugs, medications) or a general medical condition. Otherwise, depression is a heterogeneous condition diagnosed without stringent regard to etiology or response to treatment. For clarity, the term depressive disorder will be used in this chapter to denote the equivalent diagnoses of major depressive disorder and recurrent depressive disorder, excluding bipolar depression.

Table 1. DSM and ICD symptom

DSM-IV-TR	ICD-10
Depressed mood	Depressed mood
Diminished interest or pleasure	Loss of interest and enjoyment
Significant weight change	Diminished appetite
Insomnia or hypersomnia	Disturbed sleep
Psychomotor agitation or retardation	Reduced concentration and attention
Fatigue or loss of energy	Reduced energy leading to increased fatigability and diminished activity
Feelings of worthlessness or inappropriate guilt	Ideas of guilt and unworthiness
Diminished ability to think or concentrate	Reduced self-esteem and self-confidence
Recurrent thoughts of death or suicidal ideas or plan	Ideas or acts of self-harm or suicide
	Bleak and pessimistic view of the future

Fatigue-related symptoms in depression include persistent loss of energy, tiredness, and difficulty with concentration or decreased ability to think. Though fatigue is a common feature of depression and a variety of other disorders, there is no universal definition for the condition. Conceived as a multidimensional symptom, it has both physical and psychological components. Fatigue is subjectively experienced as physical exhaustion, apathy, tiring more quickly, increased effort to perform physical or mental tasks including increased difficulty concentrating. Fatigue is one of the most widespread conditions encountered among general and health care populations [10, 11]. In developed countries, about one quarter of people in community and primary care samples are fatigued with about one in five suffering chronic fatigue lasting more than six months. Cross-cultural prevalence rates of unexplained fatigue lasting at least one-month duration vary from 2–15% in primary care settings, with the higher rates in developed countries [12-18].

A central problem in assessing the clinical and research findings regarding fatigue and depression is the uncertainty about which symptoms are primary or secondary. Thus, in conditions dominated by fatigue, such as fibromyalgia or chronic fatigue syndrome (CFS), depression may be a consequence of the chronic and disabling illness. Fatigue and depression frequently accompany other non-psychiatric illnesses or their treatments, such as multiple sclerosis, cardiovascular disease, and cancer. In this chapter, fatigue will be discussed from the perspective of a symptom associated with a primary diagnosis of unipolar depressive disorder.

FATIGUE IN DEPRESSIVE DISORDERS

Why is the co-occurrence of depression and fatigue important? First, unexplained fatigue is frequently associated with an underlying undiagnosed depression. Second, most patients with depressive disorder have associated fatigue at some phase of the episode. Third, fatigue is a strong predictor of depression relapse and chronicity. Prominent fatigue and especially persistence of fatigue in depressive disorder is associated with poor long-term outcome.

Unexplained fatigue is encountered frequently in all clinical settings and is an important, but non-specific, indicator of illness. Numerous studies in both clinical and community settings have associated fatigue and psychiatric disorders, especially depression [19-24]. According to Wessely and Powell (1989) about three quarters of patients presenting to primary care with unexplained chronic fatigue have some kind of psychiatric disorder [25]. A Canadian study identified fatigue as the primary or secondary complaint in 14% of patients attending a family medicine clinic, and nearly half of the fatigued patients had a lifetime diagnosis of depression [15]. Similarly, a multinational primary care survey found that 41% of patients with unexplained fatigue had depression [17]. Many studies have confirmed the clinical observation that fatigue or loss of energy is a prominent feature of most depressive episodes. Despite the frequent correlation, depression often remains an overlooked cause of fatigue. In a study of symptom frequency in acute depression, reduced energy was reported in 97% of patients regardless of gender, age of onset, or number of episodes [26]. A pan-European community survey demonstrated that nearly three quarters of respondents have experienced tiredness or lack of energy during a depressive episode [27]. The Epidemiologic Catchment Area (ECA) study, a multi-community survey of psychiatric disorder prevalence in the United States, has also helped illuminate the relationship between fatigue and depressive disorders. In the ECA, fatigue was demonstrated to be both predictive and a consequence of depression. Participants with unexplained fatigue lasting at least two weeks had 4 times greater lifetime risk for major depression compared to non-fatigued participants. Participants with recurrent fatigue (those who reported fatigue at baseline and at the 13 year follow up) had 28 times greater lifetime risk of depression [28, 29].

Fatigue is not solely a characteristic feature of depression, but it can also be a valuable indicator of the clinical course of the disorder. It has been identified as strongly predictive of first episode onset, subsequent relapse, and chronicity of depressive disorder [20, 28, 30]. Fatigue is a common prodromal symptom of the first and subsequent episodes of major depression [31-33]. As such, it should be viewed as an early indicator of impending relapse. For many patients, full asymptomatic recovery from depression is often difficult to achieve. The persistence of residual symptoms such as fatigue, even after adequate treatment of the depressive episode, has been associated with poor long-term outcome and early re-occurrence. A large cohort study revealed patients who had asymptomatic recovery from unipolar depression relapsed on average in 157 weeks, compared to patients with residual symptoms who relapsed in only 28 weeks [34-39].

The Neurobiology of Fatigue in Depression

Different biological systems have been hypothesized to underlie depressive disorders, yet the development of a unified neurobiological theory of depression still eludes medical science. Due to the heterogeneity of depression, alterations in biological systems have not been consistently demonstrated in all patients. Similarly, it is not surprising that the neurobiology underlying fatigue in depressive disorder remains poorly understood. Neuronal circuits that mediate the symptoms of fatigue likely differ from those that mediate sadness or depressed mood. Physical fatigue symptoms are thought to be related to circuits that mediate motor function such as the striatum and cerebellum. The perception of physical tiredness may involve peripheral sensory input to descending fibers in the spinal cord. Diffuse cortical projections and prefrontal circuits appear to mediate the symptoms of mental fatigue [40-42]. The most commonly implicated pathways for fatigue in depression are diverse and include the serotonin, norepinephrine, dopamine and histamine neurotransmitter systems, the hypothalamic-pituitary-adrenal (HPA) axis, the thyroid axis, and the immune inflammatory response system.

Evidence From Imaging Studies

Structural and functional brain imaging is helping to refine understanding of the central nervous system circuitry underlying key depressive symptoms. Structural abnormalities associated with depressive disorder include volume reduction in the frontal cortex, amygdala, hippocampus, and striatum [43]. These reductions may represent chronic neurodegeneration secondary to neural death or reduced neural plasticity from repeated mood episodes [44]. Abnormalities in cerebral blood flow or glucose metabolism have been found in the prefrontal cortex, anterior cingulate cortex, amygdala and basal ganglia of depressed patients [45, 46]. Excess activation of the medial prefrontal cortex has been linked with sadness and depressed mood, whereas reduced neuronal activity in the dorsolateral prefrontal cortex may be related to the symptom of mental fatigue in depression. Prefrontal hypoactivity is believed to correlate with disturbances of motor function and effort perception commonly observed in patients with depressive disorders. Increased right thalamic perfusion in depression, similar to a comparison group of patients with CFS, is speculated to reflect an increase in vigilance towards certain tasks, which are then experienced as more effortful [47, 48].

Neurotransmitter Systems

The catecholamines norepinephrine, serotonin and dopamine have been implicated as candidate neurotransmitters in depression. This is based largely on the observations that medications that target these systems have antidepressant effects, and catecholamine system abnormalities exist in patients with depression. Current thinking emphasizes catecholamine neurotransmission in a regulatory role, mediating the symptoms of depressive disorders by modulating the activity of different brain circuits. All three neurotransmitter systems have been associated with fatigue. In addition, the histamine system has been identified as having a role in arousal, stress response, and the regulation of mental fatigue [42, 49-51].

Serotonin

Serotonin neurons originate in the midbrain raphe nucleus and project widely to the limbic system, basal ganglia, cortex and cerebellum. The serotonin system regulates many functions including the sleep-wake cycle, appetite, mood, and impulse control. Depression is associated with a functional decrease of serotonin neurotransmission [52]. Increased serotonin activity in the hypothalamus has been associated with increased fatigue [42, 53].

Dopamine

The dopamine system regulates motor and cognitive function via three neural circuits. The nigrostriatal system originates in the midbrain substantia nigra and projects to the striatum to modulate motor activity. The mesolimbic system originates in the ventral tegmental area and projects to the ventral striatum and prefrontal cortex, regulating emotion and reward response. Finally, the mesocortical system originates in the ventral tegmental area and projects to the motor cortex and dorsolateral prefrontal cortex. This system regulates movement and problem solving functions. Reduced dopamine activity observed in depressive disorder has been associated with anhedonia, loss of motivation and interest, and psychomotor slowing [54, 55]. Stimulation of striatal and prefrontal cortical dopamine pathways are believed responsible for the fatigue-reducing properties of medications such as amphetamine and levodopa, and from non-pharmacologic interventions such as physical exercise [56].

Norepinephrine

Norepinephrine neurons originate in the midbrain ventrolateral tegmental area and the locus coeruleus in the brainstem. The ventrolateral tegmental area neurons project to the hypothalamus and reticular formation, and the locus coeruleus neurons project to the thalamus, hypothalamus, cortex and prefrontal cortex. These circuits regulate functions such as sleep, feeding, energy, arousal and alertness in addition to mood regulation. Norepinephrine system dysfunction has been associated with cognitive deficits, dysphoric mood, and fatigue. Agents that enhance norepinephrine reuptake activity improve fatigue, psychomotor retardation, and sleep abnormalities [50, 57].

Histamine

Histamine neurons originate in the tuberomammillary nucleus in the hypothalamus and project widely to the central nervous system and spinal cord. One group of neurons innervate the thalamus, hippocampus, amygdala, and cortex. Descending projections innervate the cerebellum, midbrain, brainstem and spinal cord. Decreased histamine activity is associated with decreased arousal, sedation, and may be associated with mental fatigue [49, 50].

THE ENDOCRINE SYSTEM

The HPA axis has been extensively studied in depressive disorders. HPA dysregulation is a prominent feature of depression, usually represented by over-activity, with increased production of glucocorticoids, corticotrophin releasing hormone (CRH), and impaired feedback mechanisms. Hypercortisolemia, and blunted ACTH response to CRH have been associated with melancholic and psychotic types of depression. In contrast, depressive disorders with atypical features have been associated with normal or hypocortisolemic states [57-61]. The hypocortisolemia seen in atypical depression and other disorders (e.g. CFS, post-traumatic stress disorder, fibromyalgia, irritable bowel syndrome) often share the syndrome of pain, fatigue and enhanced stress sensitivity [62].

Thyroid axis dysfunction has also been demonstrated in depression. Fatigue and depression are well known attributes of hypothyroidism. Depressive disorder is associated with disturbances in thyroid metabolism including a decrease of T_3 levels, blunted TSH response to TRH, and decreased central nervous system conversion of T_4 to T_3. This suggests a central hypothyroid state even in the presence of normal peripheral thyroid status [57, 58, 63].

THE IMMUNE SYSTEM

Activation of the immune system, such as increased production of pro-inflammatory cytokines, has been associated with depression and fatigue. Although it is unclear what role cytokines play in the pathophysiology of depression, the cytokine hypothesis of major depression has evolved from several lines of evidence linking depression, fatigue, and immune system activation [59, 60, 64, 65]. Major depression has been shown to be associated with heightened inflammatory response, and increased levels of inflammatory cytokines have been associated with fatigue and depression [66, 67]. Treatment with antidepressants decreases inflammatory cytokine levels in some patients, and may modulate the central effects of pro-inflammatory immune activation [68, 69]. Therapeutic administration of the cytokine interferon can cause a syndrome of depressed mood, fatigue, and other symptoms, identical to a depressive episode. The syndrome has been experimentally reversed with cytokine antagonists [70, 71]. Cytokines acutely stimulate serotonin neurotransmission and reduce the production of serotonin. Some cytokines appear to up-regulate the serotonin transporter, thereby depleting extracellular serotonin [67, 72]. These effects on serotonergic activity may play role in the expression of depressive symptoms.

Strategies for Managing Fatigue in Depression

Currently available receptor-selective antidepressants target certain brain circuits more effectively than others. This may explain the observations that certain depressive symptoms respond more robustly to antidepressant treatment than others, and residual symptoms, including fatigue, are common even with treatment responsive depression [36, 42, 50]. To date, relatively few studies have examined antidepressant effects on fatigue specifically or the general treatment of fatigue symptoms in depression. Although fatigue will resolve for many patients when they are successfully treated for depression, a significant number will continue to suffer from residual symptoms [35, 36]. Despite the challenge it presents to the clinician and the paucity of empirical evidence currently available, residual fatigue should be aggressively treated to decrease the risk of relapse and disability. Treatment includes both pharmacologic and non-pharmacologic strategies [41, 73-78].

General Approaches

Effective management of fatigue in depression involves assessment and modification of lifestyle habits as important general measures. This approach includes attention to general health needs and lifestyle habits. Sleep disturbance is strongly associated with both fatigue and depression; therefore, educating patients regarding good sleep hygiene practices can help to improve sleep quality [79, 80]. Although not recommended as a first-line approach, short-term pharmacological treatment of insomnia may be necessary if the sleep disturbance is severe and unresponsive to other interventions. Regular physical activity is also beneficial for mood and energy. Graded aerobic exercise is thought to reduce fatigue by enhancement of central dopaminergic activity. In addition, exercise may have a protective effect for some individuals against development of mood and fatigue symptoms [56, 81]. Healthy diet and avoidance of alcohol and drugs, including excessive caffeine, are important to overall health and energy levels. Evidence supports the effectiveness of psychological therapies, such as cognitive behavior therapy (CBT), for treating mood and somatic symptoms in some patients with prominent fatigue. CBT has been shown helpful in preventing relapse and the management of residual symptoms in depressed patients [82, 83]. A wide variety of prescribed, over-the-counter medications and dietary supplements can cause fatigue. These should be evaluated for medical necessity, with use of lowest effective dose or less fatiguing alternatives when possible.

Pharmacologic Strategies

Many antidepressants have fatigue as a potential side effect. Prescribing strategies to reduce fatigue in depression include the avoidance of sedating medications, careful dose reduction, or the addition of a stimulating adjunctive agent. When choosing medication for the treatment of depressive disorder with prominent fatigue, antidepressants that increase either or both norepinephrine and dopamine activity may be advantageous [42, 50, 78, 84, 85]. Currently available, first-line antidepressants that enhance neurotransmission in these circuits include the serotonin norepinephrine reuptake inhibitors (SNRIs), norepinephrine reuptake inhibitors (NRIs), and buproprion. The use of agents with predominant serotonergic activity may be of less benefit because the enhancement of serotonin activity in certain brain areas may contribute to fatigue.[42, 53] Thus, it is not surprising that selective serotonin reuptake inhibitors (SSRIs) have not been shown to be particularly effective for the fatigue component of depressive disorder [86].

Antidepressant Monotherapy

The SNRIs include venlafaxine, duloxetine, and milnacipran. The SNRIs may be more effective in treating severe depression, as well as accompanying physical and pain symptoms [87, 88]. Buproprion is thought to activate norepinephrine and dopamine circuits. It is a non-sedating antidepressant, and it improves fatigue in depressed patients. NRIs enhance dopaminergic and noradrenergic neurotransmission in the prefrontal cortex improving executive function, energy and decreasing fatigue. Currently available NRIs include atomoxetine, a medication for attention deficit hyperactivity disorder, and reboxetine, an antidepressant [89-91].

Antidepressant Augmentation Strategies

Although the use of one medication to treat depressive disorder is preferred for several reasons, it is often difficult to achieve full symptom remission with monotherapy. Augmentation strategies are commonly used in treatment resistant or partially responsive depression, and therefore may be helpful to reduce depressive fatigue. Common strategies include adding buproprion, atomoxetine, or reboxetine to an SSRI with the rationale that this will enhance norepinephrine and dopamine neurotransmission [50, 73, 74, 78].This approach is supported by limited, but mounting, empirical evidence. A retrospective chart review suggests that atomoxetine added to conventional antidepressant therapy may be effective for residual fatigue in depression. Buproprion has been shown effective specifically in treating SSRI-related fatigue in depressed patients and in augmenting a partial response to antidepressant therapy [91-93].

Psychostimulants and Other Dopaminergic Agents

Modafinil and armodafinil are agents that promote wakefulness, possibly by modulating dopamine, norepinephrine, and histamine neurotransmission and selectively activating hypothalamic projections to the cortex [94, 95]. Approved for treating excessive sleepiness in narcolepsy, obstructive sleep apnea, and shift work sleep disorder, these medications have also been used in unapproved indications such as for treating severe fatigue that complicates non-psychiatric disorders [96, 97]. Modafinil has been studied as an augmenting agent for partially remitted depression and shown to be an effective short-term strategy to reduce residual fatigue and sleepiness in depressed patients treated with conventional antidepressant therapy. So far, results are mixed. There are some data to support synergistic serotonergic effects when modafinil is added to conventional antidepressants [98-101]. However, a recent systematic review of the literature did not show a statistically significant difference in depressive symptoms, including fatigue, in patients treated with modafinil versus placebo [102].

Agents that enhance central dopaminergic activity have been used to treat fatigue associated with a variety of disorders and may be helpful in depressive disorder. These include psychostimulants such as pemoline, methylphenidate, or amphetamine, traditionally prescribed for attention deficit hyperactivity disorder. They have broad central nervous system stimulating effects and carry the potential risk of abuse and dependence. Psychostimulants have been used to in combination with other antidepressants to augment response to older (tricyclic and monoamine oxidase inhibitors) and newer (SSRI) antidepressant agents. A number of reports suggest a potential role for psychostimulant treatment of residual fatigue in depression [102-104]. A recent systematic review of psychostimulants in depression concluded that there is evidence for the short-term use of this class of psychostimulants for the short-term treatment of residual depression symptoms, including fatigue [102].

Amantadine may enhance dopamine activity at lower doses and has been used to treat mild fatigue in patients with multiple sclerosis and theoretically could have a role in treating depression-related fatigue. Likewise, the dopamine receptor agonists pergolide and cabergoline could potentially reduce residual fatigue in depression. There is little empirical evidence to support the routine use of these medications, but pergolide has been shown to improve fatigue in patients with Parkinson's disease, and two patients with depressive disorder were reported to have improvement of fatigue and depression when cabergoline was added to a dual action antidepressant [105, 106].

Other Agents of Potential Benefit

Thyroid hormone supplementation, especially T_3, has been used as an augmenting agent for treatment resistant depression, therefore, some depressed patients with residual fatigue may respond to this strategy [107]. Improved fatigue and depression with l-thyroxine supplementation in euthyroid subjects has been demonstrated [108].

Lamotrigine, an anticonvulsant medication, has shown efficacy in treating bipolar depression and is being studied for use in unipolar depression. When added to conventional medication for depression, lamotrigine may improve treatment response and hasten onset of action [109, 110]. This medication is considered to have an activating profile and evidence suggests it could reduce fatigue and somnolence in some epilepsy patients but there are little data specific to depression and fatigue [111, 112]. Further research is needed to determine whether the favorable effects on mood and fatigue apply to individuals with depressive disorder.

Conclusion

Depressive disorder is a common and potentially debilitating illness for millions of people worldwide. Despite current treatment strategies, partial response and the persistence of residual symptoms is a common outcome. Fatigue is a core symptom of depression and can accompany any phase of the disorder - prodromal, acute, and during recovery. Most importantly, residual fatigue is a predictor of relapse, chronicity, and can contribute to severe psychosocial dysfunction. All of the key symptoms of depression merit aggressive and comprehensive treatment to improve quality of life and overall prognosis. Although there is a paucity of evidence regarding treatment approaches for specific symptoms such as fatigue in depression, a rational strategy involves combining current understanding of the underlying neurobiology of depression and fatigue with systematic use of non-pharmacological and pharmacological interventions. Future directions for study should examine the etiology of depressive disorder and the determinants of fatigue. This will guide clinicians towards more effective treatment of this common and often disabling disorder.

References

[1] Greden ,J.F. (2001). The burden of recurrent depression: causes, consequences and future prospects. *J Clin Psychiatry*, 62,5-9.

[2] Murray, C.J.L., & Lopez, A.D., eds. (1996). The Global Burden of Disease: A comprehensive assessment of mortality and disability from diseases, injuries, and risk factors in 1990 and projected to 2020. Geneva and Boston, MA: World Health Organization and Harvard University Press.

[3] Herrman, H., Patrick, D.L., Diehr, P., Martin, M.L., Fleck, M., Simon, G.E., & Buesching, D.P. (2002). Longitudinal investigation of depression outcomes in primary care in six countries: the LIDO Study. Functional status, health service use and treatment of people with depressive symptoms. *Psychol Med*, 32,889-902.

[4] Keller, M.B., & Shapiro, R.W. (1982). "Double depression" superimposition of acute depressive episodes on chronic depressive disorders. *Am J Psychiatry*, 139,438-442.

[5] Keller, M.B., & Boland R.J. (1998). Implications of failing to achieve successful long-term maintenance treatment of recurrent unipolar major depression. *Biol Psychiatry*, 44,348-360.

[6] Mueller, T.I., & Leon, A.C. (1996). Recovery, chronicity and levels of psychopathology in major depression. *Psychiatr Clin North Am*, 19, 85-102.

[7] Fava, M., Rush, A.J., Trivedi, M.H., Nierenberg, A.A., Thase, M.E., Sackeim, H.A., Quitkin, F.M., Wisniewski, S., Lavori, P.W., Rosenbaum, J.F., & Kupfer, D.J. (2003).

Background and rationale for the sequenced treatment alternatives to relieve depression (STAR*D) study. *Psychiatr Clin North Am*, 26,457-494.

[8] Diagnostic and Statistical Manual of Mental Disorders (2000). DSM-IV-TR, Fourth edition, Text revision. Washington, DC: American Psychiatric Association.

[9] The ICD-10 classification of mental and behavioural disorders: clinical descriptions and diagnostic guidelines. (1992). Geneva: World Health Organization.

[10] Wessely, S., Chalder, T., Hirsch, S., Wallace, P., & Wright, D. (1997). The prevalence and morbidity of chronic fatigue and chronic fatigue syndrome: A prospective primary care study. *Am J Public Health*, 87,1449-1455.

[11] Risdale, I., Evans, A., Jerrett, W., Mandalia. S., Osler. K., & Vora, H. (1994). Patients who consult with tiredness: frequency of consultation, perceived causes of tiredness and its association with psychological distress. *Brit J Gen Pract*, 44,413-416.

[12] Lewis, G., & Wessely, S. (1992). The epidemiology of fatigue: more questions than answers. *J Epidemiol Community Health*, 46,92-97.

[13] Wessely, S. (1995). The epidemiology of chronic fatigue syndrome. *Epidemiol Rev*, 17,139-151.

[14] David, A., Pelosi, A., McDonald, E., Stephens, D., Ledger, D., Rathbone, R., & Mann, A. (1990). Tired, weak, or in need of rest: fatigue among general practice attenders. *BMJ*, 301,1199-1120.

[15] Cathebras, P.J., Robbins, J.M., Kirmayer, L.J., & Hayton, B.C. (1992). Fatigue in primary care: prevalence, psychiatric comorbidity, illness behavior, and outcome. *J Gen Intern Med*, 7,276-286.

[16] Loge, J.H., Ekeberg, O., & Kaasa, S. (1998). Fatigue in general Norwegian population: normative data and associations. *J Psychosom Res*, 45,53-65.

[17] Skapinakis, P., Lewis, G., & Mavreas, V. (2003). Cross-cultural differences in the epidemiology of unexplained fatigue syndromes in primary care. *Brit J Psychiatry*, 182,205-209.

[18] Skapinakis, P., Lewis, G., & Mavreas, V. (2003). Unexplained fatigue syndromes in a multinational primary care sample: Specificity of definition and prevalence and distinctiveness from depression and generalized anxiety. *Am J Psychiatry*, 160,785-787.

[19] Manu, P., Matthews, D.A., & Lane, T.J. (1988). The mental health of patients with a chief complaint of chronic fatigue, a prospective evaluation and follow-up. *Arch Intern Med*, 148,2213-2217.

[20] Kroenke, K., & Price, R.K. Symptoms in the community. (1993. Prevalence, classification, and psychiatric comorbidity. *Arch Int Med*, 153,2474-2480.

[21] Pawlikowska, T., Chalder, T., Hirsch, S.R., Wallace, P., Wright ,D.J., & Wessely, S.C. (1994). Population based study of fatigue and psychological distress. *BMJ*, 308,763-766.

[22] Wessely, S., Chalder, T., Hirsch, S., Wallace, P., & Wright, D. (1996). Psychological symptoms, somatic symptoms, and psychiatric disorder in chronic fatigue and chronic fatigue syndrome: A prospective study in the primary care setting. *Am J Psychiatry*, 153,1050-1059.

[23] Hickie, I., Koschera, A., Hadzi-Pavlovic, D., Bennett, B., & Lloyd, A. (1999). The temporal stability and comorbidity of prolonged fatigue: A longitudinal study in primary care. *Psychol Med*, 29,855-861.

[24] Skapinakis, P., Lewis, G., & Meltzer, H. (2000). Clarifying the relationship between unexplained chronic fatigue and psychiatric morbidity: Results from a community survey in Great Britain. *Am J Psycyhiatry*, 157,1492-1498.

[25] Wessely, S., & Powell, R. (1989). Fatigue syndromes: a comparison of chronic "postviral" fatigue with neuromuscular and affective disorders. *J Neurol Neurosurg Psychiatry*, 52,940-948.

[26] Baker, M., Dorzab, J., Winokur, G., & Cadoret, R.J. (1971). Depressive disease: classification and clinical characteristics. *Compr Psychiatry*, 12,354-365.

[27] Tylee, A., Gastpar, M., Lepine, J-P., & Mendlewicz, J. (1999). DEPRESS II (Depression Research in European Society II): A patient survey of the symptoms, disability and current management of depression in the community. *Int Clin Psychopharmacol*, 14,139-151.

[28] Addington, A.M., Gallo, J.J., Ford, D.E., & Eaton, W.W. (2001). Epidemiology of unexplained fatigue and major depression in the community: the Baltimore ECA follow-up, 1981-1994. *Psychol Med*, 31,1037-1044.

[29] Dryman, A., & Eaton, W.W. (1991). Affective symptoms associated with the onset of major depression in the community: findings from the US National Institute of Mental Health Epidemiologic Catchment Area Program. *Acta Psych Scand*, 84,1-5.

[30] Swindle, R.W., Cronkite, R.C., & Moos, R.H. (1998). Risk factors for sustained nonremission of depressive symptoms: A 4-year follow-up. *J Nerv Ment Dis*, 186,462-469.

[31] Fava, G.A., Grandi, S., Canestrari, R., & Molnar, G. (1990). Prodromal symptoms in primary major depressive disorder. *J Affect Disord*, 19,149-152.

[32] Fava, G.A., & Kellner, R. Prodromal syndromes in affective disorders. (1991). *Am J Psychiatry*, 148,823-830.

[33] Karp, J.F., Buysse, D.J., Houck, P.R., Cherry, C., Kupfer, D.J., & Frank, E. (2004). Relationship of variability in residual symptoms with recurrence of major depressive disorder during maintenance treatment. *Am J Psychiatry*, 161,1877-1884.

[34] Faravelli, C., Ambonetti, A., Pallanti, S., & Pazzagli, A. (1986). Depressive relapses and incomplete recovery from index episode. *Am J Psychiatry*, 143,888-891.

[35] Paykel, E.S., Ramana, R., Cooper, Z., Hayhurst, H., Kerr, J., & Barocka, A. (1995). Residual symptoms after partial remission: an important outcome in depression. *Psychol Med*, 25,1171-1180.

[36] Judd, L.L., Akiskal, H.S., & Paulus, M.P. (1997). The role and clinical significance of subsyndromal depressive symptoms (SSD) in unipolar major depressive disorder. *J Affect Disord*, 45,5-17.

[37] Moos, R.H., & Cronkite, R.C. (1999). Symptom-based predictors of a 10-year chronic course of treated depression. *J Nerv Ment Dis*, 187,360-368.

[38] Fava, G.A., Fabbri, S., & Sonino, N. (2002). Residual symptoms in depression: An emerging therapeutic target. *Prog Neuropsychopharmacol Biol Psychiatry*, 26,1019-1027.

[39] Fava, M. (2003). Symptoms of fatigue and cognitive/executive dysfunction in major depressive disorder before and after antidepressant treatment. *J Clin Psychiatry*, 64,30-34.

[40] Davidson, R.J., Lewis, D.A., Alloy, L.B., Amaral, D.G., Bush, G., Cohen, J.D., Drevets, W.C., Farah, M.J., Kagan, J., McClelland, J.L., Nolen-Hoeksema, S., &

Peterson, B.S. (2002). Neural and behavioral substrates of mood and mood regulation. *Biol Psychiatry*, 52,478-502.

[41] Stahl, S.M., Zhang, L., Damatarca, C., & Grady, M. (2003). Brain circuits determine destiny in depression: a novel approach to the psychopharmacology of wakefulness, fatigue, and executive dysfunction in major depressive disorder. *J Clin Psychiatry*, 64,6-17.

[42] Demyttenaere, K., De Fruyt, J., & Stahl, S.M.(2005). The many faces of fatigue in major depressive disorder. *Int J Neuropsychopharmacol*, 8,93-105.

[43] Sheline, Y.I. Neuroimaging studies of mood disorder effects on the brain. (2003). *Biol Psychiatry*, 54, 338-352.

[44] Marchand, W.R., Dilda, V., & Jensen, C.R. (2005). Neurobiology of mood disorders. *Hospital Physician*, 41,17-26.

[45] Mayberg, H., Liotti, M., Brannan, S.K., McGinnis, S., Mahurin, R.K., Jerabek, P.A., Silva, J.A., Tekell, J.L., Martin, C.C., Lancaster, J.L., & Fox, P.T. (1999). Reciprocal limbic-corticol function and negative mood: converging PET findings in depression and normal sadness. *Am J Psychiatry*,156, 675–682.

[46] Drevets, W.C. (2000). Neuroimaging studies of mood disorders. *Biol Psychiatry*, 48,813–828.

[47] Machale, S.M., Lawrie, S.M., O'Cavanagh, J.T.O., Glabus, M.F., Murray, C.L., Goodwin, G.M., & Ebmeier, K.P. (2000). Cerebral perfusion in chronic fatigue syndrome and depression. *Brit J of Psychiatry*, 176,550-556.

[48] Lawrie, S.M., MacHale, S.M., Cavanagh, J.T.O., O'Carroll, R.E., & Goodwin, G.M. (2000). The Difference in patterns of motor and cognitive function in chronic fatigue syndrome and severe depressive illness. *Psychol Med*, 30,433-442.

[49] Brown, R.E., Stevens, D.R., & Haas, H.L. (2001). The physiology of brain histamine. *Prog Neurobiol*, 63,637-672.

[50] Stahl, S.M. (2002). The psychopharmacology of energy and fatigue. *J Clin Psychiatry*, 63,7-8.

[51] Delgado, P.L. (2004). Common pathways of depression and pain. *J Clin Psychiatry*, 65,16-19.

[52] Delgado, P.L., Miller, H.L., Salomon, R.M., Licinio, J., Krystal, J.H., Moreno, F.A., Heninger, G.R., & Charney, D.S. (1999). Tryptophan-depletion challenge in depressed patients treated with desipramine or fluoxetine: implications for the role of serotonin in the mechanism of antidepressant action. *Biol Psychiatry*, 46,212-220.

[53] Blomstrand, E. (2001). Amino acids in central fatigue. *Amino acids*, 20,25-34.

[54] Schmidt,K., Nolte-Zenker, B., Patzer, J., Bauer, M., Schmidt, L.G., & Heinz, A. (2001). Psychopathological correlates of reduced dopamine receptor sensitivity in depression, schizophrenia, and opiate and alcohol dependence. *Pharmacopsychiatry*, 34,66-72.

[55] Salamone, J.D., Correa, M., Mingote, S., & Weber, S.M. (2003). Nucleus accumbens dopamine and the regulation of effort in food-seeking behavior: implications for studies of natural motivation, psychiatry, and drug abuse. *J Pharmacol Exp Ther*, 305,1-8.

[56] Tanaka, M., Nakamura, F., Mizokawa, S., Matsumura, A., Nozaki, S., & Watanabe, Y. (2003). Establishment and assessment of a rat model of fatigue. *Neuroscience Letters*, 352,159-162.

[57] Gold, P.W., & Chrousos, G.P. (2002). Organization of the stress system and its dysregulation in melancholic and atypical depression: high vs low CRH/NE states. *Mol Psychiatry*, 7,254-275.

[58] Nemeroff, C.B. (1989). The clinical significance of psychoneuroendocrinology in psychiatry: focus on the thyroid and adrenal. *J Clin Psychiatry*, 50,13-20.

[59] Pariante, C.M., & Miller, A.H. (2001). Glucocorticoid receptors in major depression: relevance to pathophysiology and treatment. *Biol Psychiatry*, 49,391-404.

[60] Kaestner, F., Hettich, M., Peters, M., Sibrowski, W., Hetzel, G., Ponath, G., Arolt, V., Cassens, U., & Rothemundt, M. (2005). Different activation patterns of proinflammatory cytokines in melancholic and non-melancholic major depression are associated with HPA axis activity. *J Affect Disord*, 87,305-311.

[61] Stewart, J.W., Quitkin, F.M., McGrath, P.J., & Klein, D.F. (2005). Defining the boundaries of atypical depression: evidence from the HPA axis supports course of illness distinctions. *J Affect Disord*, 86,161-167.

[62] Fries, E., Hesse, J., Hellhammer, J., & Hellhammer, D.H. (2005). A new view on hypocortisolism. *Psychoneuroendocrinology*, 30,1010-1016.

[63] Lasser, R.A., & Baldessarini, R.J. (1997). Thyroid hormones in depressive disorders: a reappraisal of clinical utility. *Harv Rev Psychiatry*, 4,291-305.

[64] Schiepers, O.J., Wichers, M.C., & Maes, M. (2005). Cytokines and major depression. Prog Neuropsychopharmacol Biol Psychiatry, 29,201-217.

[65] Piche, T., Saint-Paul, M.C., Dainese, R., Marine-Barjoan, E., Iannelli, A., Montoya, M.L., Peyron, J.F., Czerucka, D., Cherikh, F., Filippi, J., Tran, A., & Hébuterne, X. (2008). Mast cells and cellularity of the colonic mucosa correlated with fatigue and depression in irritable bowel syndrome. *Gut*, 57,468-473.

[66] Hickie, I., & Lloyd, A. (1995). Are cytokines associated with neuropsychiatric syndromes in humans? *Int J Immunopharmacol*, 17,677-683.

[67] O'Brien, S.M., Scott, L.V., & Dinan, T.G. (2004). Cytokines: abnormalities in major depression and implications for pharmacological treatment. *Human Psychopharmacol*, 19,397-403.

[68] Maes, M. (2001). The immunoregulatory effects of antidepressants. *Human Psychopharmacol*, 16,95-103.

[69] Kenis, G., & Maes, M. (2002). Effects of antidepressants on the production of cytokines. Int J Neuropsychopharmacol, 5,401-412.

[70] Papanicolaou, D.A., Wilder, R.L., Manolagas, S.C., & Chrousos, G.P. (1998). The pathophysiologic roles of interleukin-6 in human disease. *Ann Intern Med*,128:127-137.

[71] Yirmiya, R., Pollak, Y., Morag, M., Reichenberg, A., Barak, O., Avitsur, R., Shavit, Y., Ovadia, H., Weidenfeld, J., Morag, A., Newman, M.E., & Pollmächer, T. (2000). Illness, cytokines, and depression. *Ann N Y Acad Sci*, 917,478-487.

[72] Miller, A.H. (1998). Neuroendocrine and immune system interactions in stress and depression. *Psychiatr Clin North Am*, 21,443-463.

[73] Bodkin, J.A., Lasser, R.A., Wines, J.D. Jr., Gardner, D.M., Baldessarini, R. J. (1997). Combining serotonin reuptake inhibitors and bupropion in partial responders to antidepressant monotherapy. *J Clin Psychiatry*, 58,137-145.

[74] Kelsey, J.K. (2002). Treatment strategies in achieving remission in major depressive disorder. *Acta Psychiatr Scand*, 106,18-23.

[75] Paykel, E.S. (2002). Achieving gains beyond response. *Acta Psychiatr Scand*, 106,12-17.

[76] Menza, M., Marin, H., & Opper, R.S. (2003). Residual Symptoms in depression: Can treatment be symptom-specific? *J Clin Psychiatry*, 64,516-523.

[77] Dittner, A.J., Wessley, S.C., & Brown, R.G. (2004). The assessment of fatigue: A practical guide for clinicians and researchers. J Psychosomatic Res, 56,157-170.

[78] Marin, H., & Menza, M.A. (2005). The management of fatigue in depressed patients. Essent Psychopharmacol, 6,185-192.

[79] Lichstein, K.L., Means, M.K., Noe, S.L., & Aguillard, R.N. (1997). Fatigue and sleep disorders. *Behav Res Ther*, 35,733-740.

[80] Fava, M. (2004). Daytime sleepiness and insomnia as correlates of depression. *J Clin Psychiatry*, 65,27-32.

[81] Glass, J.M., Lyden, A.K., Petzke, F., Stein, P. Whalen, G., Ambrose, K., Chrousos, G., & Clauw, D.J. (2004). The effect of brief exercise cessation on pain, fatigue, and mood symptom development in healthy, fit individuals. *J Psychosom Res*, 57,391-398.

[82] Fava, G.A., Ruini, C., Rafanelli, C., & Grandi, S. (2002). Cognitive behavior approach to loss of effect during long-term antidepressant treatment: A pilot study. Am J Psychiatry, 159,2094-2095.

[83] Looper, K.J., & Kirmayer, L.J. (2002). Behavioral medicine approaches to somatoform disorders. J Consult Clin Psychol, 70,810-827.

[84] Geddes, J.R., Carney, S.M., Davies, C., Furukawa, T.A., Kupfer, D.J., Frank, E., & Goodwin, G.M. (2003). Relapse prevention with antidepressant drug treatment in depressive disorders: a systemic review. *Lancet*, 361,653-661.

[85] Burt, V.K. (2004). Plotting the course to remission: The search for better outcomes in the treatment of depression. J Clin Psychiatry, 65,20-25.

[86] Nierenberg, A.A., Keefe, B.R., Leslie, V.C., Alpert, J.E., Pava, J.A., Worthington, J.J. 3rd, Rosenbaum, J.F., & Fava, M. (1999). Residual symptoms in depressed patients who respond acutely to fluoxetine. *J Clin Psychiatry*, 60,221-225.

[87] Stahl, S.M., Entsuah, R., & Rudolph, R. (2002). Comparative efficacy between venlafaxine and SSRIs: a pooled analysis of patients with depression. *Biol Psychiatry*, 52,1166-1174.

[88] Stahl, S.M., Grady, M.M., Moret, C., & Briley, M. (2005). SNRIs: Their Pharmacology, Clinical Efficacy, and Tolerability in Comparison with Other Classes of Antidepressants. *CNS Spectr*, 10,732-747.

[89] Preti, A. (2002). Tomoxetine (Eli Lilly & Co). *Curr Opin Investig Drugs*, 3,272-277.

[90] Hajos, M., Fleishaker, J.C., Filipiak-Reisner, J.K., Brown, M.T., & Wong, E.H. (2004). The selective norepinephrine reuptake inhibitor antidepressant reboxetine: pharmacological and clinical profile. *CNS Drug Rev*, 10,23-44.

[91] Ferguson, J.M., Mendels, J., & Schwart, G.E. (2002). Effects of reboxetine on Hamilton Depression Rating Scale factors from randomized, placebo-controlled trials in major depression. *Int Clin Psychopharmacol*, 17, 45-51.

[92] Green, T.R. (1997). Buproprion for SSRI-induced fatigue. *J Clin Psychiatry*, 58,174.

[93] Papakostas, G.I., Petersen, T.J., Burns, A.M., & Fava, M. (2006). Adjunctive atomoxetine for residual fatigue in major depressive disorder. *J Psychiatr Res*, 40,370-373.

[94] Scammell,T.E., Estabrooke, I.V., McCarthy, M.T., Chemelli, R.M., Yanagisawa, M., Miller, M.S., & Saper, C.B. (2000). Hypothalamic arousal regions are activated during modafinil-induced wakefulness. *J Neurosci*, 20,8620-8628.

[95] De Saint Hilaire, A., Orosco, M., Rouch, C., Blanc, G., & Nicolaidis, S. (2001). Variations in extracellular monoamines in the prefrontal cortex and medial hypothalamus after modafinil adminstration: a microdialysis study in rats. *Neuroreport*, 12,3533-3537.

[96] Morrow, G.R., Shelke, A.R., Roscoe, J.A., Hickok, J.T., & Mustian, K. (2005). Management of cancer-related fatigue. *Cancer Invest*, 23,229-239.

[97] Rosenberg, J.H., & Shafor, R. (2005). Fatigue in multiple sclerosis: a rational approach to evaluation and treatment. *Curr Neurol Neurosci Rep*, 5,140-146.

[98] DeBattista,C., Doghramji, K., Menza, M.A., Rosenthal, M.H., Fieve, R.R.; & Modafinil in Depression Study Group. (2003). Adjunct modafinil for the short-term treatment of fatigue and sleepiness in patients with major depressive disorder: a preliminary double-blind, placebo-controlled study. *J. Clin Psychiatry*, 64,1057-1064.

[99] Fava, M., Thase, M.E., & DeBattista, C. (2005). A multicenter, placebo-controlled study of modafinil augmentation in partial responders to selective serotonin reuptake inhibitors with persistent fatigue and sleepiness. *J Clin Psychiatry*, 66,85-93.

[100] Ferraro, L., Fuxe, K., Agnati, L., Tanganelli, S., Tomasini, M.C., & Antonelli, T. (2005). Modafinil enhances the increase of extracellular serotonin levels induced by the antidepressant drugs fluoxetine and imipramine: a dual probe microdialysis study in awake rat. *Synapse*, 55,230-241.

[101] Price, C.S., & Taylor, F.B. (2005). A retrospective chart review of the effects of modafinil on depression as monotherapy and as adjunctive therapy. *Depress Anxiety*, 21,149-153.

[102] Candy, M., Jones, L., Williams, R., Took,am, A. & King, M. (2008). Psychostimulants for depression. *Cochrane Database Syst Rev*, 16, CD006722.

[103] Masand, P.S., Anand, V.S., & Tanquary, J.F. (1998). Psychostimulant augmentation of second generation antidepressants: a case series. *Depress Anxiety*, 7,89-91.

[104] Ravindran, A.V., Kennedy, S.H., O'Donovan, M.C., Fallu, A., Camacho, F., & Binder, C.E. (2008). Osmotic-release oral system methylphenidate augmentation of antidepressant monotherapy in major depressive disorder: results of a double-blind, randomized, placebo-controlled trial. *J Clin Psychiatry*, 69,87-94.

[105] Abe, K., Takanashi, M., Yanagihara, T., & Sakoda, S. (2001-2002). Pergolide mesilate may improve fatigue in patients with Parkinson's disease. *Behav Neurol*, 13,117-121.

[106] Takahash, H., Yoshida, K., Higuchi, H., Shimizu, T., Inoue, T., & Koyama, T. (2003). Addition of a dopamine agonist, cabergoline, to a serotonin-noradrenalin reuptake inhibitor, milnacipran as a therapeutic option in the treatment of refractory depression: two case reports. *Clin Neuropharmacol*, 26,230-232.

[107] Joffe, R.T., & Sokolov, S.T. (2000). Thyroid hormone treatment of primary unipolar depression: a review. *Int J Neuropsychopharmacol*, 3,143-147.

[108] Cox, D.L. (1997). Experiences of fatigue and depression before and after low-dose l-thyroxine supplementation in essentially euthyroid individuals. *Res Nurs Health*, 20,389-398.

[109] Normann,C., Hummel, B., Schärer, L.O., Hörn, M., Grunze, H., & Walden, J. (2002). Lamotrigine as adjunct to paroxetine in acute depression: a placebo-controlled, double-blind study. *J Clin Psychiatry*, 63,337-344.

[110] Barbosa, L., Berk, M., & Vorster, M. (2003). A double-blind, randomized, placebo-controlled trial of augmentation with lamotrigine or placebo in patients concomitantly treated with fluoxetine for resistant major depressive episodes. *J Clin Psychiatry*, 64,403-407.

[111] Marson, A.G., Kadir, Z.A., Hutton, J.L., & Chadwick, D.W. (1997). The new antiepileptic drugs: A systematic review of their efficacy and tolerability. *Epilepsia*, 38,859-880.

[112] Ketter, T.A., Post, R.M., & Theodore, W.H. (1999). Positive and negative psychiatric effects of antiepileptic drugs in patients with seizure disorders. *Neurology*, 53,S53-67.

In: Handbook of Fatigue in Health and Disease
Editor: Howard S. Smith
ISBN 978-1-61761-920-5

Chapter 10

MANAGING FATIGUE: IS THERE ANYTHING TO DO?

Susan B. LeGrand *

The Section of Palliative Medicine and Supportive Oncology
Solid Tumor Oncology
Cleveland Clinic Taussig Cancer Institute
Cleveland, OH, USA

ABSTRACT

The management of fatigue requires first identification of the symptom. Secondly one must rule out identifiable causes including: pain, emotional distress, sleep disturbance, anemia, nutrition, activity level, medication side effects, alcohol/substance abuse and co-morbid illness. These should be treated with appropriate specific interventions if possible. Non-specific interventions can be divided into non-pharmacologic and pharmacologic interventions. Non-pharmacologic treatment includes exercise and energy conservation/ activity management (ECAM). Pharmacologic therapies include stimulants such as modafinil and methylphenidate. Other medications including hormones and nutritional supplements have been tried. The evidence for most interventions is inconsistent and limited. This chapter will review these modalities in detail.

* Address
9500 Euclid Ave. R35
Cleveland OH 44195
Phone: 216-444-4523
Fax: 216-636-3179
Email: legrans@ccf.org

Introduction

One of the key principles in symptom management is to treat the underlying cause whenever possible. Unfortunately, in the management of fatigue only a limited number of specific causes have been identified. In most circumstances, the fundamental pathophysiology is not well understood and therefore, specific therapy remains elusive. Even when the few clearly identified causes such as anemia and depression are treated, fatigue may still persist. Although this symptom is problematic in many different diseases and could, in theory, have a unifying cytokine cause; therapeutic interventions have typically been investigated in single disease states. Much of the research has been in cancer and multiple sclerosis related fatigue. In any one individual, multiple complimentary interventions might be needed for optimal management.

The National Comprehensive Cancer Network (NCCN) Guidelines [1] have identified nine conditions that are associated with fatigue. While these guidelines are cancer related, these conditions are relevant in all complaints of fatigue and should be sought and treated before resorting to non-specific interventions. The nine conditions are:

1) Pain. In cancer patients uncontrolled pain clearly contributes to fatigue [2] and this may well apply in other disease states as well.
2) Emotional distress. Depression and Anxiety.
3) Sleep disturbance.
4) Anemia
5) Nutrition. Assessment should include fluid and electrolytes, weight and calorie intake.
6) Activity level.
7) Medication side effects
8) Alcohol/substance abuse
9) Comorbidities. Problems within multiple other organ systems (endocrine, renal, pulmonary, hepatic, cardiac etc) may contribute to fatigue.

This chapter will review non-pharmacologic and pharmacologic interventions for fatigue.

Activity

Exercise is the intervention with the most study and the best evidence for efficacy in management of fatigue. This is said with the caveat that most of the studies have been in cancer patients and the majority of these have been in breast cancer during and after adjuvant therapy. Other problems exist within the studies including the difficulty of assuring compliance, substantial dropout and contamination of the control arm with those individuals initiating exercise programs also. The methodology of recent studies has improved increasing the strength of the data. There have been six systematic reviews of the exercise literature in cancer related fatigue [3-8] and readers interested in greater detail are referred here. All have come to the same conclusion, that despite some trial limitations, there is evidence to support the value of exercise in the management of fatigue in cancer patients. What remains unclear is the type of exercise (aerobic, strength or both), intensity, duration, motivational concerns, etc.

There have been several studies on exercise in the setting of high dose chemotherapy or bone marrow transplantation. In an early trial 70 patients receiving preparatory regimens for autologous bone marrow transplantation were randomized to training with a bed ergometer or a control group of standard care [9]. There was a 27% higher loss of performance ability for the untrained group. Given the expectation of loss of function and fatigue this was a positive finding. In addition, hospitalization was shorter and hematologic recovery quicker in the exercise group. In a similar study, baseline fatigue and psychological stress between the two groups were similar, but at discharge the exercise group had no change in fatigue and an improvement in psychological symptoms whereas the control group had increases in both [10]. In a randomized controlled trial 22 acute myelogenous chemotherapy patients received either standard care or a walking exercise five days weekly for three weeks. Fatigue intensity and interference plus depression, anxiety and distress improved significantly in the exercise group [11].

Fatigue is the most common symptom in the setting of advanced malignancy and there has been one pilot study of exercise in this group [12]. Patients were recruited from a home hospice service, with an Eastern Cooperative Oncology Group (ECOG) score of 1 and a life expectancy of at least 1 month. Fatigue was measured with the Multidimensional fatigue inventory (MFI), the Symptom Distress Scale (SDS), the Hospital Anxiety and Depression Scale (HADS) and Quality of Life Scale (QOL). 13/24 patients declined participation, 11 entered with 2 subsequently withdrawing. While there was no change in fatigue scores, they did not worsen and there was a trend to improvement in QOL. The results of this pilot trial demonstrate the difficulties of doing research in those with advanced disease but do not offer conclusions on the value of exercise in this setting.

Since exercise improves quality of life in those who are not ill, it is really not surprising that it would help those with illness also. The theory is an improvement in the efficiency of the muscles and heart resulting in a decrease in energy requirement for normal activities with correspondingly less fatigue [13]. There has been less research on exercise in other disease states. A recent Cochrane review of research in CFS found only 9 studies of which 5 were included but the reviewers felt the data supported the value of exercise in this setting [14]. A similar review in multiple sclerosis found no evidence for a statistically significant impact on fatigue but the majority of trials focused on muscle function rather than symptoms [15]. In a recent randomized trial 121 patients were randomized to either an exercise arm with two 30-minute exercise sessions per week or no regular physical activity. Fatigue, depression and quality of life scores improved in the exercise arm [16]. Two studies that included fatigue as an outcome measurement found trends to improvement that did not reach statistical significance [17, 18].

In conclusion, despite the limitations of the trials, different outcome measures, limited patient numbers, inability to conduct good meta-analysis etc. it is reasonable to conclude that in the setting of cancer related fatigue, exercise should be part of the therapy whenever possible. The high dose chemotherapy data would suggest that more attention to physical activity during prolonged hospitalizations is not only possible but can effectively prevent physical decline. The role in other disease states is less clear but there is certainly no evidence of harm.

Lifestyle Interventions

One of the most common recommendations to cancer and MS patients with fatigue is energy conservation and/or activity management (ECAM). ECAM is typically defined as a method to balance rest and activity by setting priorities, delegating responsibilities, pacing and scheduling activities to reflect peaks and valleys in energy levels during the day [19]. An intervention that provided information on developing a plan, monitoring via a journal and then evaluation and revision of the plan via three telephone sessions was piloted and then compared in a randomized controlled trial to three telephone sessions with nutritional counseling [19, 20]. Fatigue was measured with the short form of the Profile of Mood States (POMS-SF). In the pilot trial patients appreciated the information and planned to use it and there was some minor impact on the course of fatigue during active chemotherapy and/or radiation. In the controlled trial, study subjects were receiving active treatment; therefore the end points were to minimize the expected increase in fatigue typically seen. The intervention group used more of the techniques such as delegating and pacing than the non-intervention group. The group had significantly less fatigue compared to the control without changes in functional status. A similar strategy was piloted as the "Beating Fatigue" program in outpatients receiving chemotherapy [21]. The four elements were 1) assessing/monitoring, 2) education on fatigue, 3) coaching in self-care 4) provision of emotional support and included in-home assessment by a nurse. The small number of patients tested generally found the intervention helpful with the opportunity to talk about their symptom being a key component. Two small studies of energy conservation in multiple sclerosis have not found an impact on fatigue but did demonstrate a decreased impact of the fatigue on function [22, 23]. An additional study in MS found that the benefit on coping skills lasted at least 7-9 months [24]. With limited evidence, no strong recommendations can be made on ECAM. The opportunity to get education about fatigue and the use of specific coping strategies has seemed useful for managing the functional impact on the activities of daily living but has not shown a significant change in the symptom severity itself.

Pharmacotherapy

The exact role of medical management of fatigue is undefined. There are multiple small studies looking at the value of particular medications in cancer-related fatigue and other disease states. There have been a few randomized placebo controlled trials that will be discussed in the sections below. There have not been any comparative trials of the medications that have shown some promise.

Erythropoitin Stimulating Agents (ESA's)

Although the impact of anemia on quality of life is established [25, 26], it is also clear that maintaining near normal hemoglobin (Hgb) levels with ESAs does not prevent nor fully treat all fatigue. While there have been systematic reviews published supporting the value in the setting of cancer and renal failure [26, 27] there has recently been significant controversy with these agents. There have been several studies and a Cochrane review demonstrating a negative impact on survival particularly with Hgb levels >13g/dl [28-30]. There is similar data in renal failure for Hgb [31]. An increase in thromboembolic events has also been recognized. The FDA has suggested these agents only be used during chemotherapy and stopped when it is complete. There have not been FDA comments on their use in renal failure. Therefore despite the ability to increase Hgb, ESAs should no longer be considered a therapy for fatigue.

Modafinil

There have been randomized trials of modafinil in patients with fatigue in depression, multiple sclerosis, post polio syndrome, Parkinson's disease and general anesthesia. Modafinil has also been evaluated in sleepy pilots and other settings not discussed here. In a double-blind placebo-controlled randomized trial in nineteen Parkinson's disease patients found that 100mg daily did not improve fatigue symptoms more than placebo although physical fatigability improved [32]. No benefit was found in post-polio syndrome fatigue in a randomized, placebo-controlled crossover trial using 400mgs daily in 36 patients [33]. In a single blind placebo controlled crossover study, 72 multiple sclerosis patients were treated with 200 and then 400mg of modafinil [34]. Patients received 2 weeks each of placebo, modafinil 200mg, modafinil 400mg and placebo in that order. A statistically significant improvement was seen for the 200mg but not the 400mg dose. The authors comment that despite the lack of statistical evidence of improvement with the 400mg dose some patients preferred it.

Two studies involved depressed patients with residual fatigue and sleepiness on selective serotonin reuptake inhibitors (SSRI) [35, 36]. Together these studies randomized 450 patients with a confirmed diagnosis of major depressive disorder and a partial response to SSRI medications (≥ 8 weeks) to either placebo or modafinil for 6-8 weeks of therapy. In the first study [35] the modafinil dose varied from 100-400mg but was fixed at 200mg in the second group [36]. Pre and post therapy testing included multiple measures of fatigue -FSS, ESS, and the Brief Fatigue Inventory (BFI) - in addition to multiple measures of depression. At the conclusion of 8 weeks of treatment, there was a statistically significant improvement in the BFI rating for worst fatigue although there was no significant change in overall fatigue scores. There was an early improvement (week 1) in the FSS and ESS that was not significant at week 8 (trend in ESS).

In post-anesthesia patients [37], thirty-four patients scheduled for outpatient surgical procedures requiring general anesthesia were randomly assigned in a double blind design to either a single dose of 200mg modafinil or placebo. Medications were administered immediately prior to discharge when individuals were able to safely take oral medication. VAS scales for various symptoms (fatigue. exhaustion, sleep and others) were done pre-operatively and by phone 24 hours after dosing. Those receiving modafinil had significantly less moderate to severe (VAS ≥ 5) fatigue (65% vs. 12%) and feeling worn out (65% vs. 29%) but no difference in moderate to severe exhaustion (24% vs. 29%).

There have been several open labeled trials evaluating modafinil for fatigue. There has been a pilot study in lung cancer with 20 patients receiving 100mgs for 7 days then 200mgs for 7 days. A rapid decrease in fatigue was noted as well as improvement in daytime sleepiness, depression and anxiety [38].The drug is approved for use in narcolepsy for management of daytime sleepiness but these individuals may also have fatigue. An open-labeled study assessed the impact on fatigue, mood and health-related quality of life [39] in 151 narcolepsy sufferers. After a 14-day washout from psychostimulants, they were treated with 200mg and then if needed 400mg for 6 weeks. Fatigue was measured with the Profile of Mood States (POMS) and showed a significant improvement from baseline. >70% took 400mg daily with only 7(5%) withdrawing for adverse events. In contrast to the doses required for patients with narcolepsy two other open-labeled trials have found smaller doses effective. In the first of these a dose escalation study was done starting at 100mg/day and increasing in 100mg increments to a maximum of 400mg/day [40]. They confirmed a statistically significant benefit that persisted for the 3 months of the study. Responses were seen at 100mg (25%), 200mg (42%) and 300mg (4%). Two patients who complained of restlessness at 100mgs were dose reduced and responded to 50mg. No one required 400mgs for response. An open-labeled trial in 30 HIV patients started 50mg daily with a maximum dose of 200mg [41]. The FSS and ESS were done before treatment and after 4 weeks. Patients were allowed an additional 8 weeks of therapy if desired. 80% responded to treatment clinically and of these 83% chose to continue treatment. 2 responded to 50mg/day, 13 to 100mg/day and 9 to 200mg/day.

In addition to these trials there are case reports of improvement in pain-associated fatigue (100mg/day) [42] and chronic fatigue syndrome (200mg/day) [43]. Surprisingly there is only the one pilot study of modafinil use in cancer-related fatigue [44] or palliative medicine although it has been used in this setting with anecdotal success. In conclusion, there is conflicting evidence for modafinil in fatigue but it has been used in MS with some success. The most frequent side effects are headache, nausea and anxiety but tend to be either mild or moderate in intensity with few requiring discontinuation for toxicity. The preferred dose and the value in other disease states require additional research. The durability of the response has not been studied beyond 3 months.

Psychostimulants

There are three psychostimulants in clinical use, methylphenidate, dextroamphetamine, and pemoline. Each of these has been used in management of fatigue. Pemoline is less commonly used as it has an increased risk of liver failure and requires routine monitoring of liver function. There have been three negative randomized controlled trials in cancer fatigue. In the first 5mgs of methylphenidate was given every 2 hours as needed with a maximum of 20mgs/day for 7 days [45]. Both placebo and treatment arms had significant improvement but the authors hypothesize that the daily phone calls could have impacted the results. In a second study patients undergoing radiation therapy for primary brain tumors were prophylactically treated with up to 15mgs twice daily with methylphenidate vs. placebo [46]. There was no significant difference in quality of life or fatigue scales. In the third, women undergoing adjuvant chemotherapy for breast cancer were randomized [47]. Cognitive dysfunction and fatigue were the endpoints studied and neither improved with therapy. There have been at least two randomized, placebo-controlled trials in HIV patients. Thirty five HIV positive men with depression (major, dysthymia, sub-threshold or minor) and fatigue were randomized to either placebo or 5mg of dextroamphetamine in the morning and mid-afternoon [48]. The code was broken for non-responders who could then crossover to dextroamphetamine. There was a statistically significant improvement in depression and energy compared to placebo (73% vs. 27%) 15 patients were continued on medication up to six months with 10/15 maintaining response for the duration.

In the second study in HIV patients, randomization was to methylphenidate, pemoline or placebo [49]. Depressed patients were specifically excluded. Medication was given twice daily with starting doses of methylphenidate 7.5mg/dose and pemoline 18.75mg/dose. Both medications were equally effective and superior to placebo. Patients were only followed for 6 weeks so duration of response cannot be assessed. Side effects, predominantly hyperactivity and jitteriness, were mild and occasionally resolved with time.

There have been several open-labeled trials of methylphenidate in advanced disease settings. In a prospective pilot study of advanced cancer patients 9/11 had improvement in fatigue that was defined as having mild of none on a categorical scale [50]. The starting dose was 5mg at 8am and noon with titration if needed (8/9 responded to 10mg/day) Side effects were nausea, insomnia, dry mouth and anorexia with discontinuation for toxicity in only one patient who died one week later. In another study of a similar population, the dose was methylphenidate 5mg every 2 hours on an as needed basis (maximum 20mg/day) controlled by the patient [51]. Assessment for study completion was at day 8 but an additional 4 weeks of free drug was provided with follow-up assessment at the completion of this interval. 28/30 patients (93%) had improvement defined as a decrease of >2 on the 10 point NRS. 100% described themselves as feeling better when offered three choices (better, no different, worse) and all chose to continue the medication beyond day 8. Statistically significant improvement on fatigue scores for both the FACIT-F and the ESAS were maintained for the 21 patients available on day 28. A third study in Japan treated 16 patients with far advanced disease (11 inpatients) with 6 responders [52]. Responders tended to live longer (77 vs. 36 days) suggesting the critically ill nature of the group under study.

Although the randomized controlled trials in specific populations have been negative, pilot studies of methylphenidate in cancer related fatigue both during treatment [53] and after completion of adjuvant therapy have been published [54]. 12 Patients receiving interferon were given 20mg of sustained release methylphenidate and an exercise program. 8/12 utilized both measures (exercise and medication) and 4 stopped the medication but continued to exercise. They were compared to historical controls using the same regimen of therapy without recommendations for fatigue management. Those adding methylphenidate to their exercise regimen had less fatigue and were able to maintain their daily routine better than those who did not but the numbers are very small. In a small study of breast cancer patients >6 months but <5 years after therapy, methylphenidate at doses of 10-20mg/day had a 53% response rate with statistically significant improvements in the BFI [54]. An interesting personal report from a physician on active cancer therapy has also been published [55].

In conclusion, there is conflicting evidence that stimulants, particularly methylphenidate can be helpful in management of fatigue. Data exists in HIV patients and advanced cancer but the numbers of patients studied remain small. Randomized controlled trials in less advanced disease cancer patients have not been reported. The randomized trials in less advanced active treatment cancer patients have been negative. There are no reports in other disease states with the exception of stroke. The optimum dose, potential duration of response, and value in other disease states remains to be determined.

Amantadine

Textbooks and review articles list amantadine as a choice for management of fatigue in multiple sclerosis [56, 57]. It has also been investigated in CFS [58, 59] and in patients receiving interferon-alpha for hepatitis-C [60]. Despite this, a 2004 Cochrane review found that while it was well tolerated the existing studies did not provide strong evidence of efficacy [61] and that better trials were needed. A 1995 RCT compared amantadine, pemoline and placebo [62] in 119 MS patients. Those with severe depression on the Center for Epidemiologic Studies Depression scale were excluded. 93 patients completed the study. 79% of amantadine patients reported that they felt better on medication compared to 52% of placebo patients and 32% of pemoline patients. Amantadine has also been compared with L-Carnitine [63]. This randomized double-blind crossover trial treated 36 patients with 3 months each with medication-washout-medication-washout. Randomization determined the order of medications used. The primary fatigue measure was the FSS. 43% of amantadine patients had a decrease in the FSS scores without statistical significance.

Two studies in CFS have yielded conflicting results. In 4 patients treated in a crossover study with amantadine or placebo, the medication was well tolerated and yielded a benefit in all patients [58]. In the other study comparing amantadine and L-carnitine in 30 patients only one was able to complete 8 weeks of amantadine secondary to diarrhea [59]. An interesting trial in hepatitis C patients randomized to interferon (IFN) alfa2A alone or IFN plus amantadine [60]. The primary endpoints were viral related but there was a trend to improvement in fatigue in those treated with the combination when compared to IFN alone.

In summary, the impact of amantadine on fatigue is at best modest, tested predominantly in MS and replaced by modafinil as first line therapy. The value, if any, in other disease settings is unknown. The potential benefit in IFN treated patients suggests a possible avenue of further research.

Antidepressants

Trials of antidepressant medications for management of fatigue in non-depressed patients are few. A randomized trial of paroxetine vs. placebo in 738 individuals (74% women) receiving chemotherapy found an improvement in depression but no impact on fatigue [64]. Sustained release bupropion was given in an open-labeled series to 15 fatigued cancer patients referred for psychiatric assessment [65]. 13/15 reported improvement within 2-4 weeks of initiating therapy. Each of these individuals was also felt to have a psychiatric diagnosis so differentiating response to depressive symptoms separate from fatigue as was done in the larger trial is not possible. Citalopram was tested in idiopathic chronic fatigue [66]. The trial used the control arm of a concurrent RCT as the comparison. The primary outcome measure was the Rand Vitality Index (RVI). 31 patients were treated with "substantial improvement" in 32% vs. 18% that was not statistically significant. Subgroup analysis found statistical benefit but given the size of the study this is of marginal value.

Another study comparing testosterone, fluoxetine and placebo in HIV/AIDS patients with depression and fatigue (see below) found fluoxetine no better than placebo for fatigue although it was helpful for depression [67]. Taken together, there is no evidence that antidepressants treat fatigue that is not secondary to depression.

Testosterone

There have been two studies in HIV/AIDS patients evaluating the role of testosterone in management of fatigue [67, 68]. In the first trial (668) 108 men with clinical symptoms of hypogonadism (decreased libido plus either low mood, low energy, or involuntary weight loss) were treated with intramuscular testosterone cypionate (200mg for one dose and then 400 mg every other week). Fatigue measurement was with the CFS. 73/108 men had low energy and of this group 66 (90%) completed the study. 79% had significant improvement in fatigue as rated by the study physician using the Clinical Global Impressions Scale (CGI). There was a statistically significant improvement in the CFS from week 1 to week 12 in responders with no corresponding change in the non-responders. The second study mentioned briefly above was a RCT with fluoxetine and placebo [67] with a similar dosing schedule for the testosterone. In this study patients were specifically required to have a diagnosis of major depression, sub threshold depression or dysthymia. Rating scales were the same as in the first trial. Of those completing the trial, 70% of fluoxetine patients improved their depression at week 8 compared to 57% on testosterone and 53% on placebo. Fatigue improved in 63% of those on testosterone compared to 41% on fluoxetine and 52% on placebo. If the evaluation was limited to those with clinically significant fatigue at baseline, then the response to testosterone was statistically significant. These two studies do not suggest that testosterone supplementation is a measure that should become routine in the management of fatigue, but since hypogonadism is not uncommon and can be provoked by the use of chronic opioid medications, it may be reasonable to look for it and supplement if present.

Other

Several other medications have been tried for fatigue in different disease states with one publication each. 41 Parkinson's disease patients received either pergolide mesilate or bromocriptine with a statistically significant improvement in fatigue in those treated with the pergolide and no benefit seen with bromocriptine [69]. A placebo controlled pilot study with bromocriptine in post-polio fatigue found benefit in 3/5 patients [70]. 15 advanced lung cancer patients with weight loss, anorexia, fatigue, performance status ≥ 2 and C-reactive protein level >10μg/ml were treated with celecoxib, medroxyprogesterone and a polymeric enteral food supplement with a small but statistically significant change in fatigue [71]. Lastly there is a case report of one individual's relief from fatigue related to chronic liver disease with the use of ondansetron therapy (4mg twice daily) [72].

Supplements

Various nutritional supplements have been proposed and studied for their effect on fatigue. There are few controlled trials and the measurement of fatigue is often via non-validated tools. There is only one agent, l-carnitine with more than one published article identified.

L-Carnitine

Effective energy metabolism in the mitochondria requires adequate levels of carnitine. Deficiencies have been identified in chronic dialysis patients [73] and as a consequence of chemotherapy [74, 75]. Replacement has therefore been proposed as a mechanism of treating fatigue but it is currently unclear if the benefit is limited to deficiency syndromes. A randomized controlled trial in the elderly without determination of l-carnitine levels found improvement in physical activity and cognitive functions [76]. In CFS there have been contradictory results [77, 78]. Grau et al found no benefit to the addition of carnitine in a preliminary study focused on muscle function [77]. In contrast a randomized trial of amantadine vs. l-carnitine found clinical benefit in 12/18 patients with CFS [78]. An open labeled trial randomized 114 CFS patients to either 2 gm acetyl-l-carnitine/day (ALC), 2 gm propionyl-l-carnitine/day (PLC) or both compounds without a placebo control [78]. Patients with primary or secondary carnitine deficiencies were excluded. Fatigue measurement was with a clinical global impression of change (CGI) (very much worse-very much better), the Multidimensional Fatigue Inventory (MFI-20), the McGill Pain Inventory and others. 8 patients stopped for side effects (overstimulated and sleepless) 8 for lack of effect and 2 for unknown reasons. 89 patients were analyzed at week 8 with 59% of the ALC group, 63% of the PLC group and 37% of the combination group experiencing improvement on the CGI. Treatment was stopped after 24 weeks and 52% of ALC, 50% of PLC and 37% of combination experienced worsening of symptoms. Mental fatigue and concentration improved more in the ALC group, whereas general fatigue improved more in the groups taking PLC.

Carnitine supplementation has been used in cancer related fatigue in three trials, both in the setting of documented carnitine deficiency [79-81]. In the first study, fatigued patients with low free carnitine levels, normal hemoglobin levels, undergoing platinum or ifosfamide therapy and not taking steroids, vitamins or psychostimulants were treated with oral l-carnitine 2 gms twice daily with meals [79]. Functional Assessment of Cancer Therapy-Fatigue (FACT-F) questionnaires were completed pre-treatment and weekly until the next cycle of chemotherapy. 90% (45/50) had statistically significant improvement in the FACT-F scores. In the second, carnitine levels were assessed in a select group of fatigued patients and 83% (13/18) were found to be deficient [80]. Supplementation improved their fatigue scores on the BFI and the ESS with no change in their Karnovsky Score. In the most recent study, 21 patients with carnitine deficiency completed therapy with progressively higher doses of replacement up to 3000 mgs per day [81]. Fatigue was measured with the BFI, the ESS and the Center for Epidemiologic Studies Depression Case (CES-D) and KPS. 17/21 responded. All tests improved significantly with a dose-response relationship. There was no significant toxicity despite the high dosages. In conclusion, L-carnitine supplementation appears helpful in those with a documented deficiency. Complete resolution did not occur arguing that the deficiency is not the sole pathophysiology of the symptoms and supplementation in non-deficient states has not been tested consistently.

Other Supplements

The use of gammalinolenic acid (GLA) was reported in fatigued Sjogren's Syndrome patients [82] 30 patients were randomized in a double-blind, placebo-controlled trial to either 800 or 1600 mgs of GLA emulsion or a placebo emulsion with corn oil. VAS scales were measured pretreatment and at 3 and 6 months of therapy. No efficacy was seen. 4-aminopyridine (4-AP) was tested in a double-blind placebo-controlled crossover trial in MS that randomized to 6 months of placebo or 8 mg of 4-AP four times a day [83]. Fatigue was measured with the FSS. There was no significant difference in fatigue scores with 4-AP and placebo. Iron supplementation was given to fatigued women with normal hemoglobin and showed improved scores in those with ferritin levels < 50 mcg/l [84].

Prokarin™, [a] proprietary transdermal cream that contains histamine and caffeine has been tested for fatigue in MS patients [85]. 29 patients were treated with 7 randomized to placebo and 22 to treatment. All patients took calcium/magnesium and multivitamin with mineral supplements. Fatigue was measured with the MFIS and showed statistically significant improvement at 4 weeks that was maintained until completion of the study at 12 weeks. 45% elected to continue therapy after completion of the study interval. A homeopathic approach was tested in patients with a variety of symptoms including fatigue [86]. Over three and one-half years, 100 patients were enrolled with 56 patients completed the study. Statistically significant improvement in fatigue scores on the EORTC QLQ-30 was noted and 75% of those completing the study were satisfied with the treatment. In a study of 225 patients, 174 had used one of 56 different types of dietary supplements [87]. Using the EORTC-QLQ-30 statistically improvement in QOL for colon and breast cancer patients. No improvement was noted in lung cancer patients. In conclusion, there is some evidence of benefit from a variety of nutritional supplements but the studies are also quite limited so no strong conclusions can be made.

Other Interventions

Acupressure has been studied in end-stage renal disease in several controlled trials [88-90]. Control arms have been usual care or usual care plus a sham arm. Measurements were the PFS, a VAS, the BDI and the Pittsburg Sleep Quality Index. In each study the perception of fatigue improved and the effect was sustained throughout the intervention. Acupuncture was tested in a single arm trial in post-chemotherapy fatigue [91]. 37 patients were treated once or twice a week for four to six weeks. There was a mean improvement on the BFI of 31% with 3 patients experiencing >75% improvement. In a randomized trial of acupuncture and acupressure, acupuncture was found to be superior [92]. In a pilot randomized controlled double-blind study of acupuncture vs. sham acupuncture in 27 patients, no statistically significant changes were found between the therapies with both groups having improved fatigue, distress, QOL and depression [93].

Pulsed electromagnetic therapy was studied in multiple sclerosis patients following a pilot study that had suggested improvement [92, 93]. Each participant was treated with both placebo and the device with a two-week washout between treatment arms. Subjects were randomized to begin either with active or placebo device. Fatigue was measured with scales derived from the Multiple Sclerosis Quality of Life Inventory (MSQLI) at baseline and at the end of each four-week treatment. 51% of those treated had some improvement in fatigue compared with 36% experiencing improvement from the placebo but the clinical differences were small. In a placebo controlled study of Bio-Electro-Magnetic–Energy-Regulation (BEMER), significant differences were seen on the MFIS at 12 weeks but not at 6 [96].

Conclusion

So what does a physician faced with a fatigued patient do? The key first step in management of fatigue is recognition. NCCN Guidelines are to screen with every visit with at least the NRS (worst fatigue on a scale of 1-10) [1]. Re-evaluation would then be appropriate with any intervention. Mild fatigue [1-3] is managed with education and perhaps ECAM. Moderate or severe fatigue would start the process of evaluation for underlying cause and therapy. In most settings a relatively strong case can be made to recommend exercise and correction of any identifiable hormonal and nutritional abnormalities. If pharmacologic treatment is appropriate, then modafinil or methylphenidate would be reasonable agents to try. Insurance reimbursement may be problematic in settings other than MS where modafinil is considered a treatment of choice. Complementary approaches such as acupuncture have suggested improvement and have little associated harm. Demonstrating interest and educating patients and their families on the universality of this troublesome symptom in the setting of many diseases may be the most important thing we do in management.

References

[1] National Comprehensive Cancer Network Practice Guidelines. Cancer Related Fatigue Panel 2010 Guidelines version 1.2010, April. Rockledge (PA): *National Comprehensive Cancer Network* (http://www.nccn.org)

[2] Bower, J.E., Ganz, P.A., Desmond, K.A., Rowland, J.H., Meyerowitz, B.E., & Belin, T.R. (2000).Fatigue in breast cancer survivors: occurrence, correlates, and impact on quality of life. *Journal of Clinical Oncology*, 18, 743-753.

[3] Mock, V. (2004).Evidence-based treatment for cancer-related fatigue. *Journal of the National Cancer Institute, Monographs*, 32, 112-118.

[4] Watson, T., & Mock, V. (2004). Exercise as an intervention for cancer-related fatigue. *Physical Therapy*, 84, 736-743.

[5] Oldervoll, L.M., Kaasa, S., Hjermstad, M.J., Lund, J.A., & Loge, J.H. (2004). Physical exercise results in the improved subjective well-being of a few or is effective rehabilitation for all cancer patients? *European Journal of Cancer*, 40, 951-962.

[6] Courneya, K.S. (2003). Exercise in cancer survivors: an overview of research. *Medicine & Science in Sports & Exercise*, 35, 1846-1852.
[7] Knols, R., Aaronson, N.K., Uebelhart, D., Fransen, J., & Aufdemkampe, G. (2005). Physical exercise in cancer patients during and after medical treatment: a systematic review of randomized and controlled clinical trials. *Journal of Clinical Oncology*, 23, 3830-3842.
[8] Cramp, F., & Daniel, J. (2008). Exercise for the management of cancer-related fatigue in adults. *Cochrane Database of Systematic Reviews,* (2), CD006145.
[9] Dimeo, F., Fetscher, S., Lange, W., Mertelsmann, R., & Keul, J. (1997). Effects of aerobic exercise on the physical performance and incidence of treatment-related complications after high-dose chemotherapy. *Blood*, 90, 3390-3394.
[10] Dimeo, F., Schwartz, S., Fietz, T., Wanjura, T., Böning, D., & Thiel, E.(2003). Effects of endurance training on the physical performance of patients with hematological malignancies during chemotherapy. *Supportive Care in Cancer*, 11, 623-628.
[11] Chang, P., Lai, Y., Shun, S., Lin, L., Chen, M., Yang. Y., Tsai, J.C., Huang J.C., & Cheng, S.Y. (2008). Effects of a walking intervention on fatigue-related esperieinces of hospitalized acute myelogenous leukemia patients undergoing chemotherapy : a randomized controlled trial. *J Pain and Sympt Manag*, 35, 24-534.
[12] Porock, D., Kristjanson, L.J., Tinnelly, K., Duke, T., & Blight, J. (2000). An exercise intervention for advanced cancer patients experiencing fatigue: a pilot study. *Journal of Palliative Care*, 16, 30-36.
[13] Dimeo, F.C. (2001). Effects of exercise on cancer-related fatigue. *Cancer*, 92, 1689-1693.
[14] Edmonds, M., McGuire, H.,& Price, J.(2004). Exercise therapy for chronic fatigue syndrome. Cochrane Database of Systematic Reviews, Issue 3, Art. No.CD003200. DOI: 10.1002/14651858.CD003200, pub2.
[15] Rietberg, M.B., Brooks, D., Uitdehaag, B.M.J., & Kwakkel, G. (2005). Exercise therapy for multiple sclerosis. *Cochrane Database of Systematic Reviews*, Issue 1, Art. No.CD003980. DOI: 10.1002/14651858.CD003980.pub2.
[16] Stroud, N.M., & Minahan, C.L. (2009). The impact of regular physical activity on fatigue, depression and quality of life in persons with multiple sclerosis. *Health and Quality of Life Outcomes*, 7:68.
[17] Petajan, J.H., Gappmaier, E., White, A.T., Spencer, M.K., Mino, L., & Hicks R.W. (1996). Impact of aerobic training on fitness and quality of life in multiple sclerosis. *Annals of Neurology*, 39, 432-441.
[18] Mostert, S., & Kesselring, J. (2002). Effects of a short-term exercise training program on aerobic fitness, fatigue, health perception and activity level of subjects with multiple sclerosis. *Multiple Sclerosis*, 8, 161-168.
[19] Barsevick, A.M., Dudley, W., Beck, S., Sweeney, C., Whitmer, K., & Nail, L.(2004), A randomized clinical trial of energy conservation for patients with cancer-related fatigue. *Cancer*, 100, 1302-1310.
[20] Barsevick, A.M., Whitmer, K., Sweeney, C., & Nail, L.M. (2002). A pilot study examining energy conservation for cancer treatment-related fatigue. *Cancer Nursing*, 25, 333-341.
[21] Ream, E., Richardson, A., & Alexander-Dann, C. (2002). Facilitating patients' coping with fatigue during chemotherapy-pilot outcomes. *Cancer Nursing*, 25, 300-308.

[22] Vanage, S.M., Gilbertson, K.K., & Mathiowetz, V. (2003). Effects of an energy conservation course on fatigue impact for persons with progressive multiple sclerosis. *American Journal of Occupational Therapy*, 57, 315-323.

[23] Mathiowetz, V., Matuska, K.M., & Murphy, M.E.(2001). Efficacy of an energy conservation course for persons with multiple sclerosis. *Archives of Physical Medicine & Rehabilitation*, 82, 449-456.

[24] Sauter, C., Zebenholzer, K., Hisakawa, J., Zeitlhofer, J., Vass, K. (2008). A longitudinal study on effects of a six-week course for energy conservation for multiple sclerosis patients. *Multiple Sclerosis*; 14, 500-505

[25] Cella, D. (2002). The effects of anemia and anemia treatment on the quality of life of people with cancer. *Oncology* (Huntington), 16, 125-132.

[26] Ross, S.D., Fahrbach, K., Frame, D., Scheye, R., Connelly, J.E., & Glaspy, J. (2003). The effect of anemia treatment on selected health-related quality-of-life domains: a systematic review. *Clinical Therapeutics*, 25, 1786-1805.

[27] Bohlius,J., Langensiepen, S., Schwarzer, G., Seidenfeld, J., Piper, M., Bennet, C., & Engert, A. (2004). Erythropoietin for patients with malignant disease. *Cochrane Database of Systematic Reviews*, (3), CD003407.

[28] Leyland-Jones, B., Semiglazov, V., Pawlicki, M., Pienkowski, T., Tjulandin, S., Manikhas, G., Makhson, A., Roth, A., Dodwell, D., Baselga, J., Biakhov, J., Valuckas, K., Voznyi, E., Kiu, X., & Vercammen, E. (2005). Maintaining normal hemoglobin levels with epoetin alpha in mainly nonanemic patients with metastatic breast cancer receiving first line chemotherapy. *J of Clin Onc*, 23, 5960-5972.

[29] Henke, M., Laszig, R., Rübe, C., Schäfer, U., Haase, K.D., Schilcher,B., Mose, S., Beer, K.T., Burger, U., Dougherty, C., & Frommhold, H. (2003). Erythropoietin to treat head and neck cancer patients with anaemia undergoing radiotherapy: randomized, double-blind, placebo-controlled trial. *The Lancet*, 362, 1255-1260.

[30] Bohlius, J., Schmidlin, K., Schwarzer, G., Trelle, S., Seidenfeld, J., Zwahlen, M., Clarke, M.J., Weingart, O., Kluge, S., Piper, M., Napoli, M., Rades, D., Steensma, D., Djulbegovic, B., Fey, M,F., Ray-Coquard, I., Moebus, V., Thomas, G., Untch, M., Schumacher, M., Egger, M., & Engert, A. (2009). *Cochrane Database Syst Rev.* (3), CD007303.

[31] Cody, J., Daly, C., Campbell, M., Donaldson, C., Grant, A., Khan, I., Pennington, S., Vale, L., Wallace, S., & MacLeod, A.(2001). Recombinant human erythropoietin for chronic renal failure anemia in pre-dialysis patients. *Cochrane Database of Systematic Reviews*, (4), CD003266.

[32] Lou, J.S., Dimitrova, D.M., Park, B.S., Johnson, S.C., Eaton, R., Arnold, G., & Nutt, J.G. (2009). Using modafinil to treat fatigue in Parkinson disease: a double-blind,, placebo-controlled pilot study. *Clinical Neuropharmacology*, 32, 305-310.

[33] Vasconcelos, O.M., Prokhorenko, O.A., Salajegheh, M.K., Kelley, K.F., Livornese, K., Olsen, C.H., Vo, A.H., Dalakas, M.C., Halstead, L.S., Jabbari, B., & Campbell, W.W. (2007). Modafinil for treatment of fatigue in post-polio syndrome. *Neurology*, 68, 1680-1686.

[34] Rammohan, K.W., Rosenberg, J.H., Lynn, D.J., Blumenfield, A.M., Pollak, C.P., & Nagaraja, H.N. (2002). Efficacy and safety of modafinil (Provigil) for the treatment of fatigue in multiple sclerosis: a two centre phase 2 study. *Journal of Neurology, Neurosurgery & Psychiatry*, 72, 179-183.

[35] DeBattista, C., Doghramji, K., Menza, M.A., Rosenthal, M.H., Fieve, R.R., & Modafinil in Depression Study Group. (2003). Modafinil in Depression Study Group. Adjunct modafinil for the short-term treatment of fatigue and sleepiness in patients with major depressive disorder: a preliminary double-blind, placebo-controlled study. *Journal of Clinical Psychiatry*, 64, 1057-1064.

[36] Fava, M., Thase, M.E., & DeBattista, C. (2005). A multicenter, placebo-controlled study of modafinil augmentation in partial responders to selective serotonin reuptake inhibitors with persistent fatigue and sleepiness. *Journal of Clinical Psychiatry*, 66, 85-93.

[37] Larijani, G.E., Goldberg, M.E., Hojat, M., Khaleghi, B., Dunn, J.B., & Marr, A.T. (2004). Modafinil improves recovery after general anesthesia. *Anesthesia & Analgesia*, 98, 976-981.

[38] Spathis, A., Dhillan, R., Booden, D., Forbes, K., Vrotsou, K., & Fife, K. (2009). Modafinil for the treatment of fatigue in lung cancer: a pilot study. *Palliative Medicine*, 23, 325-331.

[39] Becker, P.M., Schwartz, J.R., Feldman, N.T., & Hughes, R.J. (2004). Effect of modafinil on fatigue, mood, and health-related quality of life in patients with narcolepsy. *Psychopharmacology*, 171, 133-139.

[40] Zifko, U.A., Rupp, M., Schwarz, S., Zipko, H.T., & Maida, E.M.. (2002). Modafinil in treatment of fatigue in multiple sclerosis. Results of an open-label study. *Journal of Neurology*, 249, 983-987.

[41] Rabkin, J.G., McElhiney, M.C., Rabkin, R., & Ferrando, S.J. (2004). Modafinil treatment for fatigue in HIV+ patients: a pilot study. *Journal of Clinical Psychiatry*, 65, 1688-1695.

[42] Fishbain, D.A., Cutler, R.B., Lewis, J., Cole, B., Rosomoff, H.L., & Steele-Rosomoff, R. (2004). Modafinil for the treatment of pain-associated fatigue: review and case report. *Journal of Pain & Palliative Care Pharmacotherapy*, 18, 39-47.

[43] Turkington, D., Hedwat, D., Rider, I., & Young, A.H. (2004). Recovery from chronic fatigue syndrome with modafinil. *Human Psychopharmacology*, 19, 63-64.

[44] Spathis, A., Dhillan, R., Booden, D., Forbes, K., Vrotsou, K., & Fife, K. (2009). Modafinil for the treatment of fatigue in lung cancer: a pilot study. *Palliative Medicine*, 23, 325-331.

[45] Bruera, E., Valero, V., Driver, L., Shen, L., Willey, J., Zhang, T., & Palmer, J.L. (2006). Patient-controlled methylphenidate for cancer fatigue: a double-blind, randomized, placebo-controlled trial. *J Clin Oncol*, 24, 2073-2078.

[46] Butler, J.M., Case, D., Atkins, J., Frizzell, B., Sanders, G., Griffin, P., Lesser, G., McMullen, K., McQuellon, R., Naughton, M., Rapp, S., Stieber, V., & Shaw, E.G. (2007). A phase III, double-blind placebo-controlled prospective randomized clinical trial of d-threo-methylphenidate HCL in brain tumor patients receiving radiation therapy. *Int J Radiation Oncology Biol. Phys*, 69, 1496-1501.

[47] Mar Fan, H.G., Clemons, M., Xu, W., Chemerynsky, I., Breunis, H.. Braganza, S., & Tannock, I.F. (2008). (A randomized, placebo-controlled double-blind trial of the effects of d-methylphenidate on fatigue and cognitive dysfunction in women undergoing adjuvant chemotherapy for breast cancer. *Support Care Cancer*, 16, 577-583.

[48] Wagner, G.J., & Rabkin, R. (2000). Effects of dextroamphetamine on depression and fatigue in men with HIV: a double-blind, placebo-controlled trial. *Journal of Clinical Psychiatry*, 61, 436-440.

[49] Breitbart, W., Rosenfeld, B., Kaim, M., & Funesti-Esch, J. (2001). A randomized, double-blind, placebo-controlled trial of psychostimulants for the treatment of fatigue in ambulatory patients with human immunodeficiency virus disease. *Archives of Internal Medicine*, 161, 411-420.

[50] Sarhill, N., Walsh, D., Nelson, K.A., Homsi, J., LeGrand, S., & Davis, M.P. (2001). Methylphenidate for fatigue in advanced cancer: a prospective open-label pilot study. *American Journal of Hospice & Palliative Care*, 18, 187-192.

[51] Bruera, E., Driver, L., Barnes, E.A., Willey, J., Shen, L., Palmer, J.L., & Escalante, C. (2003). Patient-controlled methylphenidate for the management of fatigue in patients with advanced cancer: a preliminary report. *Journal of Clinical Oncology*, 21, 4439-4443.

[52] Sugawara, Y., Akechi, T., Shima, Y., Okuyama, T., Akizuki, N., Nakano, T., & Uchitomi, Y. (2002). Efficacy of methylphenidate for fatigue in advanced cancer patients: a preliminary study. *Palliative Medicine*, 16, 261-263.

[53] Schwartz, A.L., Thompson, J.A., & Masood, N. (2002). Interferon-induced fatigue in patients with melanoma: a pilot study of exercise and methylphenidate. *Oncology Nursing Forum. Online*, 29, E85-90.

[54] Hanna, A.R., Sledge, G.W., Mayer, M.L., Einhorn, L.H., Monahan P.O., Fyffe, J., & Bhatia, S. (2003). Preliminary results of a phase II trial of methylphenidate in patient with breast carcinoma. *Proc Am Soc Clin Oncol*, 22, (abstr 2921).

[55] Wharton, R.H. (2002). Sleeping with the enemy: treatment of fatigue in individuals with cancer. *The Oncologist*, 7, 96-99.

[56] Riley, C.S., & Tullman, M.J. (2010). Multiple Sclerosis. Editors: Rowland, LP, Pedley, TA. Merritt's Neurology (12th Edition) Lippincott Williams & Wilkins.

[57] Zifko, U.A. (2004). Management of fatigue in patients with multiple sclerosis. *Drugs*, 64, 1295-1304.

[58] Bowman, M.A., Kirk, J.K., Michielutte, R., & Preisser, J.S. (1997). Use of amantadine for chronic fatigue syndrome. *Archives of Internal Medicine*, 157, 1264-1265.

[59] Plioplys, A.V., & Plioplys, S. (1997). Amantadine and L-carnitine treatment of Chronic Fatigue Syndrome. *Neuropsychobiology*, 35, 16-23.

[60] Zeuzem, S., Teuber, G., Naumann, U., Berg, T., Raedle, J., Hartmann, S., & Hopf, U. (2000). Randomized, double-blind, placebo-controlled trial of interferon alfa2a with and without amantadine as initial treatment for chronic hepatitis C. *Hepatology*, 32, 835-841.

[61] Pucci, E., Branas, P., D'Amico, R., Giuliani, G., Solari, A., & Taus, C. (2007). Amantadine for fatigue in multiple sclerosis. *Cochrane Database of Systematic Reviews*. (1):CD002818.

[62] Krupp, L.B., Coyle, P.K., Doscher, C., Miller, A., Cross, A.H., Jandorf, L., Halper, J., Johnson, B., Morgante, L., & Grimson, R.(1995). Fatigue therapy in multiple sclerosis: results of a double-blind, randomized, parallel trial of amantadine, pemoline, and placebo. *Neurology*, 45, 1956-1961.

[63] Tomassini, V., Pozzilli, C., Onesti, E., Pasqualetti, P., Marinelli, F., Pisani, A., & Fieschi, C. (2004). Comparison of the effects of acetyl L-carnitine and amantadine for

the treatment of fatigue in multiple sclerosis: results of a pilot, randomized, double-blind, crossover trial. *Journal of the Neurological Sciences*, 218, 103-108.
[64] Morrow, G.R., Hickok, J.T., Raubertas, R.F., Flynn, P.J., Hynes, H.E.,. Banerjee, T.K., Kirshner, J.J., . King, D.K., U of Rochester Cancer Center, Rochester, NY; Metro Minnesota CCOP, Minneapolis, MN; Wichita CCOP, Wichita, KS; Marshfield Medical Research Foundation CCOP, Marshfield, WI; Syracuse Hematology-Oncology CCOP, Syracuse, NY; & Greater Phoenix CCOP, Phoenix, AZ. (2001). Effect of an SSRI antidepressant on fatigue and depression in seven hundred thirty eight patients treated with chemotherapy: a URCC CCOP study. *Proc Amer Soc Clin Onc*, Abstract 1531.
[65] Cullum, J.L., Wojciechowski, A.E., Pelletier, G., & Simpson, J.S. (2004). Bupropion sustained release treatment reduces fatigue in cancer patients. *Canadian Journal of Psychiatry*, 49, 139-144.
[66] Hartz, A.J., Bentler, S.E., Brake, K.A., & Kelly, M.W. (2003). The effectiveness of citalopram for idiopathic chronic fatigue. *Journal of Clinical Psychiatry*, 64, 927-935.
[67] Rabkin, J.G., Wagner, G.J., McElhiney, M.C., Rabkin, R., & Lin, S.H. (2004). Testosterone versus fluoxetine for depression and fatigue in HIV/AIDS: a placebo-controlled trial. *Journal of Clinical Psychopharmacology*, 24, 379-985.
[68] Wagner, G.J., Rabkin, J.G., & Rabkin, R. (1998). Testosterone as a treatment for fatigue in HIV+ men. General Hospital Psychiatry, 20, 209-213.
[69] Abe, K., Takanashi, M., Yanagihara, T., & Sakoda, S. (2001-2002). Pergolide mesilate may improve fatigue in patients with Parkinson's disease. *Behavioural Neurology*, 13, 117-121.
[70] Bruno, R.L., Zimmerman, J.R., Creange, S.J., Lewis, T., Molzen, T., & Frick, N.M.(1996). Bromocriptine in the treatment of post-polio fatigue: a pilot study with implications for the pathophysiology of fatigue. *American Journal of Physical Medicine & Rehabilitation*, 75, 340-347.
[71] Cerchietti, L.C., Navigante, A.H., Peluffo, G.D., Diament, M.J., Stillitani, I., Klein, S.A., & Cabalar, M.E. (2004). Effects of celecoxib, medroxyprogesterone, and dietary intervention on systemic syndromes in patients with advanced lung adenocarcinoma: a pilot study. *Journal of Pain & Symptom Management*, 27, 85-95.
[72] Jones, E.A. (1999). Relief from profound fatigue associated with chronic liver disease by long-term ondansetron therapy. *Lancet*, 354, 397.
[73] Eknoyan, G., Latos, D.L., &Lindberg, J. (2003). Practice recommendations for the use of L-carnitine in dialysis-related carnitine disorder. National Kidney Foundation Carnitine Consensus Conference. *American Journal of Kidney Diseases*, 41, 868-876.
[74] Heuberger, W., Berardi, S., Jacky, E., Pey, P., & Krähenbühl, S.(1998). Increased urinary excretion of carnitine in patients treated with cisplatin. *European Journal of Clinical Pharmacology*, 54, 503-508.
[75] Marthaler, N.P., Visarius, T., Kupfer, A., & Lauterburg, B.H. (1999). Increased urinary losses of carnitine during ifosfamide chemotherapy. *Cancer Chemotherapy & Pharmacology*, 44, 170-172.
[76] Malaguarnera, M., Cammalleri, L., Pia Gargante, M., Vacante, M., Colonna, V., & Motta, M.(2007). L-carnitine treatment reduces severity of physical and mental fatigue and increases cognitive functions in centenarians: a randomized and controlled clinical trial. *Am J Clin Nutr*, 86, 1738-1744.

[77] Grau, J.M., Casademont, J., Pedrol, E., Fernández-Solà, J., Cardellach, F., Barros, N., & Urbano-Márquez, A. (1992). Chronic fatigue syndrome: studies on skeletal muscle. [Journal Article] *Clinical Neuropathology*, 11, 329-332.

[78] Vermeulen, R.C., & Scholte, H.R (2004). Exploratory open label, randomized study of acetyl- and propionylcarnitine in chronic fatigue syndrome. *Psychosomatic Medicine*, 66, 276-282.

[79] Graziano, F., Bisonni, R., Catalano, V., Silva, R, Rovidati, S., Mencarini, E., Ferraro, B., Canestrari, F., Baldelli, A.M., De, Gaetano, A., Giordani, P., Testa, E., & Lai, V. (2002). Potential role of levocarnitine supplementation for the treatment of chemotherapy-induced fatigue in non-anemic cancer patients. *British Journal of Cancer*, 86, 1854-1857.

[80] Cruciani, R.A., Dvorkin, E., Homel, P., Culliney, B., Malamud, S., Shaiova, L., Fleishman, S., Lapin, J., Klein, E., Lesage, P., Portenoy, R., & Esteban-Cruciani, N. (2004). L-carnitine supplementation for the treatment of fatigue and depressed mood in cancer patients with carnitine deficiency: a preliminary analysis. *Annals of the New York Academy of Sciences*, 1033, 168-176.

[81] Cruciani, R.A., Dvorkin, E., Homel, P., Malamud, S., Culliney, B., Lapin, J., Portenoy, R.K., & Esteban-Cruciani, N. (2006). Safety, tolerability and symptom outcomes associated with l-carnitine supplementation in patients with cancer, fatigue and carnitine deficiency: aphase I/II study. *J of Pain and Symptom Manage*, 32, 551-559.

[82] Theander, E., Horrobin, D.F., Jacobsson, L.T., & Manthorpe, R. (2002). Gammalinolenic acid treatment of fatigue associated with primary Sjogren's syndrome. *Scandinavian Journal of Rheumatology*, 31, 72-79.

[83] Rossini, P.M., Pasqualetti, P., Pozzilli, C., Grasso, M.G., Millefiorini, E., Graceffa, A., Carlesimo, G.A., Zibellini, G., & Caltagirone, C. (2001). Fatigue in progressive multiple sclerosis: results of a randomized, double-blind, placebo-controlled, crossover trial of oral 4-aminopyridine. *Multiple Sclerosis*, 7, 354-358.

[84] Verdon, F., Burnand, B., Stubi, C.L., Bonard, C., Graff, M., Michaud, A., Bischoff, T., de Vevey, M., Studer, J.P., Herzig, L., Chapuis, C., Tissot, J., Pécoud, A., & Favrat, B. (2003). Iron supplementation for unexplained fatigue in non-anemic women: double blind randomized placebo controlled trial. *BMJ*, 326, 1124.

[85] Gillson, G., Richard, T.L., Smith, R.B., & Wright, J.V. (2002). A double-blind pilot study of the effect of Prokarin™ on fatigue in multiple sclerosis. *Multiple Sclerosis*, 8, 30-35.

[86] Thompson, E.A., & Reillly, D. (2002. The homeopathic approach to symptom control in the cancer patient: a prospective observational study. *Palliative Medicine*, 16, 227-233.

[87] Lis, C.G., Cambron, J.A., Grutsch, J.F., Granick, J., Gupta, D. (2006). Self-reported quality of life in users and nonusers of dietary supplements in cancer. *Support Care Cancer*, 14, 193-199.

[88] Cho, Y.C., & Tsay, S.L. (2004). The effect of acupressure with massage on fatigue and depression in patients with end-stage renal disease. Journal of Nursing Research: *JNR*, 12, 51-59.

[89] Tsay, S.L. (2004). Acupressure and fatigue in patients with end-stage renal disease-a randomized controlled trial. *International Journal of Nursing Studies*, 41, 99-106.

[90] Tsay, S.L., Cho, Y.C., & Chen, M.L. (2004). Acupressure and Transcutaneous Electrical Acupoint Stimulation in improving fatigue, sleep quality and depression in hemodialysis patients. *American Journal of Chinese Medicine*, 32, 407-416.

[91] Vickers, A.J., Straus, D.J., Fearon, B., & Cassileth, B.R.(2004). Acupuncture for postchemotherapy fatigue: a phase II study. *Journal of Clinical Oncology*, 22, 1731-1735.

[92] Molassiotis, A., Sylt, P., & Diggins, H. (2007). The management of cancer-related fatigue after chemotherapy with acupuncture and acupressure: a randomized controlled trial. *Complement Ther Med*, 15, 228-237.

[93] Balk, J., Day, R., Rosenzweig, M., & Beriwal, S. (2009). Pilot, randomized, modified double-blind, placebo-controlled trial of acupuncture for cancer-related fatigue. *J Society for Integrative Oncology*, 7, 4-11.

[94] Richards, T.L., Lappin, M.S., Acosta-Urquidi, J., Kraft, G.H., Heide, A.C., Lawrie, F.W., Merrill, T.E., Melton, G.B., & Cunningham, C.A. (1997). Double-blind study of pulsing magnetic field effects on multiple sclerosis. *Journal of Alternative & Complementary Medicine*, 3, 21-29.

[95] Lappi, M.S., Lawrie, F.W., Richards, T.L., & Kramer, E.D. (2003). Effects of a pulsed electromagnetic therapy on multiple sclerosis fatigue and quality of life: a double-blind, placebo-controlled trial. Multicenter Study. Randomized Controlled Trial. *Alternative Therapies in Health & Medicine*, 9, 38-48.

[96] Piatkowski, J., Kern, S., & Ziemssen, T. (2009). Effect of BEMER magnetic filed therapy on the level of fatigue in patients with multiple sclerosis: a randomized, double blind controlled trial. *The J of Alternative and Complementary Medicine*, 15, 507-511.

INDEX

D

E

F

G

H

N

Q

W

Y